# The Whole Pediatrician Catalog

## A compendium of clues to diagnosis and management

### JULIA A. McMILLAN, M.D.

Assistant Instructor,
Department of Pediatrics,
State University of New York,
Upstate Medical Center at Syracuse

### PHILLIP I. NIEBURG, M.D.

Fellow in Infectious Diseases and
Instructor, Department of Pediatrics,
State University of New York,
Upstate Medical Center at Syracuse

### FRANK A. OSKI, M.D.

Professor and Chairman,
Department of Pediatrics,
State University of New York,
Upstate Medical Center at Syracuse

W. B. SAUNDERS COMPANY
Philadelphia • London • Toronto

W. B. Saunders Company: West Washington Square
Philadelphia, PA 19105

1 St. Anne's Road
Eastbourne, East Sussex BN21 3UN, England

1 Goldthorne Avenue
Toronto, Ontario M8Z 5T9, Canada

**Library of Congress Cataloging in Publication Data**

McMillan, Julia A.

The Whole Pediatrician Catalog

1. Pediatrics—Handbooks, manuals, etc. I. Nieburg, Phillip I.,
joint author. II. Oski, Frank A., joint author. III. Title.
[DNLM: 1. Pediatrics. WS200 M167w]

RJ48.M3          618.9'2          76-27060

ISBN          0-7216-5968-3

The front cover illustrations are before and after photographs of a child with nephrosis, from
*PEDIATRICS – The Hygienic and Medical Treatment of Children*, Volume III, Second Edition, by
Charles Hunter Dunn, M.D. Published by The Southworth Company, Troy, New York, 1920.

The Whole Pediatrician Catalog                                         ISBN  0-7216-5968-3

Last digit is the print number:     9     8     7     6     5

## DEDICATION

To all who devote time, energy and emotion to the care of children.

# INTRODUCTION

Valuable information of a practical nature is scattered in textbooks, journals, and throw-away magazines. Most physicians, particularly as students and house officers, try to collect such facts in a bulging notebook, or file it in an inaccessible or quickly forgotten spot. When confronted with a problem, a once remembered solution jogs the memory and initiates a search of reference texts, journals, or piles of unfiled reprints. Often the information that would be of most value at the moment also proves to be the most difficult to find.

How do you calculate the dose of intramuscular iron? How fast does the blood urea nitrogen fall in a dehydrated patient once intravenous therapy is started? What are the current guidelines for the prophylactic treatment of contacts of patients with meningococcal meningitis? When is the fontanel too large? How does one evaluate the infant with jaundice, the older child with conjugated hyperbili-rubinemia, and the patient with precocious puberty, failure to thrive, or just a headache?

This book is an attempt to remind the physician who cares for children about some of the clues to diagnosis and management. The topics in this book reflect the problems that we have frequently encountered and the answers we found most helpful. It also reflects the information we have frequently forgotten and wish to remember.

The title *The Whole Pediatrician Catalogue* is not meant to indicate that everything of use to a pediatrician is contained between the covers of the book. The book is not intended to be a procedure manual, a therapeutic inventory, or a collection of normal values — these, fortunately, are already available. The title *The Whole Pediatrician Catalogue* is intended to remind the reader of *The Whole Earth Catalogue*, a book full of the fun of learning and discovery and filled with the practical aspects of life in general. We hope that we have captured some of that flavor in our approach to patient management.

To make best use of this book, we suggest that the readers spend a few hours familiarizing themselves with its contents so that when the need arises for a particular fact or specific approach to diagnosis or management they will know where to find it.

We hope that you will enjoy this book. We wish to express our appreciation to the many authors from whom we borrowed wisdom. We invite any reader to tell us about omissions that they feel would make the book more useful to them.

Finally, we would like to express our thanks to Ms. Marjorie Gillette for her tireless efforts in providing us with secretarial assistance and to Mr. John Hanley of the W. B. Saunders Company for his support and encouragement of this work.

JULIA A. MCMILLAN

PHILLIP I. NIEBURG

FRANK A. OSKI

# CONTENTS

# 1
# THE HISTORY AND PHYSICAL EXAMINATION

# FONTANELS

An abnormality in size of the anterior fontanel may be a tip-off to abnormality in the infant. Figure 1–1 displays the fontanel size, defined as $\frac{\text{length} + \text{width}}{2}$, as measured with a steel tape in 201 normal infants.

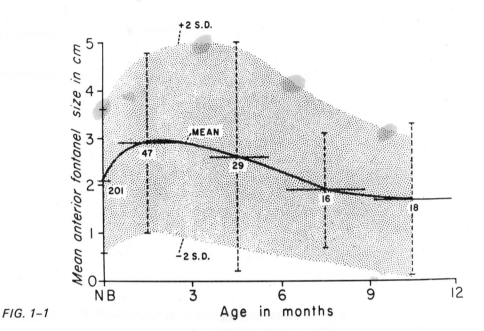

FIG. 1–1

The tables below list conditions associated with an unusually small (or prematurely closed) fontanel or with an unusually large fontanel.

*Disorders in which Premature Closure or Small Fontanel for Age May Be a Feature*

      Microcephaly

      High Ca++/vitamin D ratio in pregnancy

      Craniosynostosis

      Hyperthyroidism

      Normal variant

> *Fontanel*—From the French word *fontanelle*, which is the diminutive for *fontaine*, the word for fountain.

*Disorders in which Large Fontanel for Age May Be a Feature*

| SKELETAL DISORDERS | CHROMOSOMAL ABNORMALITIES | OTHER CONDITIONS |
| --- | --- | --- |
| Achondroplasia | Down's syndrome | Athyrotic hypothyroidism |
| Aminopterin-induced syndrome | 13 Trisomy syndrome | Hallermann-Streiff syndrome |
| Apert's syndrome | 18 Trisomy syndrome | Malnutrition |
| Cleidocranial dysostosis | | Progeria |
| Hypophosphatasia | | Rubella syndrome |
| Kenny's syndrome | | Russell-Silver syndrome |
| Osteogenesis imperfecta | | |
| Pyknodysostosis | | |
| Vitamin D deficiency rickets | | |

References: Popich, G.A., and Smith, D.W.: J. Pediatr., *80*:749, 1972. Barness, L.A.: Manual of Pediatric Physical Diagnosis. 3rd Ed. Chicago, Year Book Medical Publishers, Inc., 1966, pp. 49–50.

## THE INTRACRANIAL BRUIT

Auscultation of the head of the pediatric patient is more likely to cause confusion than to provide information to the examiner. Intracranial bruits may be found in up to 50 per cent of normal children under 5 years of age. The incidence decreases in older children. Unilateral or localized bruits do not necessarily indicate abnormality.

Though the intracranial bruit may reflect normal vascular turbulence, it is found with increased incidence in children with purulent meningitis. (See Fig. 1–2.)

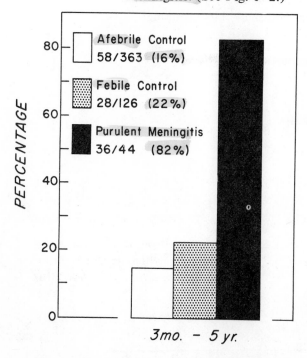

Afebrile Control
58/363 (16%)

Febile Control
28/126 (22%)

Purulent Meningitis
36/44 (82%)

PERCENTAGE

*3mo. – 5 yr.*          FIG. 1–2

The bruits in children with purulent meningitis may disappear two to three days after the initiation of therapy. *If the bruits in such patients have disappeared with treatment but then return, subdural effusion should be suspected.*

Bruits have also been associated with the following conditions:

Fever
Thyrotoxicosis
Anemia
Cardiac murmurs
Cerebral angioma
Cerebral aneurysm
Cerebral arteriovenous malformation
Intracerebral tumors
Any cause of increased intracranial pressure

Reference:  Mace, J.W., Peters, E.R., and Mathies, A.W.: N. Engl. J. Med., *278*:1420, 1968.

# HEAD CIRCUMFERENCE IN PREMATURE INFANTS

Patterns of head growth in premature infants seem to be a function of gestational age as well as of the infant's health. Mean head circumference increments for healthy premature infants are as follows:

| GESTATIONAL AGE | WEEKLY HEAD CIRCUMFERENCE INCREMENTS (CM/WEEK) | | TOTAL INCREMENT (FIRST 16 WEEKS OF LIFE) |
| --- | --- | --- | --- |
| | *Weeks 1–8 of Life* | *Weeks 9–16 of Life* | |
| 30–33 weeks | 1.1 | 0.5 | 13.2 cm |
| 34–37 weeks | 0.8 | 0.4 | 9.8 cm |

In sick premature infants, the head circumference increases at a slower rate. This increase averages 0.25 cm per week during the first 16 weeks of life. "Sick" premature infants are those requiring artificial ventilation and/or intravenous feedings for periods of two weeks or longer.

Premature infants should be suspected of having intracranial pathologic changes if:

1. They are apparently healthy but their head circumference increments do not approach these data.

2. They are sick yet have a rate of head growth approaching that of a healthy infant of the same gestational and postnatal age.

Reference:  Sher, P.K., and Brown, S.B.: Dev. Med. Child Neurol., *17*:705, 1975.

## HEAD CIRCUMFERENCE IN TERM INFANTS

Expected head circumference (HC) during infancy can be estimated by remembering that the average full-term infant will show the following increments in head growth:

| PERIOD | HC INCREMENTS | |
|---|---|---|
| First 3 months | 2 cm/month = | 6 cm |
| 4–6 months | 1 cm/month = | 3 cm |
| 6–12 months | 0.5 cm/month = | 3 cm |
| First year | | 12 cm |

## THE STANDING HEIGHT

Continuing assessment of children with short or excessive stature from any cause requires accuracy in height measurements. Tanner pointed out that casual observers without special training may offer height estimations that differ by as much as 1.5 cm; he emphasized the importance of careful measurement, using a standard technique with standard accurate instruments.

One such standard technique is the following.

The standing height should be taken without shoes, the patient standing with his heels, back and occiput in contact with an upright wall, his head so held that he looks straight forward with the lower borders of the eye sockets in the same horizontal plane as the external auditory meati. A right angle block is then slipped down the wall until the lower bottom surface touches the patient's head, and a scale fixed to the wall is read. During the measurement the patient should be told to stretch his neck to be as tall as possible, although care must be taken to prevent his heels' coming off the ground. Gentle but firm tension upward should be applied by the measurer under the mastoid processes to help the patient stretch.In this way the variation in height from morning to evening is minimized (standing height should be recorded to the nearest 0.1 cm).

Reference: Vines, R.H.: Drugs, *11*:135, 1976

## ERRORS IN THE MEASUREMENT OF CHILDREN

Great reliance is placed on the weight and length or height of our patients. These numbers are interpreted just like many laboratory tests, and just like many laboratory tests they are subject to error. A recent survey of child health clinics revealed that errors were made in almost 90 per cent of all measurements performed in children under 2 years of age and in almost 75 per cent of those performed in children over 2 years of age. Children under 2, in general, were judged to be shorter than they really were, while children over 2 were judged to be taller than they actually were. Errors were due to both faulty equipment and faulty technique. Before you trust the numbers, make sure how they are determined. The type and frequency of errors in technique are listed below.

> *Normal*—From the Latin nor-malis, which means according to a pattern; from *norma*, a carpenter's square and thus a rule or pattern.

*Frequency of Errors in Technique by Clinic Staff Weighing and Measuring Children 0 to 5 Years Old*

| ITEM | FREQUENCY AND PERCENTAGE | |
| --- | --- | --- |
| | < 2 Years | 2–5 Years |
| Number error-free | 17 (11.2%) | 40 (26.3%) |
| Number in which errors observed | 135 (88.8%) | 112 (73.7%) |
| | 152 (100%) | 152 (100%) |
| Specific weighing errors | | |
| Excessive movement | 47 (14.5%) | 10 (4.9%) |
| Clothing left on | 21 (6.5%) | 39 (19.0%) |
| Specific measuring errors | | |
| No assistance | 61 (18.8%) | — |
| Excessive movement | 45 (13.8%) | 11 (5.3%) |
| Not stretched or positioned correctly | 33 (10.1%) | 61 (29.6%) |
| Improper Frankfort plane | 33 (10.1%) | 46 (22.3%) |
| Headboard not placed against child's head | 27 (8.3%) | — |
| Child measured standing (<2) or recumbent (>2) | 25 (7.7%) | 5 (2.4%) |
| Measured with cap or shoes | 12 (3.7%) | 12 (5.8%) |
| Other | 21 (6.5%) | 22 (10.7%) |
| Total errors | 325 (100.0%) | 206 (100.0%) |
| Average errors/child | 2.1% | 1.4% |

Reference: Nutrition Surveillance, Center for Disease Control, Atlanta, Georgia, September 1975, p. 10.

## SIMPLE FORMULAS FOR APPROXIMATING HEIGHT AND WEIGHT OF CHILDREN

Not infrequently the information on the height and weight of your patient is available but you cannot find a growth grid to determine whether or not the information is normal. This is particularly true for the child from 1 to 12 years of age. The simple formulas below will enable you to calculate quickly what the 50th percentile should be.

*For Weight (in pounds)*

Ages 1 to 6 years = (age in years × 5) plus 17.
Ages 6 to 12 years = (age in years × 7) plus 5.

*For Length (in inches)*

Ages 2 to 14 years = (age in years × 2.5) plus 30.

Reference: Weech, A.: Am. J. Dis. Child., *88*:452, 1954 (as modified by Vaughan, V.C., III, and McKay, R.J. (Eds.): Nelson Textbook of Pediatrics. 10th Ed. Philadelphia, W.B. Saunders Co., 1975, p. 25).

## TESTING OCULAR MOVEMENTS

Ocular movements should always be noted. Would you know which cranial nerve was involved if those movements were not "intact"? Figure 1–3 should help you localize the abnormality.

RIGHT UPWARD GAZE

Rt. superior rectus III

Lt. inferior oblique III

LEFT UPWARD GAZE

Rt. inferior oblique III

Lt. superior rectus III

RIGHT LATERAL GAZE

Rt. external rectus VI

Lt. medial rectus III

LEFT LATERAL GAZE

Rt. medial rectus III

Lt. external rectus VI

RIGHT DOWNWARD GAZE

Rt. inferior rectus III

Lt. superior oblique IV

LEFT DOWNWARD GAZE

Rt. superior oblique IV

Lt. inferior rectus III

Remember also:

1. Sixth nerve palsies are the most common.
2. The patient with sixth (abducens) nerve weakness may rotate the head to the side of the weakened muscle to avoid diplopia.
3. Ptosis, a large pupil that reacts poorly to light, and outward and downward displacement of the eye indicate third (oculomotor) nerve palsy.
4. The head may be tilted away from the side of the weakened muscle with fourth (trochlear) nerve involvement.

Reference: Dodge, P.R.: Neurologic history and examination. *In* Farmer, T.W. (Ed.): Pediatric Neurology. New York, Harper & Row, 1975, p. 18.

## OCULAR HYPERTELORISM

The presence of ocular hypertelorism can provide a useful clue in syndrome identification. You may often find yourself suspecting that the patient's eyes appear to be widely spaced, but all too frequently you do not have access to a chart of normal values. Figures 1–4 to 1–6 may prove useful when you wish to confirm your suspicions.

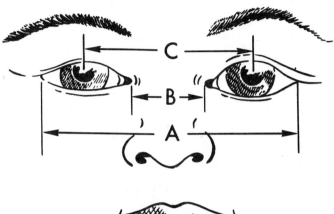

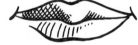

*FIG. 1–4*

*A*, Outer canthal distance. *B*, Inner canthal distance. *C*, Interpupillary distance.

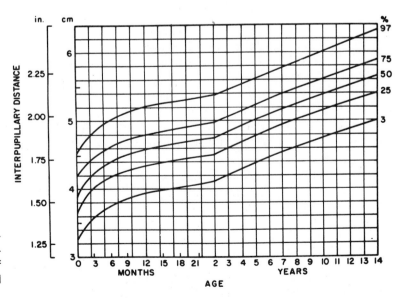

*FIG. 1–5*

The normal interpupillary distances. Lines represent smoothed means of 3rd, 25th, 50th, 75th, and 97th percentiles.

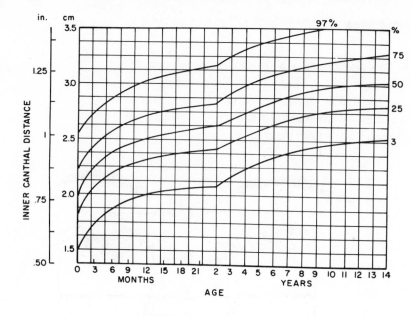

*FIG. 1–6*

The normal inner canthal distance. Lines represent smoothed means of 3rd, 25th, 50th, 75th, and 97th percentiles.

Hypertelorism relative to facial breadth is seen frequently in

Aminopterin-induced syndromes
Apert's syndrome
Hypertelorism-hypospadias syndrome
Otopalatodigital syndrome
Pyle's disease (bony wedge over bridge of nose,
    abnormal metaphyses, knock knees, and
    poor dentition)

Hypertelorism relative to facial breadth is seen occasionally in

Basal cell nevus syndrome
Cleidocranial dysostosis
Coloboma of iris—anal atresia syndrome
Conradi's syndrome
Cri-du-chat syndrome
Crouzon's disease
Hurler's syndrome
Hypercalcemia—supravalvular stenosis syndrome

---

Reference: Feingold, M., and Bossert, W.H.: Birth Defects, Original Article Series, *10* (No. 13): 7, 1974.

*"I wonder if we who have grown up will ever know on this side of the grave how much we owe to children, who seem, but only seem, to owe us so much."*

Bishop Francis C. Kelley

# CONGENITAL LACRIMAL STENOSIS

Obstruction of the lacrimal ducts (dacryostenosis), often in association with purulent dacryocystitis, is relatively common in infancy. It should be suspected in an infant with a purulent discharge from the eye whose corresponding conjunctiva appears normal. Another presentation may be recurrence of purulent discharge soon after cessation of ophthalmic antibiotic therapy for what had been thought to be conjunctivitis. The diagnosis is confirmed if pressure over the lacrimal sac produces an outpouring of mucopurulent material from the lacrimal punctum.

The goal of open passage of tears can be accomplished by an ophthalmologist using probing of the lacrimal tract, a procedure requiring general anesthesia. The goal may also be reached by a nonoperative technique easily taught to parents.

The technique is based on forcing the fluid collected in the lacrimal sac through the obstructed lacrimal drainage tract. This is accomplished by placing the tip of the thumb above the sac at the medial angle of the eye and slowly and steadily rolling the thumb caudad, thereby increasing the pressure in a downward direction (Fig. 1–7).

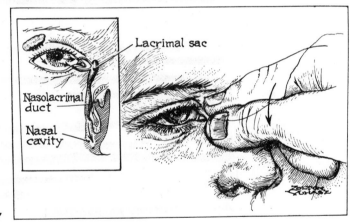

FIG. 1–7

The problem of reflux of fluid — and thus pressure — into the conjunctival sac, caused by a momentary release of thumb pressure, is easily avoidable with some practice. Care should be taken to avoid inadvertent contact between the baby's skin and the thumbnail. This technique should be used three to four times daily for a month before you decide that no improvement has occurred and referral to an ophthalmologist is made. Because the pressure generated by the thumb depends on the presence of fluid in the lacrimal sac, it can be applied only once each time; the sac takes several hours to refill. Ophthalmic antibiotics may be used to control infection caused by the obstructed tract.

Reference: Riffenburgh, R.S., and Yubasz, Z.: Pediatr. Digest, June 1971, p. 21.

## NYSTAGMUS

The commonest cause of nystagmus in an infant is a defect in vision. This must be ruled out before considering other causes, which include:

Congenital nystagmus
Side-effect of anticonvulsant therapy
Albinism
Spasmus nutans
Cerebellar disorders (ataxia, tumor, infection, malformation)
Friedreich's ataxia

*"The only trouble with all the new theories about bringing up children is that it leaves the job just as hard as ever."*

Heywood Broun

## STRABISMUS

Strabismus, or squint, is a result of one of three major pathologic processes:

1. An imbalance in the ocular muscles of the two eyes as a result of maldevelopment or innervation.
2. A difference in the refraction of the two eyes.
3. A visual defect in one eye.

Strabismus may be either paralytic or nonparalytic. Nonparalytic strabismus is seen frequently in infants during the first 6 months of life. After this age strabismus requires an explanation and treatment in order to avoid amblyopia. A paralytic squint is abnormal at any age.

When the squint is of the nonparalytic type (concomitant), all muscles move the eye normally, but they do not work in conjunction with each other. The two eyes are in the same position relative to each other, whatever the direction of gaze. The nonparalytic squint is not associated with diplopia. In young infants the presence of strabismus can easily be confirmed by shining a light at the eyes from directly in front of the patient. The reflection of the light should normally be in the center of the pupil or at a corresponding point on both corneas.

When the squint is of the paralytic type (nonconcomitant) owing to muscle paralysis, the eyes are straight except when moved in the direction of the paralyzed muscle. If full ocular movements are elicited in one eye when the other is covered, then a paralytic strabismus can be excluded.

Nonparalytic squint is seen in children with hydrocephalus, cerebral palsy, retinoblastoma, corneal opacities, and refractive errors.

Paralytic squint should suggest the presence of a brain stem lesion and increased intracranial pressure.

## WHEN TO SUSPECT HYPHEMA

Although most pediatricians would consider hyphema (bleeding into the anterior chamber of the eye) as one of the complications of blunt trauma to the eye, fewer may be aware of its spontaneous occurrence in other childhood conditions.

Hyphema should be considered whenever a patient is evaluated for or is found to have one or a combination of the following: visual disturbance, unilateral enlargement of an eye, absence of normal red reflex, and/or dilated iris vessels.

The presence of a spontaneous nontraumatic hyphema has been associated with the following pediatric conditions:

Retinoblastoma
Leukemia
Hemophilia
Retrolental fibroplasia
As a late sequel to blunt trauma (up to several months later)
Iritis of various causes
Persistent primary hyperplastic vitreous
Congenital degenerative clefts of the retina (retinoschisis)

Spontaneous hyphema in a child less than 3 years old should be regarded as evidence of retinoblastoma until demonstrated otherwise.

Reference: Howard, G.M.: Arch. Ophthalmol., *68*:615, 1962.

## VISION PROBLEMS—PREVALENCE, TYPES, AND TESTING

*Prevalence*

In preschool children, about 29 per 1000 will have a visual defect. Refractive errors are present in 89 per cent of such children, 22 per cent have muscle imbalance, and 11 per cent have amblyopia.

Visual defects are even more common in older children. It is estimated that 18 to 23 per cent of children 5 to 7 years of age have some visual defect, and about 31 per cent of children 13 to 15 years old have less than normal eyesight.

Visual defects occur with even greater frequency among children with cerebral palsy, mental retardation, or hearing deficits. It is imperative that this added handicap be recognized so that rehabilitative efforts are not compromised by unrecognized sensory problems.

Color blindness occurs with greater frequency among males (8 per cent) than among females (0.5 per cent). Red-green color blindness is more common among whites than blacks.

### Vision Screening

A careful history will often provide clues to the diagnosis of visual problems in children. About one-half of preschool children with a visual defect have either a family history of eye disease or clinical signs and symptoms suggestive of eye disease. Clinical history is frequently overlooked in this area. Any of the following place the patient at increased risk of having a visual defect:

1. Family history of visual defects (color blindness, refractive errors, strabismus, cataract, albinism, and retinoblastoma).
2. A history of congenital infections (rubella, toxoplasmosis, syphilis).
3. A history of prolonged labor.
4. A history of premature delivery.
5. A history of oxygen therapy in the neonatal period.
6. Evidence of mental retardation, cerebral palsy, or hearing difficulty.

### Testing Procedures

The minimum testing should include a test for central distance visual acuity. Whenever possible, tests for accommodative ability, muscle balance, and color vision should be performed.

Visual acuity should be tested in all children 3 to 5 years of age. Color vision, although preferably tested in the preschool child, should not be delayed beyond age 10.

Tests of visual acuity should be performed at three-year intervals and certainly in the fifth and sixth grades, as well as midway through high school.

The simplest test for the preschool child is the Snellen E test. The National Society for the Prevention of Blindness recommends that referrals to an ophthalmologist be made for the following:

Vision poorer than 20/50 in a 3 year old.
Vision poorer than 20/40 for 4 and 5 year olds.
A difference in visual acuity between two eyes, if confirmed twice, even if scores for individual eyes are within the passing range.

---

Reference: Lin-Fu, J.S.: U.S. Public Health Service Publication No. 2042, 1971.

# DETECTION OF HEARING PROBLEMS IN INFANCY

Impaired hearing during the first year of life has profound effects on language and emotional, social, and intellectual development. Detection of hearing losses during this time is important because:

1. More severe and more prolonged impairments cause greater reductions in speech and language development.

2. It is desirable to initiate therapy for hearing loss by 6 months, and it is practical to do so by 6 to 12 months.

3. Adequate hearing assessment is possible by 4 to 8 months.

4. When hearing loss is not restorable, various measures are available and indicated to promote language and speech development and to minimize the effects on emotional and social development.

Impaired hearing has been associated with several sets of perinatal circumstances, the occurrence of any of which is an indication for early (by 4 months) audiologic evaluation and for long-term follow-up.

### Conditions Associated with High Risk of Hearing Loss

1. Family history of hearing loss before approximately 50 years of age without obvious cause.

2. Maternal viral infection during pregnancy (especially rubella).

3. Defects of ears (including pinnae), nose, lips or palate.

4. Birth weight under 1500 gm.

5. Bilirubin above 20 mg/dl.

6. Prenatal treatment of mother or postnatal treatment of infant with ototoxic drugs (including kanamycin or gentamicin).

7. Multiple congenital anomalies of any kind.

Suspicion of hearing loss should be raised beyond the perinatal period in several circumstances:

| AGE | CLUE |
| --- | --- |
| Any time | Failure of infant to respond to loud environmental sounds. |
| Any time | Failure to awaken or move about in response to speech or noise when asleep in quiet room. |
| By 4–5 months | Failure to turn head or eyes toward sound source. |
| By 6 months | Failure to turn purposefully toward sound source. |
| By 8 months | No attempt to imitate sounds made by parents. |
| By 8–12 months | Lack of variety in melody and sounds during babbling. |
| By 12 months | No apparent understanding of simple phrases. |
| By 24 months | Little or no spontaneous speech. |

Occurrence of any of these clues is an indication for audiologic and otologic evaluation.

Reference: Goodman, A.C., and Chasin, W.D.: *In* Gellis, S.S., and Kagan, B.M. (Eds.): Current Pediatric Therapy. 7th Ed. W.B. Saunders Company, Philadelphia, 1976, p. 518.

## RELATION OF REFLEXES TO CENTRAL NERVOUS SYSTEM SEGMENT

Simple reflex testing may help to localize a central nervous system lesion. The table below correlates reflexes to the segment of the central nervous system being tested.

| REFLEX | SEGMENTAL LEVEL |
| --- | --- |
| *Tendon reflexes* | |
| Jaw jerk | Pons; fifth nerve |
| Biceps reflex | Cervical 5–6 |
| Radial-periosteal reflex | Cervical 5–6 |
| Triceps reflex | Cervical 6–7–8 |
| Knee reflex | Lumbar 3–4 |
| Ankle reflex | Sacral 1–2 |
| *Superficial reflexes* | |
| Corneal reflex | Pons; fifth and seventh nerves |
| Pharyngeal reflex | Medulla; ninth and tenth nerves |
| Abdominal reflex | Thoracic 8–12 |
| Cremasteric reflex | Lumbar 1–2 |
| Plantar reflex | Lumbar 5, sacral 1–2 |

Reference: Dodge, P.R.: Neurologic history and examination. *In* Farmer, T.W. (Ed.): Pediatric Neurology. New York, Harper & Row, 1975, p. 30.

## USING THE OTOSCOPE

The otoscope is a valuable diagnostic aid. It is often abused. Several points should be remembered when employing it in your examination of the ears.

1. It should be operated properly. The batteries should be fresh or the light will be yellow.

2. Always use the largest possible speculum. The speculum need never enter the canal more than one-quarter inch, or one-half inch in the older child.

3. The canal should be examined before one tries to look at the drum. Be careful not to poke the otoscope into a furuncle or vesicle at the outer edge of the canal.

4. The otoscope should be held firmly with one hand, and as the speculum is inserted, the hand holding the otoscope should rest firmly on the patient's head or face so that any motion by the patient will be accompanied by a similar movement of the otoscope.

5. Always remember the direction of the canal. In the *infant*, the canal is directed upward, so the auricle should be pulled *down* to view the drum. In the *older child*, the canal faces downward and forward, so

the tip of the auricle is pulled *up and back* for adequate visualization of the drum.

6. If pulling on the auricle elicits pain, the patient has external otitis. This maneuver does not elicit pain in patients with otitis media.

---

Reference: Barness, L.: Manual of Physical Diagnosis. 4th Ed. Chicago, Year Book Medical Publishers, 1973, p. 68.

## TEETH AND GUMS

While examining the mouth, the physician often looks past the teeth and gums directly to the pharynx. Proper oral hygiene is an essential part of preventive medicine, and it is the duty of the pediatrician, as well as the dentist, to advise the parent and child about dental care. The pediatrician should be able to recognize gingival disease that is common to the infant and child. A list of these problems, along with their clinical features and treatment, is presented below.

| DISEASE | CLINICAL FEATURES | TREATMENT |
| --- | --- | --- |
| Gingivitis<br>Early | There is slight edema of gingival margin with color change from pale pink to reddish or bluish red. | Gingivitis is caused by bacteria which form dental plaque. Treatment involves removal of that plaque. Regular tooth brushing is a necessary component of plaque removal. The type of brush used is not important nor is one particular brushing technique better than another. Brushing does not remove plaque between the teeth, however, and dental floss should be used along with brushing for this purpose.<br><br>The gingivitis should resolve within several days of the institution of the above regimen. Fibrous enlargement of the gingiva due to gingivitis must be surgically removed. |
| Moderate | Inflammation is present. The gingiva is red and glazy and bleeds with manipulation. | |
| Severe | The gingiva is red and enlarged, so that it covers more of the tooth than is normal. It may bleed spontaneously, and ulcerations may be present. | |
| Juvenile periodontitis | The gingiva may appear normal, and the only symptom is increased tooth mobility. The permanent first molars and lower incisors are primarily affected. There is extensive bone loss evident on radiologic examination. | Periodontitis may be prevented by strict attention to proper dental care. Recognition of the disease by the pediatrician is an indication for referral to a dentist. |
| Gingival hyperplasia | This is noted particularly in patients with acute myeloblastic and acute monocytic leukemia and in those treated with diphenylhydantoin. The earliest signs are beadlike enlargements on marginal and interdental areas that coalesce to form large tissue masses. These masses may cover the teeth completely in some areas. The tissue is pink and firm and does not bleed. | The hypertrophy caused by acute leukemia may be treated only by surgical removal; that caused by diphenylhydantoin therapy recedes with withdrawal of the drug. |

| | | |
|---|---|---|
| Hereditary gingival fibromatosis | This is a rare disease inherited in an autosomal dominant fashion. The gingival tissue enlarges to cover the teeth. It is of normal color and does not bleed easily. | There is no treatment except surgical removal of gingival tissue. The hypertrophic tissue will recur following removal. |
| Acute necrotizing gingivitis (Vincent's infection; trench mouth) | Bacterial cause has been assumed but never proved. There is a sudden onset of punched-out, crater-like ulcerations of the marginal gingiva. The ulcerations have a whitish pseudomembrane, and they are surrounded by erythema. Any area of the gingiva may be affected. There is spontaneous bleeding of the gingiva. The breath has a fetid odor. There may be regional lymphadenopathy, fever, and malaise. Pain is severe, and mastication is often impossible. | Treatment consists of debridement and frequent mouth rinses with hot salt water or a hydrogen peroxide solution. Systemic antibiotics may be used but are usually not necessary. |
| Acute herpetic gingivosto-matitis | The herpes simplex virus is the cause of this illness. Fever, irritability, and regional lymphadenopathy usually precede intense inflammation of the gingiva. Pain accompanies the inflammation. Small vesicles erupt and then become shallow ulcers with red, elevated margins and gray craters. The gingiva, labial or buccal mucosa, soft palate, pharynx, sublingual mucosa, and tongue may be involved. | Ulcers heal spontaneously in 7 to 14 days. The erythema persists several days more. Viscous Xylocaine may be used to provide symptomatic relief while healing takes place. |

Reference: Polson, A.M.: Pediatrics, *54*:190, 1974.


# POPSICLE PANNICULITIS

Once the popsicle was invented, could popsicle panniculitis be far behind? This form of panniculitis is produced by the sucking on cold objects, such as popsicles and ice cubes. It is characterized by the presence of a reddish-purple discoloration of the cheeks. On occasion it may feel indurated. Tenderness and warmth are unusual.

The lesions are most obvious 24 to 48 hours after the cold injury. They are most commonly confused with a cellulitis. The patients with popsicle panniculitis are afebrile and feel well. The lesions subside without treatment, leaving no permanent injury.

The next time you see a red-faced child, inquire about prolonged sucking on popsicles or ice cubes. Misdiagnosis may leave you red-faced.

Reference: Epstein, E.H., Jr., and Oren, M.E.: N. Engl. J. Med., *282*:966, 1970.

*"Happy the child that has for friend an old, sympathetic, encouraging mind, one eager to develop, slow to rebuke or discourage."*

Arthur Brisbane

## TACHE CEREBRALE

Stroking the skin can often provide diagnostic information. Two major responses may be elicited when the skin over the abdomen, back, or chest is gently stroked with the fingernail. One response is tache cérébrale, and the other is dermatographia.

In tache cérébrale, the stroking produces a red streak that is flanked by thin, pale margins. This sign develops within 30 seconds of stroking and persists for several minutes. It has been noted to be present in patients with scarlet fever, hydrocephalus, a variety of febrile illnesses, and, most particularly, in meningitis. It can be used as an early clue to the presence of meningitis, particularly in the neonatal period.

In dermatographia, the stroking produces a white or pale line with red margins. This wheal is seen in patients with fair skin, in those with vasomotor instability, or in extreme form in patients with urticaria pigmentosa.

Reference: Martin, G.I.: J. Pediatr., *87*:322, 1976.

## THE DEPTH OF RESPIRATION

In patients with alterations in the rate or characteristics of respiration, it is helpful to semi-quantitatively judge the depth of respiration. Values for normal children have been obtained simply by measuring the distance from the nose that air can be felt by the examiner's hand. Although each physician should determine his own normal values, here are some useful guidelines that were obtained while the patients were supine.

| PATIENT'S AGE | DEPTH OF RESPIRATION |
| --- | --- |
| 1 month | 2 inches |
| 3 months | 3 inches |
| 6–12 months | 4 inches |
| 2 years | 6 inches |
| 3–4 years | 8 inches |
| 5–6 years | 9 inches |
| 8–10 years | 10 inches |

Increased depth of respiration is most commonly seen in patients with metabolic acidosis, anemia, bacterial sepsis, or severe hypoxemia.

Decreased depth of respiration is most commonly observed in patients with chronic alkalosis or airway obstruction.

Reference: Barness, L.A.: Manual of Pediatric Physical Diagnosis. 4th Ed. Chicago, Year Book Medical Publishers, 1972, p. 102.

## SCRATCH-PERCUSSION AS A METHOD FOR DETERMINING CARDIAC SIZE

A precise determination of the left and right cardiac borders is a critical part of the physical examination. The use of scratch-percussion will usually detect the presence of cardiomegaly. This technique, unfortunately, is rarely employed by the pediatrician.

With the stethoscope placed over the center of the heart, longitudinal parallel scratches are made with the finger, or a tongue blade, beginning in the axillary line and moving toward the heart at about one-quarter inch intervals. As soon as the scratches are being made over the heart, a change in the intensity of the scratch sound will be detected through the stethoscope. The same procedure can then be repeated starting to the right of the sternum.

Reference: Barness, L.A.: Manual of Pediatric Physical Diagnosis, 4th Ed. Chicago, Year Book Medical Publishers, 1972, p. 114.

## THE INNOCENT THRILL

When a thrill is present, we have been taught to assume that it signifies the presence of either heart or vascular disease. This is not the case. When appropriately examined, approximately one-third of children between the ages of 2 and 15 years with a venous hum will have an accompanying thrill.

This venous hum thrill is best appreciated by placing the plantar surface of the left thumb lightly on the skin just above the right clavicle with the patient in the sitting position.

This thrill is noted only in the sitting position, is always above the right clavicle, and is continuous. Do not be fooled into thinking that you have diagnosed an arteriovenous fistula.

Reference: Bujack, W., Gioia, F., and Cayler, G.G.: J.A.M.A., *235*:2417, 1976.

## SPLENOMEGALY

Normally, the spleen's erythropoietic role ceases at birth. Its primary functions in postnatal life are the filtration of particulate matter and formed elements from the blood and the production of humoral factors required for the opsonization of infectious organisms. Splenomegaly may result from disease states in which these normal functions are required in excess. There are, however, other processes that result in splenomegaly. Reference to the following table should be of some help in making a diagnosis when the spleen is enlarged.

| MECHANISM OF ENLARGEMENT | CLINICAL EXAMPLES | OTHER FINDINGS |
|---|---|---|
| **Sequestration** | | |
| Loss of RBC deformability | Hemolytic anemias, i.e., sickle cell disease, thalassemia, RBC enzyme deficiencies | Jaundice, anemia No peripheral lymphadenopathy |
| Antibody coating of RBCs | Rh and ABO isoimmunization in the newborn. Autoimmune hemolytic anemia | Increased reticulocyte count, peripheral blood smear shows evidence of hemolysis |
| **Proliferation** | | |
| Chronic immunologic stimulation | Viral infections, i.e., infectious mononucleosis, cytomegalovirus Severe bacterial pneumonia, bacterial endocarditis, typhoid fever, indolent septicemia | Generalized lymphadenopathy Atypical lymphocytes Other findings typical of the infectious process |
| **Lipid** | | |
| Accumulation of lipid-laden macrophages in the spleen | Tay-Sach's disease Gaucher's disease Niemann-Pick disease Metachromatic leukodystrophy Gangliosidoses | Appropriate clinical and historical findings for these diseases |
| **Engorgement** | | |
| Portal hypertension | Chronic hepatitis Cystic fibrosis Wilson's disease Biliary atresia Ascending infection via umbilical vein catheter in the newborn Portal vein thrombosis | Hepatomegaly Esophageal varices Internal hemorrhoids History of liver disease Leukopenia, thrombocytopenia |
| Accumulation of blood in the splenic capsule | Splenic trauma | History of trauma |
| Acute splenic engorgement | "Sequestration crisis" of sickle cell disease | Child under 5 years Hypovolemia Anemia Findings of sickle cell disease |
| **Endowment** | | |
| Rare congenital causes of splenomegaly | Splenic hemangiomas Splenic cysts Splenic cystic hygroma | Positive spleen scan |

| iNvasion | | |
|---|---|---|
| Malignancy | Leukemia<br>Lymphoma<br>Metastatic neuroblastoma<br>Histiocytosis | Other findings consistent<br>with these diseases |
| Granuloma | Sarcoidosis<br>Tuberculosis<br>Systemic fungal infection | |

You may have noticed that the underlined letters in the headings above spell SPLEEN. Memorization of these general processes involved in splenic enlargement may help in understanding the disease state of your patient with an enlarged spleen. Remember, however, that approximately 30 per cent of normal term infants and 10 per cent of healthy infants at 1 year of age have a palpable spleen. By age 12, only 1 per cent of normal children have a spleen that may be felt as much as 1 cm below the costal margin.

Reference: Boles, E.T., Jr., Baxter, C.F., and Newton, W.A., Jr.: Clin. Pediatr., 2:161, 1963.

*"The child is surrounded by so much authority, so much school, so much dignity, so much law, that it would have to break down under the weight of all these restraints if it were not saved from such a fate by meeting with a friend."*

Dr. Wilhelm Stekel

## LIVER SIZE

The child admitted as a medical patient to a busy pediatric floor may be examined by many students and physicians. Palpation and percussion of the liver may be reflected in some write-ups as hepatic enlargement and in others as "within normal limits."

The liver size of 105 healthy children aged 5 to 12 years is depicted in Figure 1–8. Examination was by palpation and percussion in the right midclavicular line. Palpation of liver edge below the costal margin alone is an unreliable measurement, presumably because of diaphragmatic movement.

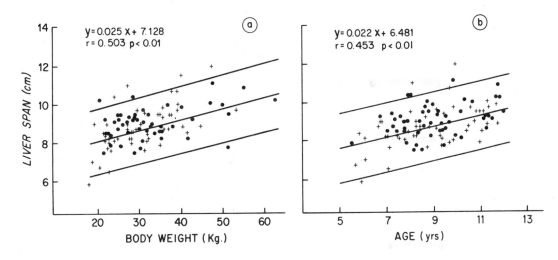

*FIG. 1–8*

Liver span (estimates of height in the right midclavicular line) in normal male and female children was obtained by palpating the lower border and percussing the upper border. The closed circles represent values for females, and the crosses represent values for males. Each mark is a *mean* of the measurements obtained by two investigators. The liver span is plotted against body weight in *A*, and against age in *B*. The middle lines are the regression lines, and the outer lines represent the 95 per cent confidence limits.

Reference:  Younoszai, M.K., and Mueller, S.: Clin. Pediatr., *14*:378, 1975.

# HEPATOMEGALY

The multiple causes of hepatomegaly in infancy and childhood may make the diagnosis of a patient with an enlarged liver difficult. There are a variety of ways of classifying the causes of hepatomegaly. The table below lists the diseases to be suspected according to the mechanism responsible for liver enlargement.

| MECHANISM | CONDITION |
| --- | --- |
| Inflammation | Infection (intrauterine and intrapartum) |
| | Viral hepatitis |
| | Hepatitis with generalized viral infection (cyto-megalovirus, mononucleosis, coxsackie A, B) |
| | Neonatal hepatitis |
| | Hepatic abscess (pyogenic, parasitic) |
| | Parasitic infection (visceral larva migrans, schistosomiasis, flukes) |
| | Toxin and drug reactions (hepatitis, cholestasis) |
| | Biliary tract obstruction |
| Kupffer cell hyperplasia | Septicemia and infection (extrinsic or intrinsic to liver) |
| | Malignant disease (extrinsic or intrinsic to liver) |

| | |
|---|---|
| | Granulomatous hepatitis (sarcoidosis, tuberculosis, etc.) |
| | Phagocyte stimulation (hypervitaminosis A, Thorotrast) |
| Congestion | Congestive heart failure, pericardial tamponade |
| | Budd-Chiari syndrome |
| | Jamaican vomiting disease |
| Infiltration | Erythroblastosis fetalis |
| | Metastatic tumors (neuroblastoma, Wilms' tumor, etc.) |
| | Histiocytosis syndromes |
| | Leukemias |
| | Lymphomas |
| Storage | Glycogen storage diseases |
| | Mucopolysaccharidoses |
| | Gaucher's disease |
| | Niemann-Pick disease |
| | Gangliosidosis $M_1$ |
| | Alpha$_1$-antitrypsin deficiency |
| | Amyloidosis |
| | Hepatic porphyrias |
| Fat accumulation | Malnutrition (kwashiorkor) |
| | Hyperalimentation |
| | Cystic fibrosis |
| | Diabetes mellitus |
| | Galactosemia |
| | Wolman's disease |
| | Reye's syndrome |
| | Tetracycline toxicity |
| Tumor, intrinsic | Congenital hepatic fibrosis–polycystic liver disease |
| | Hereditary hemorrhagic telangiectasia |
| | Hepatoblastoma |
| | Hepatoma |

Often there are accompanying signs that clarify the approach that should be taken. The following physical findings are helpful in the differential diagnosis of hepatomegaly.

| SIGN | CONDITION |
|---|---|
| *Skin* | |
| Carotenemia | Hypervitaminosis A |
| Erythema nodosum | Hepatitis with inflammatory bowel disease or tuberculosis |
| Telangiectasia | Hereditary hemorrhagic telangiectasia |
| Hemangiomas | Multinodular hemangiomatosis of liver |
| Scratch marks | Biliary obstruction |
| Eczematoid rash | Histiocytosis |

*Head*

| Microcephaly | Congenital rubella, toxoplasmosis, or cytomegalovirus infection |
| Hydrocephalus | Congenital syphilis |
| Craniotabes | Hypervitaminosis A |

*Eyes*

| Telangiectasia | Hereditary hemorrhagic telangiectasia |
| Iritis | Hepatitis with inflammatory bowel disease |
| Kayser-Fleischer rings | Wilson's disease |
| Cataracts | Wilson's disease |
| | Galactosemia |
| Papilledema | Hypervitaminosis A |

*Mouth*

| Gingival inflammation | Malnutrition |
| | Wilson's disease |
| Glossitis | Hepatitis with regional enteritis |
| | Cirrhosis of any cause |

*Chest*

| Abnormal breath sounds | Cystic fibrosis |
| | Tuberculosis |

*Abdomen*

| Enlarged cystic kidneys | Congenital hepatic fibrosis–polycystic kidney disease |
| Enlarged spleen | Storage diseases |
| | Hematologic malignancies |
| | Congenital hepatic fibrosis–polycystic liver disease |

*Genitalia*

| Testicular abnormalities | Cystic fibrosis |
| | Histiocytosis |

*Joints*

| Arthritis | Hepatitis with inflammatory bowel disease or juvenile rheumatoid arthritis |

*Neurologic Examination*

| Tremors, dystonia, dysarthria | Wilson's disease, lipid storage diseases |

The age of the patient presenting with hepatomegaly may also help in raising your level of suspicion regarding certain disease states. The list below groups diseases associated with hepatomegaly according to the age at which they are most likely to present.

### Newborn

Intrauterine and intrapartum acquired infection
Erythroblastosis fetalis
Biliary tract obstruction
Neonatal hepatitis
Congestive heart failure
Viral hepatitis
Infection, septicemia

### Infant

Cystic fibrosis
Metabolic
  glycogen storage
  galactosemia
  Gaucher's disease
  alpha$_1$-antitrypsin deficiency
  mucopolysaccharidosis
  Wolman's disease
Histiocytosis syndromes
Malnutrition
Tumors
  intrinsic (hepatoblastoma, multinodular hemangioendothelioma)
  metastatic (neuroblastoma, Wilms' tumor, gonadal tumor)

### Young Child

Toxic and drug reaction
Parasitic (visceral larva migrans)
Leukemia

### Older Child and Adolescent

Chronic active hepatitis
Liver disease with inflammatory bowel disease with juvenile
  rheumatoid arthritis
Drug and alcoholic hepatitis
Lymphoma
Wilson's disease
Hepatic porphyrias
Congenital hepatic fibrosis–polycystic liver disease
Amyloidosis
Alpha$_1$-antitrypsin deficiency

---

Reference: Walker, W.A., and Mathis, R.K.: Pediatr. Clin. North Am., *22*:929, 1975.

# ABDOMINAL MASSES

The diagnostic considerations that accompany the finding of an abdominal mass are largely determined by the age of the patient, associated symptoms, and physical findings. Many abdominal masses detected on routine physical examination ultimately prove to be:

> Fecal material
> Distended urinary bladder
> The abdominal aorta
> A pregnant uterus

*Fecal material* in the colon is usually freely movable and easily compressible. If one suspects that the mass is fecal in origin and this cannot be confirmed by rectal examination, an enema should be given to the patient and the examination repeated.

A *distended bladder* may be palpated in the newborn who has not voided within the first 24 hours of life. This delay may signify the presence of abnormalities of the urethra, such as posterior urethral valves. Other causes of bladder distention include:

> The use of anticholinergic drugs
> Spinal cord tumors
> Abnormalities of the spinal cord
> Coma
> The early postoperative period
> Bladder irritation produced by an inflammatory lesion in the pelvis,
>    such as an inflamed appendix or appendiceal abscess

If the mass is of bladder origin, it will appear to originate at a point below the symphysis pubis and may extend as high as the umbilicus. Rectal examination will usually confirm the presence of a distended bladder. If the child cannot be induced to void, catheterization may be required to confirm the diagnosis.

### Abdominal Masses in Older Infants and Children

#### GASTROINTESTINAL MASSES

Ages 3 to 6 weeks
1. Most common mass is the "tumor" of *pyloric stenosis*.
2. *Duplications* of the gastrointestinal tract, usually of the small bowel, are generally accompanied by symptoms of intestinal obstruction. May be of neurenteric origin and associated with defects in the vertebral column.

Ages 6 months to 3 years
1. *Intussusception* is the most common mass. At this age it is usually secondary to:
> Enlarged mesenteric lymph nodes
> Polyps

Meckel's diverticulum

Henoch-Schönlein purpura

2. *Mesenteric cyst.* Associated with painless abdominal enlargement. May be of months to years in duration. Freely movable in the lateral direction and sometimes associated with a fluid wave or shifting dullness.

3. *Appendiceal abscess.*

4. Abscesses and fistulas secondary to *granulomatous colitis*.

## NEOPLASMS

Most common tumors are neuroblastomas and Wilms' tumor.

### Wilms' Tumor

Clinical features include:

1. Approximately 60 per cent occur before age 5 years.
2. May be associated with fever, pain, and hypertension.
3. Hematuria present in 20 per cent of patients at diagnosis.
4. Mass may extend to midline and into the iliac fossa.
5. Intestine displaced to the opposite side.
6. Calcifications uncommon.
7. Tumor spreads locally but also metastasizes to liver, lung, and brain.
8. Occurs with increased frequency in children with sporadic (in contrast to familial) aniridia.
9. Occurs with increased frequency in patients with congenital hemihypertrophy and congenital macrosomia (Beckwith's syndrome).

### Neuroblastoma

Clinical features include:

1. About 50 per cent occur within first 2 years of life.
2. In about one-half of patients, tumor arises in the abdomen. In one-third of patients it is in the adrenal gland, and in an additional 18 to 20 per cent it arises from nonadrenal intra-abdominal sites.
3. Mass frequently crosses the midline.
4. Calcifications common on x-ray films of the abdomen.
5. Skeletal metastases common. Lung metastases uncommon.
6. Skin, hepatic, and nodal involvement may be present at time of diagnosis. Invasion of retrobulbar soft tissue frequently observed and produces proptosis of the eye as well as periorbital swelling and ecchymosis of the upper eyelid.
7. Initial signs and symptoms may reflect excessive catecholamine production by the tumor and include skin flushing, perspiration, tachycardia, hypertension, paroxysmal headaches, and intractable diarrhea.
8. Uncommon initial manifestations include signs of encephalopathy or opsoclonus.

A general list of the more common abdominal masses that may be encountered in infants and children is listed below.

### Abdominal Masses in the Older Infant and Child

Renal malformations

Hydronephrosis

Duplication cysts of the intestine
Volvulus of the gut
Intussusception
Periappendiceal abscess
Mesenteric abscess
Mesenteric cyst
Hepatic cyst or abscess
Choledochal cyst
Pancreatic pseudocyst
Hepatoma
Hemangioma of the liver or spleen
Wilms' tumor
Neuroblastoma
Lymphoma
Ovarian cyst
Ovarian tumor

Initial evaluation should include a careful rectal examination, complete blood count, urinalysis, and flat plate of the abdomen. More precise studies will be dictated by the preliminary findings.

References: Arey, J.B.: Pediatr. Clin. North Am., *10*:665, 1963. Sutow, W., Vietti, T.J., and Fernbach, D.J.: Clinical Pediatric Oncology. St. Louis, C.V. Mosby Company, 1973.

*"I remember seeing a picture of an old man addressing a small boy. 'How old are you?' 'Well if you go by what Mamma says, I'm 5. But if you go by the fun I've had, I'm 'most 100.' "*

William Lyon Phelps

# A DIAGNOSTIC APPROACH TO LYMPHADENOPATHY

Is the lymphadenopathy generalized or localized? Generalized lymphadenopathy is defined as enlargement of more than two noncontiguous node regions. Generalized lymphadenopathy is caused by generalized disease.

## GENERALIZED LYMPHADENOPATHY

What are associated signs and symptoms?
Rash?
Hepatosplenomegaly?
Thyroid enlargement?
Joint involvement?
Heart and lung abnormalities?
Pallor?
Easy bruising?

*Infections*

Exanthems
Cytomegalovirus
Infectious mononucleosis
Infectious hepatitis
Typhoid fever
Malaria

Pyogenic
Tuberculosis
Syphilis
Toxoplasmosis
Brucellosis
Histoplasmosis

*Collagen Vascular Disease*

Lupus erythematosus
Rheumatoid arthritis

## LOCALIZED LYMPHADENOPATHY

Signs of infection in the involved node?
Evidence of infection in the drainage area of node?
History of recent antigenic introduction in the node's drainage area?

*Supraclavicular* — Always consider mediastinal disease (tuberculosis, histoplasmosis, coccidioidomycosis, sarcoidosis). Always consider lymphoma. In absence of evidence of pulmonary infection, early biopsy indicated.

*Axillary* — Secondary to infections in the hand, arm, lateral chest wall, or lateral portion of the breast. May be result of recent immunization in the arm.

*Epitrochlear* — Secondary to infections on ulnar side of hand and forearm. Observed in tularemia when bite occurs on finger. Also seen in secondary syphilis.

*Immunologic Reactions*
Serum sickness, drug reactions
Granulomatous disease (sarcoid)

*Storage Disease*
Gaucher's disease
Niemann-Pick disease

*Malignancies*
Leukemia
Lymphoma
Histiocytosis
Neuroblastoma, metastatic

*Hyperthyroidism*

*Inguinal* — Infection in lower extremity, scrotum, penis, vulva, vagina, skin of lower abdomen, perineum, gluteal region, or anal canal. May be seen in lymphogranuloma venereum. May represent metastatic disease from testicular tumors or bony tumors of the leg. Immunization in leg.

*Cervical* — Generally the result of localized infection. See accompanying table for differential diagnosis.

## Causes of Cervical Adenitis

| CAUSE | COMMENT |
|---|---|
| Viral upper respiratory infections | Most common cause. Nodes soft, minimally tender, and not associated with evidence of redness and warmth of overlying skin. |
| Bacterial infection | Streptococcus and staphylococcus most common etiologic agents. Usually secondary to previous or associated infection in drainage area of node. More frequently unilateral. Signs of infection — tenderness, warmth, and redness generally present. Look for primary focus of infection in scalp, mouth, pharynx, and sinuses. |
| Tuberculosis | *Mycobacterium tuberculosis* infections generally bilateral, involve multiple nodes. Associated with evidence of chest disease and systemic signs. Atypical mycobacteria infections more commonly unilateral initially. Not associated, in general, with other foci of disease. With either agent, evidence of local warmth and redness uncommon. |
| Infectious mononucleosis | Fever, malaise, preceding upper respiratory infection often noted. Splenomegaly common. Atypical lymphocytes present. Epstein-Barr virus titers required for diagnosis in younger children. |
| Cytomegalovirus Toxoplasmosis | Indistinguishable clinically from Epstein-Barr virus infections. Requires serologic studies to make the diagnosis. |
| Cat-scratch disease | History of contact with young cat. May be preceded by history of fever and malaise. Adenopathy restricted to area drained by initial cat scratch. |
| Sarcoidosis | Disease bilateral. Chest x-ray almost always abnormal. May have keratitis, iritis and evidence of bone disease. |
| Hodgkin's disease | Common presenting symptom. Frequently unilateral at time of initial manifestation. Node is rubbery, nontender, and not associated with signs of inflammation. Make certain that supraclavicular involvement is not present. When present, strongly suspect lymphoma. |

Non-Hodgkin's lymphoma

Bilateral at time of initial presentation in approximately 40 per cent of patients. Cervical and submaxillary nodes commonly involved together.

## MANAGEMENT

*If nontender*

Complete blood count
Epstein-Barr virus antibody tests
Skin test for both *Mycobacterium tuberculosis* and atypical mycobacteria
Chest x-ray

*If warm and tender*
Aspirate for smear and culture

If all studies are normal, presume to be dealing with deep-seated bacterial infection. Measure node carefully. Measure node carefully, then treat with penicillin or penicillin derivative for 2 to 4 weeks in large doses. If the node has not decreased in size or changed in character, or has gotten painlessly larger, then node excision and biopsy should be performed.

*"Children work a greater metamorphosis in men than any other condition of life. They ripen one wonderfully and make life ten times better worth having than it was."*

T. H. Huxley

## THE TESTES—SITUS INVERSUS

Usually the left testis hangs lower in the scrotum than does the right. When both testes are descended and the right testis is lower than the left, always suspect that the patient may have situs inversus.

## SCROTAL SWELLING

Although most children with swelling of the scrotum have either a hernia or hydrocele, other conditions must be considered. A thorough history and physical examination can often point to a specific diagnosis prior to or obviating the need for surgical exploration.

*Conditions Associated with Scrotal Swelling*

| CONDITION | CLINICAL CLUES |
| --- | --- |
| Hernia, direct | Uncommon, usually does not transilluminate; reducible unless incarcerated; usually tender. |
| Hernia, indirect | History of intermittent swelling in the inguinal region; fluid sometimes present (therefore, transillumination may be positive); usually tender; reducible unless incarcerated; peristalsis may be audible on auscultation. |
| Hydrocele | Frequent under 2 years of age; transillumination usually positive; nontender; not reducible; associated testicular enlargement is suggestive of tumor. |
| Torsion of testis or appendage | Acute onset of pain, followed shortly by swelling and discoloration; elevation of mass *increases* pain; surgical emergency. |
| Epididymo-orchitis | May be accompanied by signs of urethritis (e.g., dysuria); can be gonococcal in origin; associated fever common; painful; elevation of testis *decreases* pain; torsion can be ruled out only by surgical exploration. |
| Orchitis (true) | May be history of recent parotid swelling or other clues to mumps or enteroviral infection; painful; elevation of testis decreases pain. |
| Trauma | History usually positive; hematoma may be seen. |
| Edema, generalized | History and physical examination will often provide clues to primary process, as well as demonstrate edema of eyelids, sacrum, ankles, or other sites. |

| | |
|---|---|
| Edema, local | Examination may reveal source of local problem (e.g., insect bite or diaper dermatitis characteristic of detergent sensitivity); testis is nontender and normal in size. |
| Leukemia | Other systemic signs of illness usually present. |
| Anaphylactoid purpura | Characteristic rash usually present or beginning. |
| Filariasis | Peripheral eosinophilia. |
| Testicular tumor | Painless; may have associated hydrocele; sexual precocity or gynecomastia have been associated. |
| Cyst or angioma | May transilluminate; painless; not reducible; examination may disclose lesions elsewhere. |

# UNILATERAL ANOMALIES OF PAIRED STRUCTURES

Symmetrical morphogenesis is a natural phenomenon that is best appreciated when it does not occur. There may be unilateral defects in human beings that are the result of anomalous morphogenesis. It is interesting that some of the frequent unilateral anomalies tend to occur on one side more than the other, while others occur equally on either side.

| AREA | DEFECT | LEFT (%) | RIGHT (%) |
|---|---|---|---|
| Craniofacial | Cleft lip | 68 | 32 |
| | Agenesis of maxillary incisor | 55 | 45 |
| | Hemifacial microsomia | 38 | 62 |
| Thoracoabdominal | Renal agenesis | 56 | 44 |
| | Supernumerary nipples | 55 | 45 |
| | Poland's anomaly | 32 | 68 |
| | Pulmonary agenesis | 43 | 57 |
| | Cryptorchidism | 40 | 60 |
| | Inguinal hernia | 33 | 67 |
| Limb | Postaxial polydactyly | 77 | 23 |
| | Congenital dislocated hip | 62 | 38 |
| | Clubfoot | 45 | 55 |
| | Radial aplasia | 42 | 58 |
| | Fibular aplasia | 35 | 65 |
| General | Hemihypertrophy | 38 | 62 |
| | Hemiatrophy, isolated | 73 | 27 |
| | Hemiatrophy, as a feature in Russell-Silver syndrome | 70 | 30 |

| Neoplastic | Neuroblastoma | 55 | 45 |
|---|---|---|---|
| | Wilms' tumor | 50 | 50 |
| | Retinoblastoma | 45 | 55 |

Congenital hemihypertrophy is the grossest of these unilateral inequities, but bodily asymmetry may represent the failure of growth on one side rather than the acceleration of development on the other. Asymmetry may be due to any of the following:

Hemiatrophy

Hemidysplasia
   Intrauterine growth retardation
    Russell-Silver syndrome
    Chromosomal mosaicism
   Chromosomal abnormalities
   Hemifacial microsomia
   Cerebral palsy

Hemihypertrophy
   Idiopathic congenital hemihypertrophy
   Syndromes
    Neurocutaneous syndromes
     Neurofibromatosis
     Tuberous sclerosis
     Sturge-Weber disease
     Lindau-von Hippel disease
    Beckwith-Wiedemann syndrome

Skin and vascular abnormalities
   Angiodysplasias
    Arteriovenous malformations
    Venous malformations
    Hemangiomatosis
   Lymphatic abnormalities
    Lymphangioma
    Lymphedema
   Lipomatosis

Hemiatrophy is probably a postnatal process with onset in preadolescence in 75 per cent of cases. Atrophy usually involves subcutaneous tissues and fat and is often associated with neurologic disorders.

Idiopathic hemihypertrophy, on the other hand, is congenital, though it may not be detected until late infancy or childhood. Abnormalities associated with idiopathic hemihypertrophy are listed below. These associated abnormalities may be ipsilateral or contralateral.

*Anomalies Associated with Idiopathic Hypertrophy*

Renal abnormalities
  Benign nephromegaly
    Unilateral
    Bilateral
  Medullary sponge kidney
  Wilms' tumor

Tumors
  Common
    Wilms' tumor
    Adrenocortical tumors
      Carcinoma
      Adenoma
      Hyperplasia
    Hepatoblastoma
  Rare
    Gonadoblastoma
    Neuroblastoma
    Sarcoma

Skin abnormalities
  Edema
  Ichthyosis
  Coarse hair
  Hypertrichosis
  Calor
  Nevi
  Hemangiomas
  Telangiectasia
  Prominent veins
  Café-au-lait spots
  Dystrophic nails
  Minor dermatoglyphic pattern changes

Other
  Mental retardation (15–20 per cent)
  Enlarged pupil
  Polydactyly
  Bronchiectasis
  Congenital heart disease
  Supernumerary nipples
  Hypogonadism
  Hypospadias
  Cryptorchidism

Because of the risk of intra-abdominal tumors, children with hemihypertrophy should have close follow-up, including periodic intravenous pyelogram and liver-spleen scan.

---

References: Kirks, D.R., and Shackelford, G.D.: Radiology, *115*:145, 1975. Schnall, B.S., and Smith, D.W.: J. Pediatr., *85*:509, 1974.

## LOCALIZED EDEMA—A SIGN OF SYSTEMIC DISEASE

Some generalized disorders may produce characteristic localized signs. One such sign is the presence of unusual edema. Listed below are some sites of localized edema and the disease process that should be considered.

| | |
|---|---|
| Edema of the eyelids | Early finding of both roseola infantum and infectious mononucleosis |
| Edema of the forehead | Henoch-Schönlein purpura |
| Edema of the glottis | Angioneurotic edema |
| Edema of the neck | Diphtheria. Accompanied by lymphadenopathy |
| Edema over the sternum | Mumps |
| Edema of the hands and feet in the newborn period | Turner's syndrome Milroy's disease |
| Edema of the hands and feet in the older infant and child | Sickle cell disease ("hand-foot syndrome"). Edema usually accompanied by warmth and tenderness |
| Scrotal edema | Early manifestation of Henoch-Schönlein purpura |
| Pretibial edema | Hypothyroidism |

## BUT DOCTOR, WHAT ABOUT MY CHILD'S FEET?

This question is frequently asked and all too often prompts an ambiguous answer from the physician. Two of the more common concerns are for "flatfeet" or "pigeon toes." Before dealing specifically with these problems, some definitions and general principles are required.

### Definitions

| | |
|---|---|
| Adduction | Displacement toward the midline of the body. |
| Abduction | Displacement away from the midline of the body. |

| | |
|---|---|
| Varus | Bending inward toward the midline (like a flexible bow). |
| Valgus | Bending away from the midline of the body (synonymous with the term "valgus of the foot" is the term "pronation"). |
| Inversion of foot | Usually implies the simultaneous motions of: <br>     plantar flexion at the ankle (toes down) <br>     varus at the heel <br>     adduction of the forefoot <br> Fixed inversion is characteristic of the clubfoot. |
| Eversion of foot | Usually refers to the simultaneous motions of: <br>     dorsiflexion at the ankle (toes up) <br>     valgus of the heel <br>     abduction of the forefoot <br> Fixed eversion is characteristic of the calcaneovalgus foot. |

### Principles of the Foot Examination

1. Foot deformities must always be evaluated from the standpoint of all three interdependent joint movements and not from the obvious problem at the heel or forefoot.

2. When examining for a potential foot problem, never limit your examination to the foot.

3. All bony relationships in the infant's foot should be palpated.

4. The infant's foot should also be examined from the undersurface to evaluate deformities in the forefoot and hindfoot.

5. Always invert and evert the foot to detect any rigidity or limitation of motion.

6. Look for tibial torsion or bowing.

7. Check for range of motion at the knee.

8. Check for abnormalities of hip motion.

9. Examine the spine for evidence of scoliosis, dimpling, or other evidence of spinal deformity.

10. In the older infant and child, always observe the patient walking without shoes.

11. Inspect the shoes for evidence of abnormal wear. Normal heel-toe gait wears the shoes more on the outer border of the heel and the inner border of the toe.

12. Test reflexes at the ankle and knee. Check for an "anal wink."

13. Look for asymmetry of muscles or muscle weakness.

### Flatfeet

Flatfeet may be categorized as flexible or rigid. Only 2 per cent of flatfeet are rigid flatfeet as a result of bony abnormalities. In flexible flatfeet, the abnormality is evident only upon weight-bearing, while in rigid flatfeet the abnormality is obvious at all times.

In evaluating a patient for a flat or pronated foot, remember the following:

1. In the pre–weight-bearing period, the foot does not have any real arch and the positions of the developing bones are concealed in a thick layer of adipose tissue.

2. When the child first begins to stand, he assumes a wide-based stance with the weight-bearing line falling toward the inner side of the foot.

3. Between the ages of 12 and 30 months, slight pronation is normal, but beyond this period it is significant.

4. When pronation is present, as the child stands, the pronated foot tends to roll outward. The arch disappears and the medial border of the foot becomes prominent. This is best observed from the rear, and in the usual case the medial side of the foot drops downward and inward. Figures 1–9 and 1–10 should allow you to recognize the true flat or pronated foot.

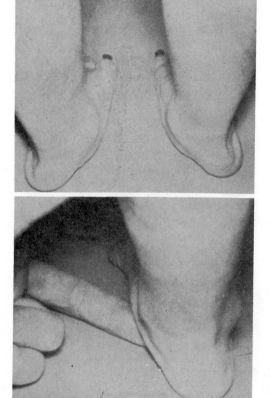

FIG. 1–9

*A*, Depression of longitudinal arch. Note eversion of heel and curve in line of Achilles tendon. *B*, Note how evaluation of longitudinal arch corrects heel valgus.

FIG. 1–10

A, In the normal foot, weight is borne slightly on the medial side of the heel as seen from the rear. On side view, the normal arch has adequate talar support from the calcaneus, and weight is transmitted to the os calcis and metatarsal heads. B, Flatfeet are characterized by a turning out of the calcaneus from under the talus as seen from the rear. On side view, the loss of talar support (arrow) is evident as weight is borne on the entire medial border of the foot.

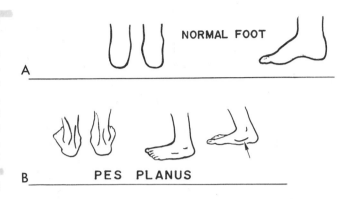

## Pigeon Toes

Toeing-in may be caused by many conditions in the foot, tibia, femur, or a combination of these. Most commonly, it arises in the foot as a metatarsus adductus or adductovarus. It is characterized by adduction through the tarsometatarsal joint, a tendency to walk on the lateral side of the foot, an increase in the height of the longitudinal arch, and an increase in the space between the first and second toes. Figure 1–11 illustrates some of these features.

FIG. 1–11

A, Pigeon toes due to metatarsus adductus are characterized by a convex lateral border of the foot and prominent base of the fifth metatarsal. Anteroposterior x-ray views show adduction of the forefoot and widening of the space between the first and second metatarsals. The talocalcaneal angle is increased as the calcaneus is turned out from under the talus, while the talus remains relatively fixed by the ankle. On lateral x-ray view, the metatarsals appear to be stacked on one another owing to the turned-in position of the forefoot (adductovarus). B, Toeing-in from tibial torsion is characterized by a posterior position of the medial malleolus relative to the lateral malleolus. X-ray examination frequently shows bowing of the tibia, which magnifies the apparent internal rotation. Increased medial cortical density seen in the bowed tibia and fibula is due to compressive stress.

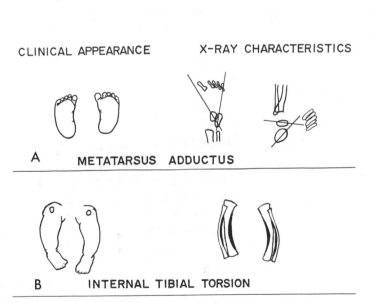

In evaluating patients for pigeon toes, remember:

1. Metatarsus adductus is usually present at birth.

2. The most reliable method of detecting this deformity is by examining the foot from the undersurface, as illustrated in Figure 1–11.

3. In the normal foot, a definite concavity can be seen and felt along the lateral border at the base of the fifth metatarsal. Forefoot adduction reverses this concavity to a convexity and is associated with a prominent base of the fifth metatarsal.

4. The majority of feet with forefoot adduction will correct spontaneously by age 3 years if the child has a flexible foot.

5. The flexibility of the foot can best be demonstrated by stroking along the lateral border of the foot and ankle to stimulate the peroneal muscles. If the child straightens out the forefoot adduction, generally the foot will correct spontaneously, and cast treatment will not be required.

References: Connolly, J., Regen, E., and Hillman, J.W.: Pediatr. Clin. North Am., *17*:291, 1970. Funk, F.J., Jr.: Pediatr. Clin. North Am., *14*:571, 1976.

## TOE-WALKING

Remember, some normal children walk on their toes. The most common cause of toe-walking is cerebral palsy. These children have the spastic form of the disease. A simple neurologic examination will reveal the cause of the toe-walking in this circumstance. Less common causes of toe-walking include:

Congenital shortening of the Achilles tendon
Dystonia musculorum deformans
Early muscular dystrophy
Infantile autism

## ALOPECIA

Parental complaints of childhood hair loss are not uncommon. An important cause of such hair loss is alopecia areata.

### Characteristics of Alopecia Areata

*Scalp examination* shows pattern of hair loss in smooth, white shiny bald patches without erythema, edema, scaling, or scarring; eyelashes and/or eyebrows may be involved.

*Microscopic examination* reveals diagnostic "exclamation point" morphology of hair at border of patch.

*Associated findings* can include pitting, ridging, and/or thickening of nails.

*Natural history* is that of hair loss followed by appearance of vellus hair and subsequently by normal terminal hair; new patch may appear as earlier one fills in.

*Etiology* is unknown.

*Therapy* in any form is ineffective; reassurance of eventual outcome will help parents and patient; wig may be indicated.

*Prognosis* is good if terminal hair appears within a year; 2 to 5 per cent of patients develop total hair loss (alopecia totalis), but incidence may be greater in younger children.

The characteristics of other types of hair loss are shown in the accompanying table.

| TYPE OF HAIR LOSS | ASSOCIATED CONDITIONS | DIFFERENTIAL POINTS |
|---|---|---|
| Traumatic | Trichotillomania; excessive massaging, brushing, combing, braiding, pressure from bands. | Pattern of loss irregular or bizarre; broken-off hair usually seen; "exclamation point" hair *not* seen. |
| Congenital alopecia | None or progeria, ectodermal dysplasia, aminoacidopathy, monilethrix, pili torti. | Hair sparse, fine, thin, rather than totally absent. Other findings of primary condition usually found. Monilethrix — hair shows beading under microscope. Pili torti — hair shaft shows twisting under microscope. |
| Telogen effluvium | Severe fever, intoxication, or anemia; malnutrition. | Hair loss diffuse rather than patchy; smooth, white shiny scalp *absent*. |
| Drug-induced | Antimitotic agents, thallium, anticoagulants, thyroid compounds, excessive vitamin A, chloroquine, trimethadione. | Hair loss diffuse rather than patchy; smooth, white shiny scalp *absent*. |
| Endocrine disturbances | Hypopituitarism, hypothyroidism, hyperthyroidism, hyperadrenocorticism/precocious puberty. | Findings of primary disorder will be present. |
| Inflammatory diseases | Lupus vulgaris, leprosy, syphilis, pediculosis, varicella-zoster virus infections; multiple insect bites or tick bites. | Inflammatory involvement usually obvious. |
| Alopecia with scaling | Fungus infection. | Culture usually positive, Wood's lamp exam often positive; microscopic exam of scales and hair are diagnostic. |
| Alopecia with scarring | Trauma, x-irradiation, morphea, scleroderma, sarcoid, discoid lupus erythematosus, necrobiosis lipoidica, lichen planopilaris, incontinentia pigmenti, ichthyosis, congenital erythroderma, Darier's disease. | Scarring; total absence of hair follicles, atrophic epidermis; skin biopsy may be helpful; findings of primary disorder may be present. |

Reference: Wilgram, G.F.: *In* Gellis, S.S., and Kagan, B.M. (Eds.): Current Pediatric Therapy. 6th Ed. Philadelphia, W.B. Saunders Company, 1973, p. 510.

# CHRONIC FATIGUE

The tired physician frequently tires of hearing about patients with chronic fatigue. Although lassitude is a complaint of adults, it is not unusual for parents to complain that their child "has no pep."

Listed on the following page are some things to consider:

Normal developmental feature (common among children
2 to 5 years of age)
Insufficient sleep
Puberty
Psychological factors, including personality and insecurity
Chronic infection, such as pyelonephritis, lung abscess,
tuberculosis
Rheumatic fever
Rheumatoid arthritis
Medications
Myasthenia gravis
Collagen vascular diseases
Gilbert's disease
Subacute bacterial endocarditis
Addison's disease
Chronic renal disease with azotemia
Iron deficiency anemia

A careful history coupled with a physical examination, complete
blood count, urinalysis, and sedimentation rate is generally sufficient in
an initial sorting out of the problem.

## SCHOOL PHOBIA

Vague physical complaints are frequently heard in the pediatrician's
office. When combined with normal physical and laboratory findings
*and* poor school attendance because of the complaints, the child is
often found to have "school phobia," a descriptive term for anxiety
over leaving home in the 6 to 10 year old group.

Once a significant child-teacher conflict or fear of harassment by
other children has been ruled out, the physician's immediate goal
should be the return of the child to full school attendance. Steps in this
direction to be discussed during the visit are listed below.

1.  Do a thorough physical examination and pertinent laboratory studies as
soon as possible. The child should then be given an unequivocal "clean bill of
health." The findings should be conveyed to the parents along with a brief but
sympathetic explanation about the reality of symptoms caused by anxiety or
depression.

2.  The parents should be gently but firmly convinced that *immediate* return
of the child to school is essential. The parents must insist on the child's return to
school for this step to be effective. Delay in return to school makes it increasingly
difficult for the child to go back.

3.  What to expect and what to do on school mornings should be reviewed
with the mother. She should *not* ask the child how he feels. If he is up he should go
to school, even if he is late or has missed the school bus. If he comes home at lunch
he should be returned. If the child says he is ill, the mother should do one of two
things. If questionably or mildly ill, he can be sent to school. If the mother feels the
child is truly ill, he should be seen by the physician *early that same morning. The
child is not to stay at home without seeing a physician.*

4.  The person to be in charge of taking the child to school if he refuses to go
should be clarified. This may be one of the parents, another relative, school social
worker, or other responsible adult.

5. The school principal should be contacted by the physician, who can ask the school's cooperation in helping the child return to school. This is especially important if the child has a real or imaginary fear regarding some condition at school. The school nurse should also be contacted if she has been sending the child home for minor illness. She should be asked to have the child rest in her office for a time rather than send him home.

6. Weekly visits for several weeks are important for follow-up. A final visit several months later will allow long-term assessment.

Failure of this program, if conscientiously carried out by parents, physician and school personnel, suggests the necessity of psychiatric referral to explore the severe dependency problems that are often present.

Prevention of school phobia and related dependency problems can be aided by the encouragement of independence at appropriate times during infancy and preschool problems. The following milestones of independence may be useful guidelines.

| WHEN | CHILD SHOULD |
|------|-------------|
| By 6 months | be left with baby sitter while parents have evenings out. |
| By 2 years | be left home, while awake, with baby sitter. |
| By 3 years | experience being left somewhere other than his home. |
| As soon as ready | be allowed to feed, dress, and wash himself. |
| By 3–4 years | be allowed to play in yard by himself. |
| By 4–5 years | be allowed to play in neighborhood by himself. |

Reference: Schmitt, B.D.: Pediatrics, *48*:433, 1971.

*"The real child does not confuse fact and fiction. He simply likes fiction. He acts it, because he cannot as yet write it or even read it; but he never allows his moral sanity to be clouded by it. To him no two things could possibly be more totally contrary than playing at robbers and stealing sweets."*

G. K. Chesterton

# PHOTOPHOBIA

Although the illnesses associated with photophobia are often obvious and relatively easily diagnosed (e.g., viral conjunctivitis, measles, or bacterial meningitis), there are other, more subtle conditions that must be considered when the primary diagnosis is not so obvious. Some of these associations are listed below.

| *More Common Associated Infections* | *Noninfectious Associations* |
|---|---|
| Measles | Infantile glaucoma |
| Coxsackie B infection | Albinism |
| Lymphocytic choriomeningitis | Vitamin A deficiency |
| Viral conjunctivitis | Keratitis (e.g., Reiter's |
| Arbovirus infection | syndrome) |
| Bacterial meningitis | Erythropoietic porphyria |
| | Acute cerebellar ataxia |
| | Chédiak-Higashi syndrome |
| *Less Common Associated Infections* | Aniridia |
| | Cystinosis |
| Phlyctenular conjunctivitis | Migraine |
| Yellow fever | Corneal ulcer |
| Psittacosis infections | Hysteria (in older child) |
| Rickettsial infections | Arsenic poisoning |
| | Mercury poisoning |
| | Drug toxicity |
| | Trimethadione |
| | Ethosuccimide |
| | PAS |

References: Wintrobe, M.M., Thorn, G.W., Adams, R.D., et al. (Eds.): Harrison's Principles of Internal Medicine. 7th Ed. New York, McGraw Hill Book Company, 1974. Illingworth, R.S.: Common Symptoms of Disease in Children. 5th Ed. Oxford, Blackwell Scientific Publications, 1975, p. 184. Barnett, H.L. (Ed.): Pediatrics. 15th Ed. New York, Appleton-Century-Crofts, 1972.

## THE EYELASH SYNDROME

All adults appreciate the fact that a foreign body in the eye is both annoying and painful. The most common foreign body to produce such discomfort indoors is the eyelash. We frequently forget that eyelashes may get into the eyes of infants as well. The next time you are confronted with an irritable, crying baby for which you cannot find a suitable explanation, be sure to check the eyes for a foreign body. If you find it, you can produce an instant cure.

## COLIC

Colic can best be defined as paroxysms of irritability and crying that may progress to agonized screaming, in which an infant, during the first 3 to 4 months of life, appears to be in abdominal pain. During the attacks, the infant often draws up his knees against his abdomen and may pass flatus. The attacks generally occur in the late afternoon or early evening on an almost daily basis and may last from 15 minutes to 4 to 6 hours. These attacks may commence within the first week of life and usually subside by 4 months of age.

The fact that colic is so common and yet so poorly understood in terms of its cause bears a not so silent testimony to our medical ignorance.

Colic should be distinguished from other causes of fussiness. Among those would be included:

Anal fissure
Incarcerated hernia
Glaucoma
Lash in the eye
Corneal abrasion
An open safety pin
Testicular torsion
Caffey's disease
Mercury poisoning
Hypervitaminosis A
Otitis media

Management should include the following:

1. A prompt response to the parent's concern.
2. A careful physical examination.
3. An explanation to the parents of the natural course of colic and our lack of medical knowledge that can produce a specific treatment.
4. If mother is breast-feeding, an inquiry as to whether she is eating shellfish, nuts, or chocolate. Rarely, they may be responsible.
5. Discuss the possibility that it may represent an allergy to cow milk. This is also unusual, but a trial of a soy protein may be justified.
6. Encourage the institution of abdominal warmth or rhythmic rocking or singing to soothe the child. Sometimes placing the child in an infant seat on top of an automatic clothes washer in full cycle produces both slight vibration and warmth and may relieve the attack.
7. Any trial should be prescribed for a brief and finite time so that you may see the mother again to check on results and then try something new.
8. Encourage the parents to get out of the house on occasion to gain surcease from the crying.
9. Bolster the mother's confidence so that these attacks do not destroy her confidence or instill negative feelings about her baby which may engender guilt.
10. As a last resort, attempt a brief trial of a mild anticholinergic agent such as Bentyl (dicyclomine hydrochloride).

---

References: Honig, P.J.: Curr. Probl. Pediatr., 5:22, 1975. Illingworth, R.S.: Lancet, 2:119, 1959.

*"They dwell and flourish in their own natures, preternaturally practical and crafty pygmies in the world of dull and tyrannous giants into which it has pleased God to call them."*

Walter de la Mare

## THE BEST OF BARNESS

Despite the introduction of computerized axial tomography, the SMA–12, the bone scan, ultrasonography, and similar technologic advances, the detailed history and careful physical examination still remain the bedrock of the diagnostic process. The text entitled *Manual of Pediatric Physical Diagnosis* by Lewis A. Barness is a testimony to what can be learned by examination of the infant and child. On every page are multiple facts and helpful suggestions to guide you in performing a physical examination. Some of the pointers we like best are excerpted below.

Physical examinations are performed in children by taking full advantage of opportunities as they present themselves. . . . The order of an adequate examination, therefore, is more or less determined by the child rather than the physician.

A rectal examination is done whenever the patient has any symptom referable to the gastrointestinal tract.

Modesty should be respected in a child regardless of age.

The child with paradoxical hyperirritability may lie quietly on the examining table only to scream when picked up by the mother. This is a valuable sign since most children are calmed when picked up, and may indicate a serious disturbance in the central nervous system, particularly meningitis, or pain in motion such as occurs with scurvy, fracture, cortical hyperostosis, or acrodynia; or it may represent a serious disturbance in response to painful stimuli.

A musty or mousy odor is found in children with phenylketonuria or diphtheria.

Slight pulsations of the anterior fontanel occur in normal infants. Marked pulsations, however, may be a sign of increased intracranial pressure, venous sinus thrombosis, obstruction of the venous return from the head, or increased pressure due to an arteriovenous shunt, patent ductus arteriosus, or excitement.

Macewen's sign is one that many examiners like to elicit, but usually it has little significance in childhood. On percussing the skull with one finger, a resonant "cracked-pot" sound is heard. As long as the fontanel is open, this type of sound is physiological. After closure of the fontanel, the sound indicates increased intracranial pressure or a dilated ventricle.

Unilateral paralysis of the face, including the muscles of the forehead and eyelid, indicates a peripheral facial nerve lesion and may be due to trauma, otitis media, or other peripheral lesions. Recovery from the peripheral nerve palsy may occur in the upper portion of the face first, and at this time may resemble a supranuclear weakness.

---

*Pediatrics*—Derived from the Greek *pais* or *paido*, which means child, and *iatria*, which means medical treatment.

Children's pupils should react to light quickly. Reaction of the pupil on which the light shines is the direct reaction; of the opposite pupil, consensual reaction. The pupils of newborn infants are constricted until about the third week of age so that light reaction, while always sluggish in an infant with congenital glaucoma, is not a good test of glaucoma in the newborn.

Gray stippling around the optic disc is a sign of lead poisoning.

Unilateral papilledema with contralateral optic atrophy may be due to a frontal lobe tumor, Foster Kennedy syndrome.

A white disc may indicate optic atrophy, as occurs with osteopetrosis causing compression of the nerve, or with neurofibroma of the optic nerve. It also occurs following optic neuritis which affects the nerve far back of the eyeball, as with multiple sclerosis or methyl alcohol poisoning.

Patients with discharge and crusting below or on the edges of the alae nasi, particularly with redness of the surrounding skin, usually have infections with β-hemolytic streptococci.

With circumoral pallor the immediate area around the mouth appears white, while a strip just below the nose, the surface of the checks, and lower chin are red. This appearance may occur with any febrile disease, but is particularly noted in children who have just exercised or who have scarlet or rheumatic fever or hypoglycemia.

A palpatory thud (or audible slap) may be felt or heard over the trachea and may indicate the presence of a foreign body free in the trachea.

Children below the age of 3 years with upper airway obstruction rarely breathe faster than 50 per minute, while those with lower airway obstructive disease, such as bronchiolitis, frequently breathe at rates of 80 to 100.

It is occasionally difficult to distinguish the third heart sound from a gallop rhythm which indicates a failing heart. Occasionally, the three beats of the gallop can be felt on palpation; the third heart sound can never be felt as an impulse.

Free fluid may give one the impression of a non-tense abdomen even though peritonitis is present.

Intra-abdominal tenderness can be distinguished from muscle tenderness by asking the child to raise his head and then palpating. Intra-abdominal tenderness is lessened, while superficial tenderness is increased, by this maneuver.

A thrill over an enlarged liver is found with hydatid echinococcal cysts in the liver; a gurgling sound may be heard in the same area.

Auscultation over the femoral artery may reveal a booming sound or "pistol shot" characteristic of aortic insufficiency or other causes of increased pulse pressure. A double sound is indicative of the same.

Occasionally, a prostate will be palpated as a flat mass several centimeters up and on the midline anterior wall of the rectum. Any prostate felt larger than 1 cm before the age of 10 years may indicate precocious puberty or congenital adrenal hyperplasia.

Spina bifida occulta can occasionally be determined by pressing carefully over the area under suspicion when the trunk is flexed. The spinous processes above and below the spina bifida will feel thin and well formed, while that of the defective vertebra may feel split.

A painful limp, especially in the morning, is usually seen in children with tuberculosis of the hip.

Associated movements, or voluntary movement of one muscle accompanied by involuntary movement of another muscle, may sometimes be noted. These movements are regulated by the cerebellum. They occur as mirror movements in the Klippel-Feil syndrome, in diseases with increased intracranial pressure, and in patients whose handedness has been changed. Reciprocal movements occur normally in infants 2 to 4 months of age and usually decrease by 4 to 6 months; failure of these movements to appear or disappear at the proper times is an indication of brain damage.

A "reverse" Moro reflex consists of extending and externally rotating the arms, with rigidity following the usual stimulus. Such a reflex is seen in children over 5 days of age who have basal ganglia disease, including kernicterus of erythroblastosis fetalis.

Sweating is rare in the newborn, but may be present in babies with brain cortex irritation, anomalies or injuries of the sympathetic nervous system, or in babies whose mothers were morphine addicts.

Reference: Barness, L.A.: Manual of Pediatric Physical Diagnosis. 4th Ed. Chicago, Year Book Medical Publishers, 1972.

# SYMPTOMS OF IMPORTANCE— ILLINGWORTH'S BAKER'S DOZEN

Failure to take note of these may have disastrous results.

1. Jaundice on the first day of life.
2. Vomitus containing bile in the newborn period, or vomiting with abdominal distention.
3. Vomitus containing streaks of blood in a baby, because it suggests hiatus hernia or reflux, and calls for investigation.
4. Diarrhea in any infant or young child, because of the rapidity with which dehydration may occur.
5. Stridor of acute onset.
6. Cough of really sudden onset, without an upper respiratory infection, because it suggests an inhaled foreign body.
7. Ear pain, because if it is due to otitis media, it requires immediate antibiotic treatment (and not drops in the ear).
8. Neck stiffness (in flexion), because it may signify meningitis.
9. Fits with fever, because although febrile convulsions are the most likely diagnosis, they may be due to pyogenic meningitis. Hence a lumbar puncture must be performed.
10. The onset of drowsiness with an infection, because it may represent pyogenic meningitis.

11.  Loss of weight.

12.  A severe attack of asthma, not responding to the usual treatment, because it may be fatal. A child with such an attack should be sent to the hospital.

13.  Poisoning of any kind, because hospital investigation and treatment are needed. The dangerous latent period, between the time of ingestion of the poison and the onset of symptoms, is a particular hazard.

---

Reference: Illingworth, R.S.: Common Symptoms of Disease in Children. 3rd Ed. Oxford, Blackwell Scientific Publications, 1971, p. 309.

# THE VULNERABLE CHILD SYNDROME

Parents of a child who was expected to die, or parents of an only child, or parents who have experienced the death of a child often react in a manner that produces a disturbance in the psychosexual development of their offspring. Learn to recognize the circumstances that produce "the vulnerable child" syndrome and its manifestations. The psychosexual disturbance manifests itself most commonly in the following ways:

1.  *Difficulty with separation.*  Child may be briefly entrusted to the care of grandparents, but baby sitters are rarely used. In extreme instances, mother and child never separate. Sleep problems are common. The child frequently sleeps with parents or in parents' room. Mother or father wakes frequently during the night to check on the status of the child.

2.  *Infantilization.*  Parents are unable to set disciplinary limits. Parent is overprotective, overindulgent, and oversolicitous. Child is overly dependent, disobedient, irritable, argumentative, and uncooperative. Children may be physically abusive to parents. Feeding problems are common.

3.  *Bodily overconcerns.*  Hypochondriacal complaints, recurrent abdominal pain, headaches, and infantile fears are prominent. School absence is common. Mothers express concern about minor respiratory infections, stool habits, "poor color," circles under the eyes, and blueness when crying.

4.  *School underachievement.*  Unspoken agreement that the child is only safe with mother may produce separation anxiety that results in poor school performance.

## Predisposing Factors in the Production of the Vulnerable Child

1.  Child is first-born to older parents who had resigned themselves to being childless.

2.  Parents cannot have additional children as a result of a hysterectomy or other sterilization procedure.

3.  The patient was born with a congenital anomaly.

4.  The patient was born prematurely.

5.  The patient has an acquired handicap, e.g., epilepsy.

6.  The child has had a truly life-threatening illness, such as erythroblastosis, nephrosis, or severe asthma.

7. During pregnancy the mother was told that the fetus might die.

8. Mother had a postpartum depression.

9. Mother has ambivalent feelings about child, such as instances where child was born out of wedlock.

10. Parents have unresolved grief reaction as a result of loss of another child.

11. A hereditary disorder is present in the family, such as cystic fibrosis or muscular dystrophy.

12. There is a psychological need on the part of the parents to find something physically wrong with the child in order to displace unacceptable feelings about the patient. Child is frequently brought to physicians because of parents' suspicion of leukemia, brain tumor, rheumatic fever, or other serious illness.

### Treatment

1. Recognize the circumstances that may produce a vulnerable child and try to reassure parents about the health of the infant or child before symptoms appear.

2. Make authoritative statements about the child's well-being based on a thoughtful, cumulative history, physical examination, and pertinent measurements and laboratory findings.

3. Point out to the parents and get them to accept the reasons for their unnecessary concern, the child's responsive behavior, and the mutual reinforcement that is present.

Do not produce the syndrome yourself with comments such as "I thought for sure he was going to die," or "If she hadn't gotten here when she did we wouldn't have been able to save her," or "You are very lucky parents that we saved your child."

Reference: Green, M., and Solnit, A.J.: Pediatrics, *34*:58, 1964.

*"All the little ones of our time are collectively the children of us adults of the time, and entitled to our general care."*

Thomas Hardy

# THE CHRONIC OR RECURRENT HEADACHE

The chronic, or recurrent, headache always produces concern in parents, as well as in older children and adolescents. All fear that the headache signifies the presence of a brain tumor. Obviously, most recurrent headaches in older children and adolescents are not caused by brain tumors but are usually a result of stress and tension. Equally obvious is the fact that a serious disorder may be present; an orderly approach to the problem is required to allay the concerns of the patient and family, as well as your own.

As a general rule, most headaches in children under the age of 4 to 5 years have an organic basis, while headaches in children over 5 do not.

The location of the headache and its associated signs and symptoms provide important clues as to the cause.

LOCATION

Frontal

*Frontal sinusitis;* may be unilateral or bilateral. Pain on palpation of frontal sinuses may be present. Often exhibits a diurnal pattern.

*Tumor of cerebral origin;* may be unilateral or bilateral. Generally worse after a period of recumbency. May be associated with vomiting.

*Ethmoid sinusitis;* pain may be referred to area over the eyes.

*Migraine;* generally unilateral; may be seen during the first 4 years of life; cyclic vomiting prominent feature in young child; attacks more common in the morning or may awake patient from sleep; scotomas occur more commonly in older child; transient loss of vision may be reported; photophobia; unilateral neurologic deficit of transient nature. Family history of other affected individuals.

*Hypertension;* headache commonly reported as throbbing; may be associated with epistaxis.

*Ocular disturbances.*

Occipital and suboccipital

*Cerebellar tumors;* may be accompanied by frontal pain as well. Head tilting may be present; periodic vomiting.

*Sphenoid sinusitis.*

*Tension.* On examination, pain and tenderness may be present in muscles at base of skull and neck. Usually accompanied by a "feeling of pressure." Worse at end of day; does not cause arousal from sleep. May be a history of similar headaches in other family members. Patients may have a long history of nonspecific abdominal pain or other gastrointestinal complaints.

Many diseases have an increased incidence of intracerebral complications that may produce headaches. Some of these disorders include:

| | |
|---|---|
| Cyanotic heart disease | Cerebral abscess; cerebral vessel occlusion. |
| Sickle cell anemia | Large vessel occlusion; small vessel hemorrhage. |
| Neurofibromatosis | Meningiomas and other intracranial tumors. |
| Hemophilia | Cerebral hemorrhage. |
| Leukemia | Meningeal or cerebral infiltrates. |
| Sturge-Weber syndrome | Cerebral hemorrhage |

The diagnostic process should include:

A detailed history of nature of headaches; life stresses and history of other family members. Always ask about *pica* in younger children.
A blood pressure measurement.
An examination of the eye grounds.
A complete neurologic examination.
Palpation of the skull; auscultation of the skull for bruits.
Examination of the teeth as a source of infection.
Palpation and transillumination of the sinuses.
Urinalysis.

If history or neurologic examination suggests the presence of intracranial disease, then additional diagnostic procedures to consider would include skull films, electroencephalogram, brain scan, CT scan, and lumbar puncture.

## DYSMENORRHEA

Primary dysmenorrhea is a symptom complex without demonstrable associated pelvic disease that may include any of the following:

Irritability
Emotional lability
Premenstrual tension
Abdominal cramps
Nausea
Vomiting
Loss of appetite
Weight gain
Constipation
Fluid retention
Sweating
Pallor
Light headed feeling
Syncope

Up to 90 per cent of all adolescent girls may experience one or more of these symptoms, and dysmenorrhea is a major cause of school absenteeism in this age group. Secondary dysmenorrhea may include many of these symptoms, but it is an acquired entity associated with pelvic disease.

The cause of primary dysmenorrhea is unknown. Recent theories implicate a hormonal imbalance resulting from an alteration in the estrogen-progesterone ratio during the early years of menstruation. Another hypothesis points to effects of prostaglandins on the myometrium, causing increased smooth muscle contraction. Whatever the cause, the discomfort is associated with the menses from menarche or shortly thereafter.

The pain associated with this symptom complex usually has its onset during the 24 hours prior to the menses and subsides within 24 to 48 hours following the beginning of the menstrual flow. It is most frequently suprapubic, but it may radiate to the back, down the thighs, or to the vagina.

Many of the symptoms of dysmenorrhea disappear within months to years after the onset of the menses. A decrease in painful periods is noted particularly with parity.

Confirmation of the diagnosis involves ascertaining the appropriate history and performing a careful abdominal and rectal or vaginal examination to rule out the presence of lesions associated with acquired dysmenorrhea (discussed below).

The most important part of treatment is reassurance. The patient may have many misconceptions about menstruation and the changes her body is undergoing. It is essential that the physician deal with the emotional aspects of this problem. In addition, the patient may be reassured that her present discomfort is transient and should decrease with age. Treatment should not include restriction of activities. Medication may include pain relievers such as aspirin, phenacetin, and acetanilid. Codeine may be necessary in some cases. Relief of depression and edema may be achieved with antidepressants and diuretics. Estrogen and progesterone alone or in cyclic combination may be used with or without the suppression of ovulation. Surgical measures have included dilatation and the insertion of a stem pessary, which acts as a foreign body and decreases the effects of the circular musculature around the os. The pessary is retained for two to three cycles.

Secondary or acquired dysmenorrhea results from demonstrable pelvic or systemic disease. It is much less frequent during the adolescent years than in adult women. The more common causes include complications of pregnancy, endometriosis, pelvic inflammatory disease, or ovarian cyst or neoplasm. Some clue that the pain is secondary to a pathologic condition may be derived from a history that is not completely typical for primary dysmenorrhea. Pain that begins several days before the onset of the menses and continues after cessation of flow may suggest an abnormality. Menstrual cramps that appear for the first time two or more years after the menarche should strongly suggest the presence of organic disease. Acute onset of low abdominal pain with vomiting and shocklike symptoms may indicate torsion of an ovarian cyst or tumor.

Reference: Oriatti, M.D.: Pediatr. Ann., 4:60, 1975.

# 2
# NUTRITION

# CLASSIFICATION OF NUTRITIONAL STATUS

*Marasmus*—From the Greek word *marasmos*, which means wasting or withering.

**2**

Is your patient obese, or merely overweight? Conversely, is your patient mildly or severely malnourished? Figure 2–1 depicted below serves as a convenient and simple means of accurately classifying the nutritional status of patients under 5 years of age.

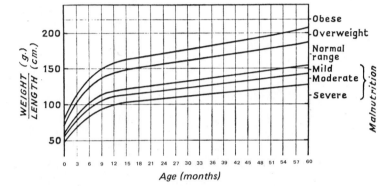

FIG. 2–1

To determine the nutritional status of a subject at a given age, the weight in grams is divided by the length in centimeters, and a mark is placed on the graph where the quotient coincides with the appropriate vertical age lines.

Reference: McLaren, D.S., and Read, W.C.: Lancet, *2*:219, 1975.

# CALORIC EXPENDITURES IN INFANCY

How does the infant spend the energy that he derives from his caloric intake? As the infant grows, more is consumed by activity and less is required for growth.

*Calorie Intake and Usage by Infant Boys*

| | | USAGE (kcal/kg) | | | |
|---|---|---|---|---|---|
| WEIGHT (kg) | INTAKE (kcal/kg) | *Basal Metabolism* | *Growth* | *Activity* | *Stool Losses* |
| 3 | 120 | 46 | 56 | 8 | 10 |
| 4 | 120 | 50 | 53 | 8 | 10 |
| 5 | 118 | 54 | 46 | 8 | 10 |
| 6 | 114 | 56 | 38 | 10 | 10 |
| 8 | 106 | 56 | 28 | 12 | 10 |
| 10 | 98 | 54 | 22 | 13 | 9 |

Reference: Holt, L.E., and Fales, H.L.: Am. J. Dis. Child., *21*:1, 1921.

## THE DAILY MILK INTAKE

How much milk will be taken by the normal term infant during the first half year of life? The data in the table below were compiled from a study of infants in whom milk was the sole source of nutrition. All were thriving. Note the marked variation that was observed in these babies.

| | VOLUME OF MILK TAKEN PER DAY (ml/kg) | | | | |
| | *Intake Percentiles* | | | | |
| AGE | 10th | 25th | 50th | 75th | 90th |
| --- | --- | --- | --- | --- | --- |
| 5–12 days | 105 | 120 | 145 | 180 | 195 |
| 1 week–1 month | 172 | 184 | 199 | 220 | 224 |
| 1–2 months | 164 | 174 | 189 | 205 | 220 |
| 2–3 months | 145 | 155 | 174 | 190 | 199 |
| 3–4 months | 134 | 148 | 158 | 170 | 180 |
| 4–5 months | 132 | 138 | 149 | 158 | 172 |

Reference: Fomon, S.J., Owen, G.M., and Thomas, L.N.: Am. J. Dis. Child., *108*:601, 1964.

## HOW TO ENCOURAGE BREAST-FEEDING

Although most physicians, as well as many potential mothers, recognize the physiologic, immunologic, and psychologic virtues of human milk feeding, these alone appear to be insufficient to motivate the physician to encourage, and the mother to accept, breast-feeding.

There are several ways to remedy this situation. The physician should familiarize himself with the scientific facts about breast-feeding and then try to employ the following procedures.

*Prenatally*

1. Plan to meet and discuss the decision about breast-feeding with the expectant mother.

2. Do not say that it is "very easy and natural" or that it is "very hard and fraught with difficulties." The highly motivated, goal-oriented woman will be discouraged by the first approach, while the anxious mother will be dismayed by the second approach. State that it has a "reasonable probability of success."

3. Allow the expectant mother to meet and discuss breast-feeding with other women who have breast-fed their children, or provide her with an opportunity to witness mothers feeding their children. The incidence of successful breast-feeding is much higher among women who have had friends or relatives who have breast-fed their infants.

4. Explain prenatal breast care. Avoid soap on the nipples. The nipples may be prepared by briskly rubbing with a Turkish towel. Other excellent preparatory techniques include:

    a. Exposing the breasts to room air as much as possible.

    b. Allowing the nipples to rub against the clothing by going braless periodically.

    c. Exposing breasts to ultraviolet rays. Sun-bathing or a sun lamp are both suitable. Start slowly — avoid burns.

    d. Have breasts stimulated manually or orally. Employ nipple rolling several times per day. This is accomplished by taking nipple between thumb and forefinger and pulling it out firmly — just enough so that it can be felt but not enough so that it really hurts.

5. Explain that the criterion of adequate breast-feeding is weight gain by the infant. Excessive crying or frequent feeding does not indicate that her milk supply is inadequate or that the quality is poor.

## Postnatally

1. Avoid sedation of the mother during labor. Oversedation of the mother will produce a sleepy infant with a decreased capacity for vigorous sucking during the first several days of life.

2. Place the baby to the mother's breast as soon after birth as possible. Optimally, this should be done within the first hour of life.

3. Encourage rooming-in. Try to pair the new mother with another woman who is breast-feeding.

4. If rooming-in is not possible, or desired, place the baby on a "demand" feeding schedule. If the baby is allowed to cry excessively before being brought to his mother, he will be exhausted. If he is brought while asleep, sucking may be unsatisfactory. Do not allow the infant to be fed in the nursery.

5. Have the mother suckle her infant for five minutes at each breast during each feed on the first day of life, ten minutes per breast on the second day, and 15 minutes per breast on the third day. Alternate the initial breast at each feeding.

6. Provide positive reinforcement in terms of weight gain. Explain that weight gain should not be anticipated during the first few days of life.

7. Plan to see or talk to the mother within three to seven days after discharge from the hospital.

8. Again remind the mother to clean her nipples with water — not soap. Avoid A and D ointment — it is irritating. If nipples are painful, suggest the application of anhydrous lanolin and not petrolatum. Try to keep nipples dry. Expose nipples as frequently as possible.

9. Remember that mastitis is not an indication to discontinue breast-feeding. The incidence of breast abscess is higher among women who discontinue breast-feeding than among women who do not.

Recommend that the expectant mother or the nursing mother read *The Complete Book of Breastfeeding* by Marvin S. Eiger and Sally W. Olds (Workman Publishing Company, New York). Read it yourself.

---

Reference: Weichert, C.: Personal communication.

# EFFECT OF BREAST-FEEDING ON THE SIZE OF THE BREAST

A great deal of both mythology and misinformation concerns the cosmetic consequences of breast-feeding. Textbooks make categorical statements that suggest that breast-feeding has no ultimate effect on the size of the breast. If one asks women who have been pregnant, a different impression emerges. The following conclusions were obtained from a survey of 750 women.

| GROUP | PERCENTAGE REPORTING CHANGE 6 MONTHS AFTER DELIVERY OR TERMINATION OF NURSING |
|---|---|
| Non–breast-feeding | 27.9 |
| Breast-feeding, 0–2 weeks | 26.3 |
| Breast-feeding, 2–6 weeks | 27.0 |
| Breast-feeding, 6 weeks–6 months | 48.7 |
| Breast-feeding, more than 6 months | 48.4 |

## Type of Changes

Non-breast-feeders or those breast-feeding for less than 2 weeks and noting a change:

| | |
|---|---|
| Increase in breast size | 60 per cent |
| Decrease in breast size | 24 per cent |
| No change in size, less tone | 16 per cent |

Breast-feeding for more than 2 weeks and noting a change:

| | |
|---|---|
| Increase in breast size | 14 per cent |
| Decrease in breast size | 50 per cent |
| No change in size, less tone | 36 per cent |

Only three women among the group noting a change in breast size following breast-feeding did not feed their subsequent children. All felt the cosmetic consequences were of little significance when contrasted with the psychological and nutritional benefits of nursing.

---

Reference: Oski, F.A.: Program, American Pediatric Society, 1968, p. 58.

# INFANT FOODS—
# CALORIES AND THEIR DISTRIBUTION

**2**

When you begin to add strained foods or junior foods to the infant's diet, you should be aware of the number of calories you are providing and where they are coming from. The table below provides estimates derived from analysis of a variety of products in each category.

## Strained Foods

| CATEGORY | KCAL/100 GM | PERCENTAGE OF CALORIES | | |
| --- | --- | --- | --- | --- |
| | | Protein | Fat | Carbohydrates |
| Juices | 65 (45–98) | 2 | 2 | 96 |
| Fruits | 85 (79–125) | 2 | 2 | 96 |
| Vegetables | | | | |
| Plain | 45 (27–28) | 14 | 6 | 80 |
| Creamed | 63 (42–94) | 13 | 13 | 74 |
| Meats | 106 (86–194) | 53 | 46 | 1 |
| Egg yolks | 192 (184–199) | 21 | 76 | 3 |
| High meat dinner | 84 (63–106) | 29 | 45 | 29 |
| Desserts | 96 (71–136) | 4 | 7 | 89 |
| Cereal | 360 (349–393) | 39 | 12 | 49 |
| Cereal-fruit | 85 (76–98) | 18 | 6 | 76 |

## Junior Foods

| | | | | |
| --- | --- | --- | --- | --- |
| Fruits | 85 (69–116) | 2 | 2 | 96 |
| Vegetables | | | | |
| Plain | 46 (27–71) | 12 | 7 | 81 |
| Creamed | 64 (45–72) | 13 | 17 | 70 |
| Meats | 103 (88–135) | 56 | 43 | 1 |
| Soup-dinner | 61 (39–100) | 15 | 27 | 58 |

Reference: Fomon, S.J.: Infant Nutrition. 2nd Ed. Philadelphia, W.B. Saunders Company, 1974, p. 410.

*"It is through the idealism of youth that man catches sight of truth, and in that idealism he possesses a wealth which he must never exchange for anything else."*

Albert Schweitzer

## THE MILK PROTEIN-FREE DIET

Infants who exhibit severe milk allergy must have milk, milk products, and proteins derived from cattle eliminated from their diets. Here is a list of foods that are safe for such infants.

*Beechnut Products*

High-protein cereal
Strained or junior vegetables
Beans, sweet potatoes
Ham, lamb, or liver
Turkey-rice dinner
Egg yolks
Egg yolks and bacon

*Gerber Products*

Cereals: high-protein, barley, mixed grains, oatmeal, or rice
All baby juices and fruits
All fruits, baby, strained, or junior foods
Turkey-rice dinner
Chicken, ham, lamb, turkey, liver, and bacon
Banana pudding (junior only), cherry-vanilla pudding, fruit dessert, and peach cobbler

*Heinz Products*

Cereals: barley, mixed, oatmeal, rice
All juices and fruits
Chicken, lamb, pork
Carrots
Tomatoes

Soybean milks, goat's milk

---

Reference: Gryboski, J.: Gastrointestinal Problems in Infants. Philadelphia, W.B. Saunders Company, 1975. p. 766.

## THE CALCIUM CONTENT OF SOME COMMONLY USED PREPARATIONS

Calcium compounds employed for either intravenous or oral supplementation differ widely in their actual calcium content. The list below describes the actual calcium by weight of some of these compounds.

| CALCIUM SALT | PER CENT CALCIUM BY WEIGHT |
|---|---|
| Calcium carbonate | 40.04 |
| Calcium chloride | 27.26 |
| Calcium glycerophosphate | 19.07 |
| Calcium lactate | 13.00 |
| Calcium gluconate | 9.30 |

Example: When you administer a 10 per cent calcium gluconate solution, you are not providing 10 grams of calcium per 100 ml of solution, but only 930 mg.

# SIMPLIFIED PREDICTION OF RENAL SOLUTE LOAD

On occasion, it is important to know if the urine osmolality is appropriate for the infant on a particular diet.

A simple estimate of renal solute load may be based on dietary intake of nitrogen and of three minerals: sodium, potassium, and chloride. Each gram of dietary protein can be considered to yield 4 milliosmols of renal solute load (assumed to be all urea), and each milliequivalent of sodium, potassium, and chloride is assumed to contribute 1 milliosmol.

Estimated renal solute load from various feedings is listed in the table below.

*Dietary Intake of Protein, Sodium, Chloride, and Potassium, and Estimated Renal Solute Load from Various Feedings*

| FEEDINGS (1000 ML) | DIETARY INTAKE | | | | ESTIMATED RENAL SOLUTE LOAD | | |
|---|---|---|---|---|---|---|---|
| | Protein (gm) | Na (mEq) | Cl (mEq) | K (mEq) | Urea (mosm) | Na + K + Cl (mosm) | Total mosm |
| Whole cow milk | 33 | 25 | 29 | 35 | 132 | 89 | 221 |
| Human milk | 12 | 7 | 11 | 13 | 48 | 31 | 79 |
| Boiled skim milk | 46 | 35 | 40 | 49 | 184 | 124 | 308 |
| Similac (20 kcal/oz) | 15.5 | 11 | 17 | 19 | 62 | 47 | 109 |
| Isomil (20 kcal/oz) | 20 | 13 | 15 | 18 | 80 | 46 | 126 |

The estimated renal solute load and minimum urinary osmolality of a hypothetical 6 kg infant from various feedings are analyzed below.

*Estimated Renal Solute Load and Minimum Urinary Osmolality*
*of a Hypothetical 6 kG Infant from Various Feedings*

| FEEDING | ESTIMATED RENAL SOLUTE LOAD | OSMOLALITY OF 730 ML URINE |
|---|---|---|
| Whole cow milk | 221 mosm | 303 mosm/liter |
| Human milk | 79 mosm | 108 mosm/liter |
| Boiled skim milk | 308 mosm | 422 mosm/liter |
| Similac (20 kcal/oz) | 109 mosm | 149 mosm/liter |
| Isomil (20 kcal/oz) | 126 mosm | 172 mosm/liter |

Reference: Ziegler, E.E., and Fomon, S.J.: J. Pediatr., *78*:561, 1971.

## EXPENDITURE OF ENERGY IN THE HOSPITALIZED PATIENT

The hospitalized patient has a caloric expenditure somewhat below that estimated for normal activity, but above that needed to maintain the basal metabolic rate. The patient's energy expenditure may be related to weight in the following table.

| EXPENDITURE OF ENERGY (cal) | WEIGHT OF BODY (kg) | EXPENDITURE OF ENERGY (cal) | WEIGHT OF BODY (kg) |
|---|---|---|---|
| 100 | 1 | 1,600 | 25 |
| 200 | 2 | 1,700 | 30 |
| 300 | 3 | 1,800 | 35 |
| 400 | 4 | 1,900 | 40 |
| 500 | 5 | 2,000 | 45 (average adult female) |
| 600 | 6 | 2,100 | 50 |
| 700 | 7 | 2,200 | 55 |
| 800 | 8 | 2,300 | 60 |
| 900 | 9 | 2,400 | 65 |
| 1,000 | 10 | 2,500 | 70 (average adult male) |
| 1,100 | 12 | 2,600 | 75 |
| 1,200 | 14 | 2,700 | 80 |
| 1,300 | 16 | 2,800 | 85 |
| 1,400 | 18 | 2,900 | 90 |
| 1,500 | 20 | 3,000 | 95 |

2

The simple calculations below will alleviate the need to refer to this table.

0–10 kg — 100 cal/kg
10–20 kg — 1000 cal + 50 cal/kg for each kg over 10
20 kg and up — 1500 cal + 20 cal/kg for each kg over 20

Reference: Segar, W.E.: Curr. Probl. Pediatr., *3*:3, 1972.

## EATING PROBLEMS

Most feeding difficulties result from problems in feeding management. Treatment of feeding problems should include suggestions to parents that will help promote the child's appetite at mealtime. Your advice may include the following:

1. Portions on the child's plate may be too large. The child given extremely small portions may be free to ask for more, while the child whose plate is too full looks at quantities of food that frustrate the appetite.

2. Children appreciate food that is simple and attractively served. They may prefer raw vegetables to cooked ones. If a child likes spicy foods, there is no reason he should not eat them.

3. Mealtime battles may ensue because children reject certain foods, especially vegetables. Nutritional equivalents may be found for almost all foods. Fruits may be substituted for vegetables. The negative associations provoked by parental insistence that the child eat particular foods may prevent the child from eventually developing a taste for a variety of foods.

4. Development of good manners is important, but if insistence on good manners interferes with the child's appetite, manners may be neglected until the appetite improves.

5. Battles over hand washing should be avoided. Washing may be made more pleasant by use of a bar of soap in the shape of an animal. The help or accompaniment of a parent at the sink may make this task more pleasant.

6. Mealtime may be so late or last so long that the child's appetite is lost. It may be desirable to feed the children before their parents. Once the child's meal is finished, he should be excused.

7. The child should be included in conversation at the table. Disputes over eating may be the only means the child has of getting attention.

8. The dinner table is not the place for discussion of disciplinary problems or the meting out of punishments.

9. Between-meal snacks should be given midway between meals and should be offered in small quantities.

10. Use of candy and desserts as rewards for good behavior simply increases the child's devotion to them. Dessert should not be denied to the child who does not eat the meal. Children who are denied a meal as punishment may attach unpleasant associations to mealtime. Other disciplinary devices should be sought.

11. Do not expect children to eat anything their parents do not like.

Rarely, feeding difficulties may reflect profound problems of adjustment for the child. Anxiety about loss of love, such as during the arrival of a new baby in the household, may result in anorexia. The pediatrician should be aware of these possibilities and question parents appropriately.

Reference: Schwartz, A.S.: Pediatr. Clin. North Am., *5*:595, 1958.

## FEELING FIT TO COMPETE IN ATHLETICS

It always helps to have a "light" feeling in the abdomen before strenuous physical exercise. This can be facilitated by avoiding foods of high residue for several days before competition. High residue foods include the following:

Raw fruits and vegetables
Dried fruits such as raisins and apricots
Nuts
Whole grain cereal products
Milk

You can avoid "water logging" before an event by refraining from foods with high salt content that produce fluid retention. These include:

Sauerkraut
Potato chips, corn chips, and other salted snacks
Pretzels
Smoked fish and smoked meats
Bacon
Chipped and corned beef
Bologna
Hot dogs
Relish, pickles
Soy sauce
Worcestershire sauce
Sausage

If you have to eliminate all the fun foods in life, you may think twice about getting to top competitive form!

Smith, N.J.: J.A.M.A., *236*:149, 1976.

*"He who helps a child helps humanity with an immediateness which no other help given to a human creature in any other stage of life can possibly give again."*

**Phillip Brooks**

# GAINING WEIGHT—LOSING WEIGHT FOR ATHLETICS

2

High-school students may request guidance in weight reduction or weight gaining programs so that they more optimally compete in athletics. Some helpful guidelines include the following:

1. A kilogram of fat represents approximately 7000 calories. If an individual wishes to lose a kilogram by exercise, he must expend this amount of energy. This is very difficult. A net reduction of 7000 calories, below the individual's requirements, over any period of time will result in the loss of a kilogram of body weight.

2. When weight loss is desired, it should not exceed one kilogram per week.

3. It takes approximately 5000 calories in excess of normal needs to gain one kilogram of lean body mass. Increasing intake in association with daily exercise can increase lean body mass. If the increase is not associated with exercise, it will result in an increase in body fat.

4. Diets modified for either weight gain or weight reduction should contain an optimal intake of all essential nutrients. If this goal cannot be attained, vitamin and mineral supplements should be provided. Approximately 15 to 50 per cent of all adolescent females are iron deficient. Iron status of all females contemplating athletic competition should be evaluated, and iron supplements provided for those with reduced iron stores regardless of whether they are anemic or not.

5. Individuals in excellent physical condition should have no more than 5 to 10 per cent of their body weight as fat. The level of body fatness can be estimated by measuring skin-fat folds with a skin caliper. The skin-fat fold is measured at four sites; they are:

> The subscapular area
> An area over the triceps
> The area above the iliac crest
> The anterior abdominal wall

When the body weight and the estimated percentage of body weight that is fat are known, a simple calculation can be made to determine how much fat weight should be lost to achieve optimum condition. Consulting an article by Tcheng and Lipton in Medicine, Science and Sports, 5:1–10, 1973, can provide you with accurate formulas to assist in making recommendations.

---

Smith, N.J.: J.A.M.A., *236*:149, 1976.

# 3

# GROWTH AND DEVELOPMENT

# ERUPTION OF DECIDUOUS TEETH

The eruption of the first tooth in an infant is accompanied by parental pride in the fact that yet another milestone is reached. Figure 3–1 indicates the age and the order in which deciduous teeth erupt. The dot represents the mean age, while the wavy line demonstrates normal variation. Exceptions to the sequence of eruption are uncommon. Late eruption is unlikely to be of significance; however, it has been associated with both hypothyroidism and rickets.

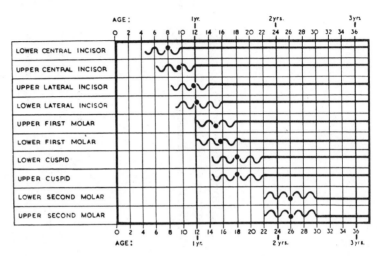

FIG. 3–1

Reference: MacKeith, R., and Wood, C.: Digestion and absorption. *In* Infant Feeding and Feeding Difficulties. London, J. & A. Churchill, 1971, p. 19.

*"Adam and Eve had many advantages, but the principal one was that they escaped teething."*

Mark Twain

# LANGUAGE DEVELOPMENT

The methods by which a child learns to use language are very poorly understood; however, the sequence of language development and the relationship of cerebral hemispheric dominance to that development are well known. The table below lists the stages of language development along with corresponding central nervous system lateralization and maturation at those stages.

*Language Development, CNS Maturation and Lateralization*

| AGE | USUAL LANGUAGE DEVELOPMENT | EFFECTS OF ACQUIRED, LATERALIZED LESIONS | PHYSICAL MATURATION OF CNS | LATERALIZATION OF FUNCTION | EQUIPOTENTIALITY OF HEMISPHERES | EXPLANATION |
|---|---|---|---|---|---|---|
| *Months* 0–3 | Emergence of cooing | | | | | Neuroanatomic and physiologic prerequisites become established |
| 4–20 | From babbling to words | No effect on onset of language in half of all cases; other half has delayed onset but normal development | About 60 to 70% of developmental course accomplished | None: symptoms and prognosis identical for either hemisphere | Perfect equipotentiality | |
| 21–36 | Acquisition of language | All language accomplishments disappear; language is reacquired with repetition of all stages | Rate of maturation slowed down | Hand preference emerges | Right hemisphere can easily adopt sole responsibility for language | Language appears to involve entire brain; little cortical specialization with regard to language, although left hemisphere beginning to become dominant toward end of this period |

**3**

| Years | | | | | | |
|---|---|---|---|---|---|---|
| 3–10 | Some grammatical refinement; expansion of vocabulary | Emergence of aphasic symptoms; disorders tend to recover without residual language deficits (except in reading and writing). During recovery period, two processes active: diminishing aphasic interference and further acquisition of language | Very slow completion of maturational processes | Cerebral dominance established between 3 and 5 years, but evidence that right hemisphere may often still be involved in speech and language functions. About one-fourth of early childhood aphasias due to right hemisphere lesions | In cases where language is already predominantly localized in left hemisphere and aphasia ensues with left lesion, it is possible to reestablish language, presumably by reactivating language functions in right hemisphere | A process of physiologic organization takes place in which functional lateralization of language to left is predominant. "Physiologic redundancy" is gradually reduced, and polarization of activities between right and left hemisphere is established. As long as maturational processes have not stopped, reorganization is still possible |
| 11–14 | Accents characteristic to region or country emerge | Some aphasic symptoms become irreversible (particularly when acquired lesion was traumatic) | An asymptote is reached on almost all parameters. Exceptions are myelinization and EEG spectrum | Apparently firmly established, but definitive statistics not available | Marked signs of reduction in equipotentiality | Language markedly lateralized, and internal organization established irreversibly for life. Language-free parts of brain cannot take over except where lateralization is incomplete or had been blocked by pathologic conditions during childhood |
| *Midteens to Adulthood* | Acquisition of second language becomes increasingly difficult | Symptoms present 3 to 5 months postinsult are irreversible | None | In about 97% of the entire population, language is definitely lateralized to the left | None for language | |

*The normal development of the child's ability to hear and understand language occurs as follows:*

*Newborn:* The infant responds only to loud noises by crying or startling.

*2 weeks:* The infant assumes listening attitudes to the sound of the human voice.

*2 months:* The infant changes activity or attends to the human voice and no longer startles to familiar loud noises.

*4 months:* The infant turns head in search of sound or voice as he develops localizing skill to position sound and a sense of space in relation to himself.

*5 to 6 months:* The infant can distinguish friendly from angry tone in talking.

*8 months:* The infant may respond to his name.

*12 months:* The infant can follow a few simple commands, responds to "no-no" and to "patty cake" and "bye-bye" with gestures.

*18 months:* The toddler can point to his nose, eyes, hair on command.

*24 months:* The child is able to understand simple questions and commands, and recognizes 120 to 175 words.

*30 months:* The child understands about 400 words and is beginning to identify objects by their use as well as their name, e.g., "show me the one that goes on your foot," "the one you use to drink milk."

*36 months:* The child understands about 800 words and can respond to requests involving his understanding of comparisons and quality or degree, such as "give me the one that runs the fastest, that is strongest, that you eat most often."

*3 to 4 years:* The child understands up to 1500 words by age 4 years. He comprehends complex sentences and simple questions.

*4 to 5 years:* The child can carry out complex commands involving two or three actions.

*5 to 6 years:* The child understands 2500 to 2800 words. He can respond correctly to more complicated sentences, but often is still confused by involved sentences.

*Development of language expression in the normal child is outlined below:*

*13 to 14 months:* The child usually uses one or two recognizable words in relation to familiar objects present in his immediate vision or grasp.

*15 months:* Two to 6 recognizable words are used appropriately by the child. He understands many more words than this and is beginning to understand and obey simple commands.

*18 months:* The child uses 6 to 20 recognizable words related to his own "here and now." He still indicates desires by pointing accompanied by words. He echoes words and phrases and enjoys nursery rhymes.

*21 months:* Primitive sentences of 2 to 3 words are used meaningfully. The toddler also begins questioning with voice inflection, e.g., "Daddy gone car?"

*24 months:* The child speaks 50 or more words and uses simple sentences. He talks as he plays. He asks many "what," "where," and "who" questions and begins to use the verbal negative, e.g., "That not car."

*30 months:* The child demonstrates a greatly increased vocabulary and uses pronouns and most prepositions. He can repeat nursery rhymes and enjoys simple stories read from picture books.

*36 months:* A vocabulary of 250 or more words is in the child's possession. He uses plurals, and asks "why," "how," and "when" questions.

*48 months:* The child can describe and give a connected account of recent experiences and events. He tells long stories but can confuse fact and fantasy. He asks the meaning of new words, including abstract ones.

Reference:  Gofman, H.P., and Allmond, B.W., Jr.: Curr. Probl. Pediatr., *1*:3, 1971.

# EVALUATION OF ARTICULATION DISORDERS

The following test is designed to detect articulation disorders in the 2½ to 6 year old child.

The child's ability to articulate the underlined italicized sounds in the words below should be determined.

| | | |
|---|---|---|
| 1. *t*able | 9. *th*umb | 17. gu*m* |
| 2. shi*rt* | 10. too*th*brush | 18. *h*ou*se* |
| 3. *d*oor | 11. *s*ock | 19. pen*c*il |
| 4. tru*n*k | 12. vac*uu*m | 20. *f*i*sh* |
| 5. *j*umping | 13. *y*arn | 21. *l*ea*f* |
| 6. zip*per* | 14. *m*o*th*er | 22. ca*rr*ot |
| 7. *gr*apes | 15. *tw*inkle | |
| 8. *fl*ag | 16. *w*ago*n* | |

Evaluation should be made according to the following normal scores.

| Age in Years | Normal Number of Sounds Articulated Correctly |
|---|---|
| 2½–3 | 7 or more |
| 3–3½ | 15 or more |
| 4–4½ | 16 or more |
| 4½–5 | 18 or more |
| 5–5½ | 22 or more |
| 5½–6 | 24 or more |
| 6 and older | 25 or more |

The child should also be evaluated for intelligibility as words or phrases are put together. The child who is 2½ to 3 years old should be understood half the time or more. The child who is over 3 years of age should be readily understood.

An abnormal score on this simple test should provoke a complete neurologic assessment, an evaluation of the general development and intelligence, a physical examination of the oropharyngeal cavity, lateral head x-ray examination to determine degree of velopharyngeal closure, and a complete audiologic examination. Failure to determine the abnormality should lead to evaluation by a speech pathologist.

Reference: Silver, H.K.: *In* Kempe, C.H., Silver, H.K., and O'Brien, D. (Eds.): Current Pediatric Diagnosis and Treatment. Los Altos, California, Lange Medical Publications, 1976, p. 30.

# DEVELOPMENTAL WARNING SIGNS

Complete neurologic examination and Denver developmental tests are rarely carried out at the time of the well child check-up. There are certain warning signs, however, that should provoke further evaluation of the infant. Awareness of these easily observed abnormalities will make even the briefest examination more complete.

### Warning Signs at Different Ages

| AGE* | WEIGHT (kg) / SKULL CIRC. (cm) 3rd–97th percentiles | | GENERAL | HEARING AND SPEECH | VISION | ARMS | LEGS | PELVIS |
|---|---|---|---|---|---|---|---|---|
| 6 weeks | 3.4–5.9 | 35–41 | Any major maternal anxiety. "Fits," "spasms," or "colic" of uncertain origin at any time, especially first six months. | Absence of auditory "alertness." | Lack of fixation or following at 9 to 12 inch distance. Cataract. | Excessive head lag on pulling to sitting position. Asymmetry in movements, tone, or neonatal responses. | Immobility or undue extension. | Definite click or instability of hips. Absent femoral pulses. |
| 6 months | 5.9–9.4 | 40–45 | Persistence of heart murmur. Lack of smiling. Fits or spasms as above. Persistence of hand regard. | Failure to localize to soft sound on either side. | Failure to fix and follow both near and far objects around 180°. Persistent squint. | Failure to reach out or transfer (both hands). Persistent fisting or preference for one hand. | Increased adductor tone. Increased reflexes. Clonus. | Limited abduction of hips. (x-ray necessary) |
| 10 months | 7.2–11.0 | 43–49 | Absence of chewing. Lack of imitation. | Absence of babble. | Squint or nystagmus. | Abnormal hand posture or ataxia. | Absence of weight-bearing while held. | Failure to sit without support. |
| 18 months | 8.8–13.6 | 45–50 | Absence of constructive play. Persistence of casting, drooling or mouthing. | Lack of spontaneous vocalization. | Any apparent visual defect. | Abnormal grasp, abnormal hand posture, no pincer grip. | Inability to stand without support. | |
| 2 years | 9.6–14.9 | 46–51 | Hyperkinesia, failure to concentrate. | Absence of recognizable words. | Failure to match toys. | Tremor or ataxia with bricks. | Lack of walking without aid. | |

*Conceptual rather than chronologic age.

Reference: Wood, B. (Ed.): A Pediatric Vade-Mecum. London, Lloyd-Luke (Medical Books) Ltd., 1974, p. 7.

# EMOTIONAL AND COGNITIVE DISTURBANCES IN THE YOUNG CHILD

3

The alert and sensitive physician may detect abnormalities in the behavior or history of the young child that will allow early identification of emotional and cognitive disturbances. The child between the ages of 3 and 5 years is old enough to demonstrate disordered behavior. The child with gross mental retardation has usually been discovered before this age, but the mildly disturbed child of less than 5 years of age is rarely seen by an educational, mental health, or medical professional, except in the physician's office.

The following chart provides a list of observational data and major and minor historical indicators that will aid the physician in evaluating the 3 to 5 year old child. The observational data accumulated will increase in value as the particular child is seen for return visits and as the physician practices these observations of many children over a period of time.

### *Office and Waiting Room Observation*

Motor function      Integration of knowledge
Speech level      Interaction with children, adults
Independence and trust      Understanding; cooperation

### *Major Indicators*

(Two or more episodes should arouse suspicion.)

Behavior dangerous to self or others
Bizarre behavior
Night terrors at age 5
Bowel incontinence (daytime regression after control)
Loss or lack of speech
No personal interaction
Severe separation anxiety (terror)

*Minor Indicators*

(Clusters of minors, or minor + major, should arouse suspicion.)

| CONSTITUTIONAL DATA | INTRAPERSONAL OR INTRAPSYCHIC DATA | INTERPERSONAL DATA |
|---|---|---|
| Precursors or Increased Risk<br> Perinatal illness of mother and child<br> Prematurity or low birth weight<br> Serious infantile illness, especially of central nervous system<br> Seizure disorder<br><br>Symptoms<br> Hyperkinesis<br> Selective visual loss<br> Selective auditory loss<br> Minor aphasias<br> Mixed cerebral dominance<br> Slow speech development<br> Extremes of temperament: passivity, aggression<br> Clumsiness<br> Short attention span | Symptoms<br> Regressive habit patterns that arise repetitively in new events (nightmares, nose-picking, nail-biting, daytime enuresis)<br> De novo repetitive rituals (tics, checking locks or gas jets<br> Unrealistic persistent fears<br> Anxiety without obvious cause<br> Multiple ingestions<br> Head banging<br> Continuous rocking<br> Recurrent masturbation<br> Recurrent night terrors at ages 3 and 4 | Precursors or Increased Risk<br> Excessive demands on child by parents or school<br> Poor sibling or peer relationships<br> Disruption of family (single parent, poor living conditions; parent absent physically or emotionally; mental illness; alcoholism or drug abuse in family; financial problems; pending divorce or separation)<br><br>Symptoms<br> Mild to moderate separation anxiety<br> Temper tantrums<br> Breath-holding spells<br> Infantile speech<br> Negativistic behavior<br> Stuttering, stammering, indistinct speech |

Reference: Gabriel, H.P.: Pediatr. Clin. North Am., *18*:179, 1971.

## CREEPING AND CRAWLING

These two forms of locomotion are frequently confused. An infant generally crawls before he creeps. Crawling is accomplished by moving across the ground with the abdomen hugging the floor. A snake and other reptiles crawl. Creeping is locomotion accomplished by moving on your hands and knees. American jargon has helped add to this confusion. The term "creep" should not be regarded as the ultimate insult; "crawl" is a more primitive behavior and thus should be substituted for "creep" as the more pejorative term.

## PREDICTION OF ADULT STATURE

Increasing numbers of pediatric patients are treated with hormones, anabolic steroids, or other agents that may alter rates of skeletal elongation or maturation. Prediction of adult stature may be important in these patients. The following method provides the most accurate system currently available for prediction of adult stature, and it allows the prediction to be made on the initial visit.

**3**

Measurements used in the calculation include:

1. Recumbent length in centimeters. If only the standing height measurement is available, 1.25 cm should be added to this figure.
2. Nude weight in kilograms.
3. Measurement of stature of each parent. The stated stature of one parent may be used if necessary. If even this is not available, the sex-appropriate value for the population may be employed, though there will be some loss of accuracy. These values for the United States are 174.5 cm for the father, and 162.0 cm for the mother.
4. Skeletal age of left-hand wrist using the Greulich-Pyle atlas. If more than one-half of these bones are adult in maturity, this method of height prediction should not be applied. Prior to age 13 years in boys and age 8 years in girls, chronologic age may be substituted for skeletal age. If this is done, the chronologic age that is substituted must be multiplied by the skeletal age weight in the tables below.

The following tables are used in making the necessary calculations.

*Monthly Weights for the Prediction of Adult Stature in Boys**

| AGE (yr) | (mo) | $\beta rl$ | $\beta w$ | $\beta mps$ | $\beta sa$ | $\beta o$ |
|------|------|------|------|------|------|------|
| 1 | 0 | 0.966 | 0.199 | 0.606 | −0.673 | 1.632 |
| 1 | 3 | 1.032 | 0.086 | 0.580 | −0.417 | −1.841 |
| 1 | 6 | 1.086 | −0.016 | 0.559 | −0.205 | −4.892 |
| 1 | 9 | 1.130 | −0.106 | 0.540 | −0.033 | −7.528 |
| 2 | 0 | 1.163 | −0.186 | 0.523 | 0.104 | −9.764 |
| 2 | 3 | 1.189 | −0.256 | 0.509 | 0.211 | −11.618 |
| 2 | 6 | 1.207 | −0.316 | 0.496 | 0.291 | −13.114 |
| 2 | 9 | 1.219 | −0.369 | 0.485 | 0.349 | −14.278 |
| 3 | 0 | 1.227 | −0.413 | 0.475 | 0.388 | −15.139 |
| 3 | 3 | 1.230 | −0.450 | 0.466 | 0.410 | −15.729 |
| 3 | 6 | 1.229 | −0.481 | 0.458 | 0.419 | −16.081 |
| 3 | 9 | 1.226 | −0.505 | 0.451 | 0.417 | −16.228 |
| 4 | 0 | 1.221 | −0.523 | 0.444 | 0.405 | −16.201 |
| 4 | 3 | 1.214 | −0.537 | 0.437 | 0.387 | −16.034 |
| 4 | 6 | 1.206 | −0.546 | 0.431 | 0.363 | −15.758 |
| 4 | 9 | 1.197 | −0.550 | 0.424 | 0.335 | −15.400 |
| 5 | 0 | 1.188 | −0.551 | 0.418 | 0.303 | −14.990 |
| 5 | 3 | 1.179 | −0.548 | 0.412 | 0.269 | −14.551 |
| 5 | 6 | 1.169 | −0.543 | 0.406 | 0.234 | −14.106 |
| 5 | 9 | 1.160 | −0.535 | 0.400 | 0.198 | −13.672 |
| 6 | 0 | 1.152 | −0.524 | 0.394 | 0.161 | −13.267 |
| 6 | 3 | 1.143 | −0.512 | 0.389 | 0.123 | −12.901 |
| 6 | 6 | 1.135 | −0.499 | 0.383 | 0.085 | −12.583 |
| 6 | 9 | 1.127 | −0.484 | 0.378 | 0.046 | −12.318 |

*The abbreviations are as follows: $\beta rl$, regression weights for recumbent stature; $\beta w$, weight; $\beta mps$, midparent stature; $\beta sa$, skeletal age; and $\beta o$, the intercept of the regression equation.

| AGE | | | | | | |
| (yr) | (mo) | $\beta rl$ | $\beta w$ | $\beta mps$ | $\beta sa$ | $\beta o$ |
| --- | --- | --- | --- | --- | --- | --- |
| 7 | 0 | 1.120 | −0.468 | 0.373 | 0.006 | −12.107 |
| 7 | 3 | 1.113 | −0.451 | 0.369 | −0.034 | −11.948 |
| 7 | 6 | 1.106 | −0.434 | 0.365 | −0.077 | −11.834 |
| 7 | 9 | 1.100 | −0.417 | 0.361 | −0.121 | −11.756 |
| 8 | 0 | 1.093 | −0.400 | 0.358 | −0.167 | −11.701 |
| 8 | 3 | 1.086 | −0.382 | 0.356 | −0.217 | −11.652 |
| 8 | 6 | 1.079 | −0.365 | 0.354 | −0.270 | −11.592 |
| 8 | 9 | 1.071 | −0.349 | 0.353 | −0.327 | −11.498 |
| 9 | 0 | 1.063 | −0.333 | 0.353 | −0.389 | −11.349 |
| 9 | 3 | 1.054 | −0.317 | 0.353 | −0.455 | −11.118 |
| 9 | 6 | 1.044 | −0.303 | 0.355 | −0.527 | −10.779 |
| 9 | 9 | 1.033 | −0.289 | 0.357 | −0.605 | −10.306 |
| 10 | 0 | 1.021 | −0.276 | 0.360 | −0.690 | −9.671 |
| 10 | 3 | 1.008 | −0.263 | 0.363 | −0.781 | −8.848 |
| 10 | 6 | 0.993 | −0.252 | 0.368 | −0.878 | −7.812 |
| 10 | 9 | 0.977 | −0.241 | 0.373 | −0.983 | −6.540 |
| 11 | 0 | 0.960 | −0.231 | 0.378 | −1.094 | −5.010 |
| 11 | 3 | 0.942 | −0.222 | 0.384 | −1.211 | −3.206 |
| 11 | 6 | 0.923 | −0.213 | 0.390 | −1.335 | −1.113 |
| 11 | 9 | 0.902 | −0.206 | 0.397 | −1.464 | 1.273 |
| 12 | 0 | 0.881 | −0.198 | 0.403 | −1.597 | 3.958 |
| 12 | 3 | 0.859 | −0.191 | 0.409 | −1.735 | 6.931 |
| 12 | 6 | 0.837 | −0.184 | 0.414 | −1.875 | 10.181 |
| 12 | 9 | 0.815 | −0.177 | 0.418 | −2.015 | 13.684 |
| 13 | 0 | 0.794 | −0.170 | 0.421 | −2.156 | 17.405 |
| 13 | 3 | 0.773 | −0.163 | 0.422 | −2.294 | 21.297 |
| 13 | 6 | 0.755 | −0.155 | 0.422 | −2.427 | 25.304 |
| 13 | 9 | 0.738 | −0.146 | 0.418 | −2.553 | 29.349 |
| 14 | 0 | 0.724 | −0.136 | 0.412 | −2.668 | 33.345 |
| 14 | 3 | 0.714 | −0.125 | 0.401 | −2.771 | 37.183 |
| 14 | 6 | 0.709 | −0.112 | 0.387 | −2.856 | 40.738 |
| 14 | 9 | 0.709 | −0.098 | 0.367 | −2.922 | 43.869 |
| 15 | 0 | 0.717 | −0.081 | 0.342 | −2.962 | 46.403 |
| 15 | 3 | 0.732 | −0.062 | 0.310 | −2.973 | 48.154 |
| 15 | 6 | 0.756 | −0.040 | 0.271 | −2.949 | 48.898 |
| 15 | 9 | 0.792 | −0.015 | 0.223 | −2.885 | 48.402 |
| 16 | 0 | 0.839 | −0.014 | 0.167 | −2.776 | 46.391 |

*The abbreviations are as follows: $\beta rl$, regression weights for recumbent stature; $\beta w$, weight; $\beta mps$, midparent stature; $\beta sa$, skeletal age; and $\beta o$, the intercept of the regression equation.

*Monthly Weights for the Prediction of Adult Stature in Girls* *

| AGE (yr) | (mo) | $\beta$rl | $\beta$w | $\beta$mps | $\beta$sa | $\beta$o |
|---|---|---|---|---|---|---|
| 1 | 0 | 1.087 | −0.271 | 0.386 | 0.434 | 21.729 |
| 1 | 3 | 1.112 | −0.369 | 0.367 | 0.094 | 20.684 |
| 1 | 6 | 1.134 | −0.455 | 0.349 | −0.172 | 19.957 |
| 1 | 9 | 1.153 | −0.530 | 0.332 | −0.374 | 19.463 |
| 2 | 0 | 1.170 | −0.594 | 0.316 | −0.523 | 19.131 |
| 2 | 3 | 1.183 | −0.648 | 0.301 | −0.625 | 18.905 |
| 2 | 6 | 1.195 | −0.693 | 0.287 | −0.690 | 18.740 |
| 2 | 9 | 1.204 | −0.729 | 0.274 | −0.725 | 18.604 |
| 3 | 0 | 1.210 | −0.757 | 0.262 | −0.736 | 18.474 |
| 3 | 3 | 1.215 | −0.777 | 0.251 | −0.729 | 18.337 |
| 3 | 6 | 1.217 | −0.791 | 0.241 | −0.711 | 18.187 |
| 3 | 9 | 1.217 | −0.798 | 0.232 | −0.684 | 18.024 |
| 4 | 0 | 1.215 | −0.800 | 0.224 | −0.655 | 17.855 |
| 4 | 3 | 1.212 | −0.797 | 0.217 | −0.626 | 17.691 |
| 4 | 6 | 1.206 | −0.789 | 0.210 | −0.600 | 17.548 |
| 4 | 9 | 1.199 | −0.777 | 0.205 | −0.582 | 17.444 |
| 5 | 0 | 1.190 | −0.761 | 0.200 | −0.571 | 17.398 |
| 5 | 3 | 1.180 | −0.742 | 0.197 | −0.572 | 17.431 |
| 5 | 6 | 1.168 | −0.721 | 0.193 | −0.584 | 17.567 |
| 5 | 9 | 1.155 | −0.697 | 0.191 | −0.609 | 17.826 |
| 6 | 0 | 1.140 | −0.671 | 0.190 | −0.647 | 18.229 |
| 6 | 3 | 1.124 | −0.644 | 0.189 | −0.700 | 18.796 |
| 6 | 6 | 1.107 | −0.616 | 0.188 | −0.766 | 19.544 |
| 6 | 9 | 1.089 | −0.587 | 0.189 | −0.845 | 20.489 |
| 7 | 0 | 1.069 | −0.557 | 0.189 | −0.938 | 21.642 |
| 7 | 3 | 1.049 | −0.527 | 0.191 | −1.043 | 23.011 |
| 7 | 6 | 1.028 | −0.498 | 0.192 | −1.158 | 24.602 |
| 7 | 9 | 1.006 | −0.468 | 0.194 | −1.284 | 26.416 |
| 8 | 0 | 0.983 | −0.439 | 0.196 | −1.418 | 28.448 |
| 8 | 3 | 0.960 | −0.411 | 0.199 | −1.558 | 30.690 |
| 8 | 6 | 0.937 | −0.384 | 0.202 | −1.704 | 33.129 |
| 8 | 9 | 0.914 | −0.359 | 0.204 | −1.853 | 35.747 |
| 9 | 0 | 0.891 | −0.334 | 0.207 | −2.003 | 38.520 |
| 9 | 3 | 0.868 | −0.311 | 0.210 | −2.154 | 41.421 |
| 9 | 6 | 0.845 | −0.289 | 0.212 | −2.301 | 44.415 |
| 9 | 9 | 0.824 | −0.269 | 0.214 | −2.444 | 47.464 |
| 10 | 0 | 0.803 | −0.250 | 0.216 | −2.581 | 50.525 |
| 10 | 3 | 0.783 | −0.233 | 0.217 | −2.710 | 53.548 |
| 10 | 6 | 0.766 | −0.217 | 0.217 | −2.829 | 56.481 |
| 10 | 9 | 0.749 | −0.203 | 0.217 | −2.936 | 59.267 |

*The abbreviations are as follows: $\beta$rl, regression weights for recumbent stature; $\beta$w, weight; $\beta$mps, midparent stature; $\beta$sa, skeletal age; and $\beta$o, the intercept of the regression equation.

| AGE | | | | | | |
|---|---|---|---|---|---|---|
| (yr) | (mo) | $\beta$rl | $\beta$w | $\beta$mps | $\beta$sa | $\beta$o |
| 11 | 0 | 0.736 | −0.190 | 0.216 | −3.029 | 61.841 |
| 11 | 3 | 0.724 | −0.179 | 0.214 | −3.108 | 84.136 |
| 11 | 6 | 0.716 | −0.169 | 0.211 | −3.171 | 66.093 |
| 11 | 9 | 0.711 | −0.159 | 0.206 | −3.217 | 67.627 |
| 12 | 0 | 0.710 | −0.151 | 0.201 | −3.245 | 68.670 |
| 12 | 3 | 0.713 | −0.143 | 0.193 | −3.254 | 69.140 |
| 12 | 6 | 0.720 | −0.136 | 0.184 | −3.244 | 68.966 |
| 12 | 9 | 0.733 | −0.129 | 0.173 | −3.214 | 68.061 |
| 13 | 0 | 0.752 | −0.121 | 0.160 | −3.166 | 66.339 |
| 13 | 3 | 0.777 | −0.113 | 0.144 | −3.100 | 63.728 |
| 13 | 6 | 0.810 | −0.105 | 0.127 | −3.015 | 60.150 |
| 13 | 9 | 0.850 | −0.085 | 0.106 | −2.915 | 55.522 |
| 14 | 0 | 0.898 | −0.083 | 0.083 | −2.800 | 49.781 |

*The abbreviations are as follows: $\beta$rl, regression weights for recumbent stature; $\beta$w, weight; $\beta$mps, midparent stature; $\beta$sa, skeletal age; and $\beta$o, the intercept of the regression equation.

Use of the tables may be explained by an example of a boy whose chronologic age is 6 years, 3 months. His recumbent length is 108.7 cm, his nude weight is 17.4 kg. Midparent height (the average of the height of the two parents) is 169.0 cm, and his skeletal age is 5.4 years. Each of these variables is multiplied by the weight given for the appropriate measurement at the patient's chronologic age. The intercept of the regression equation, $\beta$o, is listed below as the constant.

| | | | PRODUCTS | |
|---|---|---|---|---|
| VARIABLE | VALUE | WEIGHT | Positive | Negative |
| Recumbent length | 108.7 | 1.143 | 124.044 | |
| Weight | 17.4 | −0.512 | | −8.909 |
| Midparent stature | 169.0 | 0.389 | 65.741 | |
| Skeletal age | 5.4 | 0.123 | 0.664 | |
| Constant | | | | −12.901 |
| | | Subtotals.........190.449 | | −21.810 |
| | | Prediction............168.639 cm | | |

The positive and negative values are added algebraically to give the predicted value, and the value is rounded to one decimal point. Figure 3–2 provides the values that should be added to and subtracted from the predicted value to give the upper and lower limits between which actual adult statures will lie for 90 per cent of children. For the boy who is 6 years, 3 months, for example, 4.7 cm should be added to and subtracted from the predicted value to achieve 90 per cent error limits.

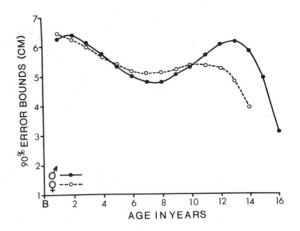

*FIG. 3-2*

It should be noted that these figures were determined from measurements of "normal" Caucasian American children.

Reference: Roche, A.F., Wainer, H., and Thissen, D.: Pediatrics, *56*:1026, 1975.

## TIPS ON TOILET TRAINING

Bowel control is not a simple physiologic reflex; it is a complicated behavior pattern profoundly influenced by maturity factors that are both neurologic and psychologic. For reasons that are difficult to understand, society has placed undue emphasis on early toilet training. This is often translated into a belief that "practice makes perfect." We ask our children to carry our cultural burden at a very early age; the child must do his "duty." We are prepared to extend liberties to our dogs that we will not extend to our children.

The facts of growth and maturity must be explained to parents. Most mistakenly believe that all infants should be toilet trained by 2 years of age, and that failure in this regard is a form of either perversity or, worse still, disobedience.

### Steps in Normal Bowel Control

*16 weeks:* By this age the gastrocolic reflex has weakened somewhat, and there is a delay between feeding and defecation. A vigilant mother may note this delay and take the opportunity to place the child on the toilet. Success leads her to believe that the child is already trained.

*28 weeks:* Bowel movements become more irregular. They may occur unrelated to either waking or eating. Infants are generally indifferent to soiling.

*40 weeks:* The capacity to sit is usually well developed. Child may sit on toilet seat and look at mother and make imitative grunting movements. Occasionally a stool may be passed.

*52 weeks:* A higher order of neurologic maturation is taking place with the assumption of the upright posture. Child is usually not interested in sitting on toilet and making facial grimaces at this time.

*15 months:* If standing and walking have been achieved, the child may actually like to go to the toilet. Some children may instinctively assume a squatting position.

*18 months:* If the child has incorporated meaningful words like "toidy" into his growing vocabulary, and can relate it to bowel control and is ambulating without difficulty, he may be ready for toilet "training." The child must still understand the social significance of the act.

*24 months:* Most children by this age are "trainable." The child should be permitted to take over this responsibility. The child should have his own toilet seat. The seat should allow the child to place his feet squarely on the ground or on a bar so that he may develop the necessary intra-abdominal pressure. He may need help in removing his clothes.

*30 months:* Children of this age frequently display extremes and exaggerations of behavior. Bowel movements may become less regular.

*36 months:* Child has developed increased ability to withhold and postpone. Daily bowel movements may occur late in the day. The child is ready to accept the cultural burden.

*48 months:* The bowel movement has become a private affair. The child has a healthy "childlike" interest in the physical properties of the stool. He is frank, forthright, and independent.

The training process, therefore, requires a neurologically mature nervous system, a psychologically prepared child, and a healthy cultural setting. "Intestinal fortitude" is not a requirement.

The process may be facilitated but not expedited by:

1. An educated and relaxed attitude on the part of the parents.
2. The provision of a toilet seat or chair for the child.
3. Providing an opportunity for imitative behavior.
4. The avoidance of punishment or excessive rewards.
5. The avoidance of training during periods of stress in a child's life, such as a new sibling or a new home.
6. Providing training pants when appropriate.

---

References: Brazelton, T.: Pediatrics, *29*:121, 1962. Stehbens, J.A.: Pediatrics, *54*:493, 1974.

## USE OF BONE AGE DETERMINATION IN THE DIAGNOSIS OF SHORT STATURE

The cause for short stature may often be determined by careful history and physical examination. Nutritional or emotional deprivation, chronic disease, or a history of short stature in other family members may provide an explanation for decreased height. Facial appearance may suggest a genetic or chromosomal abnormality. Organ enlargement may lead to a diagnosis of a storage disease.

Often, however, the diagnosis is not readily apparent. In these cases, it is helpful to begin with a comparison of skeletal maturation (bone age) to height age and chronologic age. The table lists the diagnoses that should be suggested by such a comparison, and the clinical features accompanying each diagnosis.

| MEASUREMENT | DIAGNOSIS SUGGESTED | CLINICAL FEATURES |
|---|---|---|
| Bone age equal to or slightly behind chronologic age | Primordial short stature | Birth weight and length below normal for gestational age. Subsequent growth parallel to, but below, 3rd percentile Normal onset and progression of puberty. Minor skeletal abnormalities. Includes genetic and chromosomal aberrations, e.g., Down's syndrome and Turner's syndrome. Short stature as adult. |
| | Familial short stature | Normal length and weight for first 1 to 2 years of life. Height falls below 3rd percentile at 5 to 10 years of age. Puberty not delayed. "Normal" adult height not attained. |
| Bone age retarded in relation to chronologic age, but less retarded than height age | Constitutional short stature | Appropriate weight and length for gestational age at birth. Slow growth during childhood. Delayed onset of puberty. Other family members may remember similar growth pattern. Important to differentiate from hypothyroidism and growth hormone deficiency. Ultimately reach "normal" adult height. |
| | Metabolic disorders, e.g.: Hypophosphatemic rickets Hypophosphatasia Mucopolysaccharidoses Glycogen storage diseases Renal tubular acidosis Bartter's syndrome Vasopressin-resistant diabetes insipidus | Clinical and laboratory findings consistent with these disorders |

*(Continued)*

| MEASUREMENT | DIAGNOSIS SUGGESTED | CLINICAL FEATURES |
|---|---|---|
| | Organic acidemias and acidurias<br>Hemolytic anemias<br>Disorders of mineral metabolism<br>Immunoglobulin or white blood cell abnormality<br>Others | Clinical and laboratory findings consistent with these disorders. |
| | Chronic disease, e.g.:<br>Chronic infection<br>Hepatic disease<br>Pulmonary disease<br>Renal disease<br>Malabsorption<br>Malignancy<br>Collagen vascular disease<br>Others | Clinical and laboratory findings consistent with the disease; initial clue may be increased erythrocyte sedimentation rate.<br>May exhibit variable growth rate over several years. |
| Bone age equal to or advanced in comparison with height age | Familial short stature | See above |
| | Sexual precocity with androgen excess | Increased linear growth early in life with early closure of epiphyses.<br>Clinical signs of androgen excess (facial, axillary, and pubic hair, penile or clitoral enlargement). |
| | Sexual precocity with estrogen excess | Early closure of epiphyses without prior augmentation of linear growth.<br>Clinical signs of estrogen excess (breast enlargement, galactorrhea in females, and so on). |
| Bone age greatly decreased and less than or equal to height age | Hypothyroidism | Degree of growth retardation depends upon age of onset.<br>Congenital hypothyroidism is associated with severe growth failure.<br>In juvenile hypothyroidism, the growth retardation is more insidious.<br>Delayed dental age. |

3

| | |
|---|---|
| Cushing's syndrome (most often iatrogenic) | Truncal obesity, moon facies, violaceous striae, hirsutism, muscle weakness, hypertension. |
| Hypopituitarism and growth hormone deficiency. Causes include: Congenital absence of pituitary Infection Reticuloendothelioses Vascular infarcts and anomalies Trauma Irradiation Surgical resection Malnutrition | Delayed dental age. Puberty often delayed. May have neurologic abnormalities. |
| Maternal deprivation | May have impaired motor and intellectual development. May or may not be associated with malnutrition. May have growth hormone deficiency. |

Reference: Gotlin, R.W., and Mace, J.W.: Curr. Probl. Pediatr. 2:3, 1972.

# THE EVALUATION OF A CHILD WITH FAILURE TO THRIVE

Pediatricians are commonly required to evaluate infants and children who have "failed to thrive." This frequently encountered problem has many causes, although simple malnutrition is responsible for 75 to 90 per cent of all cases in the United States. Infants with genetic short stature and those with central nervous system deficits account for many of the remainder. An orderly approach to investigation coupled with careful history, physical examination, and simple observation can reduce both unnecessary laboratory investigation and the length of hospitalization.

A few useful general rules:

1. The malnourished infant or child will display a weight reduction out of proportion to his length reduction. His head circumference will be normal or near normal.

2. The infant of short stature will have a length reduction in proportion to or more than his weight reduction. His head circumference will be normal or even increased relative to his length.

3. In the child with a central nervous system deficit, both weight and length will be reduced proportionally, and the head circumference will generally be subnormal.

4. Chronic illness generally produces a proportional reduction in both length and weight, although the weight may be reduced more than the length.

5. Physical signs of neglect usually indicate malnutrition as the cause of the failure to thrive. These signs include: dirty nails, diaper rash, skin infections, flat occiput and "bald spot."

## Initial laboratory tests should include:

| | |
|---|---|
| *Complete blood count* | *Macrocytic anemia* (hypothyroidism, folic acid, or vitamin $B_{12}$ deficiency, which may indicate disease of the small bowel) |
| | *Microcytic anemia* (iron deficiency, gastrointestinal blood loss as a result of milk allergy, chronic infection) |
| | *Polycythemia* (chronic lung disease, heart disease, dehydration) |
| | *Neutropenia* (pancreatic insufficiency and bone marrow hypoplasia syndrome) |
| | *Leukocytosis* (occult infection) |
| | *Thrombocytosis* (neuroblastoma with metastases, granulomas of liver and bone marrow) |
| *Urinalysis* | *Reducing substance* (diabetes, renal tubular disease, disaccharide intolerance) |
| | *Urine pH* ($>6.5$ — renal tubular acidosis?) |
| | *Sediment* (WBCs — urinary tract infection; RBCs — nephritis) |
| | *Proteinuria* (renal disease, renal tubular disease, aminoaciduria) |
| | *Ferric chloride* |
| | *Specific gravity* ($<1.010$ — diabetes insipidus) |
| *Stool examination* | *Reducing substance* (disaccharide intolerance) *Stool pH* (below 6.0, disaccharide intolerance) *Occult blood* (cow milk intolerance) *Ova and parasites* |
| *Tine test* | |
| *Blood urea nitrogen, serum sodium, potassium, chloride, and carbon dioxide* | |

3

If the initial history, physical examination, and simple laboratory tests are all normal, then the infant should be placed on a "therapeutic trial" of feeding. The infant's requirements for fluids, calories, and protein should be calculated, and intake and weight gain carefully recorded on a daily basis.

After several days of observation, the following conclusions may be drawn:

1. *Intake adequate* (120 cal/kg/day) and *weight gain* ensues.
   Conclusion: Inadequate feeding at home; maternal neglect or unsatisfactory parent-child relationship.
2. *Intake inadequate — no weight gain*
   Consider:
   Poor swallowing     — neurologic or neuromuscular disorder
   Eats small amounts — cardiorespiratory disease, severe debilitation, chronic infection, hypothyroidism
   Eats vigorously     — psychological disorder, gastrointestinal anomalies, but spits, vomits,     increased intracranial pressure, chronic subdural or ruminates     hematoma, metabolic abnormality
3. *Intake adequate — No weight gain.* Increase caloric intake to what would be optimal for patient's normal weight. If no weight gain after increase in diet, then malabsorption of some cause must be considered.

Abnormal physical findings or initial laboratory tests may provide you with clues to the diagnosis. Disorders that may produce failure to thrive may be broadly grouped into the classification listed below.

### Inadequate Intake

Economic deprivation
Social deprivation
Psychic anorexia
Mechanical feeding problems
  Cleft palate
  Aerophagia
  Nasal obstruction
Avitaminosis C
Diabetes insipidus

### Failure to Assimilate

Cystic fibrosis
Celiac disease
Milk allergy
Parasites
Postdiarrheal recovery phase
Portal hypertension

### Increased Metabolism

Chronic infection
Malignancy
Collagen disease
Hyperthyroidism
Cerebral palsy–athetoid

### Failure to Utilize (Sick Cells)

Renal acidosis
Renal alkalosis
Renal insufficiency
Hypercalcemia
Hepatic insufficiency — cirrhosis
Diabetes
Storage disease
  Glycogen storage disease
  Hurler's syndrome
Galactosemia

Aminoacidopathies
Hypoxemia
  Cardiac
  Pulmonary insufficiency

*Bone Diseases*

  Chondrodystrophia
  Ellis–van Creveld
  Morquio's

*Failure of Stimulation*

  Cretinism
    Pituitary
    Primordial
    Constitutional
  IUGR (intrauterine growth retardation)
  Gonadal dysgenesis
  Mental retardation
    CNS anomalies and tumors
    Subdural hematomas

## THE DIENCEPHALIC SYNDROME—ANOTHER CAUSE OF FAILURE TO THRIVE

One of the possible diagnoses included near the bottom of the list when an infant presents with "failure to thrive" is the diencephalic syndrome. Although the syndrome is encountered rarely, its recognition can lead to the successful treatment of some children whose average survival time without treatment would be approximately 12 months.

The cause of the diencephalic syndrome is one of a variety of tumors. Histologic diagnosis is not always possible, but tumors identified include a variety of gliomas, ependymomas, gangliogliomas, and dysgerminomas. The tumor may be located at the optic nerve chiasm, in the third ventricle, or in the fourth ventricle.

Mean age of onset of symptoms is 6 months, though some children present as late as 3 to 4 years. Clinical features include the following:

| CLINICAL FEATURES | PER CENT |
|---|---|
| Emaciation | 100 |
| Alert appearance | 87 |
| Increased vigor and/or hyperkinesis | 72 |
| Vomiting | 68 |
| Euphoria | 59 |
| Pallor | 55 |
| Nystagmus | 55 |
| Irritability | 32 |
| Hydrocephalus (clinical and pneumoencephalographic) | 33 |
| Optic atrophy | 24 |
| Tremor | 23 |
| Sweating | 15 |
| Large hands/feet | <5 |
| Large genitals | <5 |
| Polyuria | <5 |
| Papilledema | <5 |
| Positive pneumoencephalogram | 98 |
| Endocrine anomalies (of those adequately recorded) | 90 |
| CSF protein | 64 |
| CSF abnormal cells | 23 |

Two findings that are especially helpful in distinguishing this syndrome from other causes of failure to thrive are (1) the "alert" appearance characteristic of these patients secondary to lid retraction (Collier's sign), and (2) the abnormal cells and/or increased protein present in the cerebrospinal fluid in 70 per cent of those affected.

Localization of the tumor may be aided by the knowledge that vomiting is generally an early sign of posterior fossa (fourth ventricle) tumors, while tremor, optic atrophy, and nystagmus occur earlier in tumors located more anteriorly.

Endocrine abnormalities are variable, and pneumoencephalography may not be diagnostic.

Reference: Burr, I.M., Slonim, A.E., Danish, R.K., et al.: J. Pediatr., *88*:439, 1976.

## DEVELOPMENT IN DOWN'S SYNDROME CHILDREN RAISED AT HOME

For some time it has been clear that the child with Down's syndrome who is raised at home is likely to be superior mentally and socially to his institutionalized counterpart. On the other hand, parents should not be led to expect normal development in children whose capabilities are limited. The table below lists realistic ages at which developmental milestones may be reached in children with Down's syndrome who are not institutionalized.

| ATTRIBUTE | UNIT OF MEASUREMENT | AGE RANGE | AVERAGE AGE | AGE IN NORMAL CHILDREN |
|---|---|---|---|---|
| *Developmental* | | | | |
| Holds head up (when held vertically) | Week | 1–18 | 3.95 | 6–17 |
| Rolls over | Months | 1–60 | 6.38 | 2–5 |
| Sits up unsupported (boys) | Months | 5–72 | 12.52 | 5–8 |
| Sits up unsupported (girls) | Months | 5–36 | 11.14 | 5–8 |
| Creeps (on hands and knees) | Months | 4–24 | 12.19 | 7–10 |
| Stands up (boys) | Months | 8–84 | 22.17 | 5–10 |
| Stands up (girls) | Months | 7–72 | 18.97 | 5–10 |
| Walks unassisted (boys) | Months | 7–74 | 26.09 | 11–15 |
| Walks unassisted (girls) | Months | 8–72 | 22.72 | 11–15 |
| Toilet-trained | Months | 8–108 | 34.78 | 24–27 |
| *Speech* | | | | |
| Speaks first word (boys) | Months | 6–72 | 26.59 | 9–13 |
| Speaks first word (girls) | Months | 6–84 | 21.82 | 9–13 |
| Speaks first phrase | Months | 12–96 | 41.82 | 14–24 |
| Speaks first sentence | Months | 17–132 | 52.05 | 18–30 |

Reference: Melyn, M.A., and White, D.T.: Pediatrics, *52*:542, 1973.

# 4

# METABOLISM

# PREDICTABLE FALL OF BUN
# IN A DEHYDRATED CHILD

Children admitted to hospital with diarrhea and dehydration often have elevated blood urea nitrogen (BUN) levels. Usually this elevation is assumed to be prerenal and the abnormality is ignored, at least until just before discharge. Brill and coworkers found that the rate of fall of BUN in a dehydrated child with normal renal function was predictable. They plotted BUN levels against time on semilogarithmic graph paper. BUN had fallen to one-half the admission level in 24 hours or less in all children with uncomplicated dehydration and diarrhea.

Line A in Figure 4–1 represents the slope along which the BUN should fall in a child without renal disease or excess nitrogen load (e.g., gastrointestinal bleed). Lines B and C represent 2½ standard deviations on either side of that rate of fall.

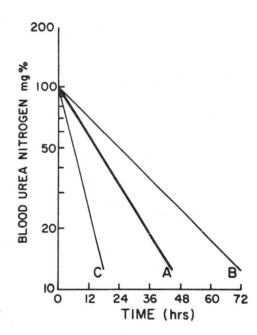

FIG. 4–1

Complicating disease should be sought in the dehydrated child whose BUN does not fall at a rate parallel to line A or within 2½ standard deviations from that rate.

Reference: Brill, C.B., Uretsky, S., and Gribetz, D.: J. Pediatr., *52*:197, 1973.

*"In bringing up a child, think of its old age."*

Joubert

## SERUM OSMOLALITY

It is often important to estimate serum osmolality before the laboratory measurement becomes available. The following formula will make that estimation more accurate.

The short cut approach is

$$\text{Serum Osmolality} = \{Na(mEq/L) + K\,(mEq/L)\} \times 2 + \frac{\text{Glucose}}{18} + \frac{\text{BUN}}{3}$$

The normal value is 280.

## HYPOGLYCEMIA

The symptoms and signs of hypoglycemia are due to epinephrine secretion and the effects of low blood sugar on the central nervous system.

| Epinephrine Secretion | CNS Effect of Low Blood Sugar |
|---|---|
| Anxiety | Disturbed mentation |
| Sweating | Incoordination |
| Pallor | Ataxia |
| Weakness | Visual disturbances |
| Tremulousness | Dysarthria |
| | Convulsions |
| | Coma |

Insulin reaction in the diabetic patient is probably the most well recognized cause of hypoglycemia. Other causes are listed below.

*Pancreatic*

Hyperplasia of the islet cells
Islet cell tumor (nesidioblastoma) — very rare in children, but cases have
    been described in infants
Functional hyperinsulinism

*Adrenal Insufficiency*

Cortical
  Primary
  Secondary (to corticotropin insufficiency)

*Pituitary Insufficiency*

(as primary effect due to deficiency of growth hormone; or as secondary
    effect due to deficiency of corticotropin)

## Hepatic

Toxins — e.g., carbon tetrachloride, chloroform, *Amanita phalloides,*
  drug reactions
Hepatitis
  Viral
  Bacterial — cholangitis, pylephlebitis
Fatty change
Cirrhosis
Chronic passive congestion in heart failure
Glycogen storage disease (von Gierke's hepatorenal type)
Galactosemia

## Chronic Malnutrition

(e.g., starvation, celiac disease, tuberculous mesenteric adenitis)

## Spontaneous Infantile Hypoglycemia

Leucine-sensitive type
Hereditary intolerance to fructose
Postprandial hypoglycemia
Maple sugar urine disease
Epinephrine refractive type
Growth hormone deficiency
Jamaican vomiting sickness and Reye's syndrome
Ketotic hypoglycemia
In infants of toxemic mothers
In infants of diabetic mothers
In infants delivered by cesarean section
Symptomless hypoglycemia of the newborn

Reference: Jenkins, R.B.: Nutritional disorders. *In* Farmer, T.W. (Ed.): Pediatric Neurology. New York, Harper & Row, 1975. p. 231.

# THE DIAGNOSIS OF HYPOGLYCEMIA

Beyond the neonatal period, the diagnosis of hypoglycemia can be complex. Like so many other problems in differential diagnosis, an individualized approach based on the clues provided by the history and the physical examination should be employed.

In the history, details such as age of onset, frequency, temporal relationship to meals, drug ingestion, and facts concerning carbohydrate intolerance or diabetes in other members of the family should be elicited.

In the physical examination, the size of the liver should be noted as well as evidence of macrosomia, cataracts, signs of hypothyroidism, or abdominal masses. The height and weight should be carefully recorded and the blood pressure obtained.

Diagnostic procedures should be conducted in a facility where plasma insulin assays can be obtained.

The flow sheet illustrates one means of evaluating a patient with a history of hypoglycemia. The table provides a list of the numerous diagnostic possibilities.

*Diagnostic Approach to Childhood Hypoglycemia*

1. History
2. Physical Examination
3. Complete Urinalysis
4. Liver Function Screen
5. Fasting Blood Glucose and Serum Insulin

---

**REACTIVE HYPOGLYCEMIA**

5-hour glucose tolerance test

**FASTING HYPOGLYCEMIA (WITHOUT KETONURIA)**

1. Prolonged fast with frequent blood glucose, serum insulin, growth hormone, corticoid, and glucagon determinations
2. Leucine tolerance test
3. Glucagon tolerance test
4. Intravenous or oral glucose tolerance test
5. Tolbutamide tolerance test
6. Pancreatic arteriogram

---

**KETONURIA (WITHOUT HEPATOMEGALY)**

1. Prolonged fast as tolerated with frequent blood glucose, serum insulin, and alanine levels
2. Growth hormone, corticoids, and glucagon levels at beginning and end of fast
3. Glucagon tolerance test at beginning and end of fast
4. Roentgenograms for bone age and sella size

---

**ABNORMAL LIVER FUNCTION OR HEPATOMEGALY**

1. Glucagon tolerance test
2. Galactose tolerance test
3. Fructose tolerance test
4. Liver biopsy
5. Tissue enzyme analysis

---

**SHORT STATURE OR OTHER CLINICAL EVIDENCE OF HORMONE DEFICIENCY**

1. Arginine tolerance test
2. Metyrapone test
3. Thyroid evaluation

---

Information gained from the initial history, physical examination, and laboratory studies defines specific areas of carbohydrate metabolism that require further investigation.

*Classification of Disorders Associated with Hypoglycemia*

## TRANSIENT NEONATAL HYPOGLYCEMIA

Low birth weight infant
"Hyperinsulinism"
   1. Infant of diabetic or gestational diabetic mother
   2. Infant with erythroblastosis
Stresses in infant that may be associated with hypoglycemia

## PERSISTENT HYPOGLYCEMIA OF INFANCY AND CHILDHOOD

Inability to release adequate endogenous glucose
   1. Hereditary enzyme deficiencies
      a. glycogen storage diseases
         (1) glucose 6-phosphatase (type I)
         (2) debrancher enzyme complex (type III)
         (3) phosphorylase abnormalities (type VI)
      b. glycogen synthetase deficiency
      c. fructose intolerance (decreased fructose 1-phosphate aldolase)
      d. fructose 1, 6-diphosphatase deficiency
      e. galactose intolerance (galactose 1-phosphate uridyl transferase deficiency)
      f. amino acid disorders (cystinosis, maple syrup urine disease, tyrosinemia, argininosuccinic aciduria)
   2. Ketotic hypoglycemia
   3. Hormone abnormalities
      a. panhypopituitarism
      b. isolated growth hormone deficiency
      c. glucocorticoid deficiency
         (1) congenital adrenal hyperplasia
         (2) Addison's disease; ACTH unresponsiveness
         (3) isolated adrenocorticotropin deficiency
      d. catecholamine abnormalities
      e. thyroid hormone deficiency
   4. Liver disease
      a. Reye's syndrome
      b. hepatitis, cirrhosis
      c. malnutrition
Increased or inappropriate insulin release
   1. Beta cell hyperplasia
   2. Nesidioblastosis
   3. Islet cell adenoma
   4. Functional hyperinsulinism (?)
   5. Reactive hypoglycemia
   6. Beckwith-Wiedemann syndrome

## MISCELLANEOUS DISORDERS ASSOCIATED WITH HYPOGLYCEMIA

Extrapancreatic tumors
   1. Fibrosarcoma
   2. Wilms' tumor
   3. Hepatoma
   4. Neuroblastoma
Malabsorption
Poisons or toxins
   1. Salicylates
   2. Oral hypoglycemics
   3. Insulin
   4. Jamaican vomiting sickness

5. TRIS buffer
6. Propranolol
7. Alcohol

---

Reference: Bacon, G.E., Spencer, M.L., and Kelch, R.P.: A Practical Approach to Pediatric Endocrinology. Chicago, Year Book Medical Publishers, 1975.

## THE HYPERLIPIDEMIAS

The pediatrician should become familiar with the manifestations of the hyperlipidemias. Type I and Type II hyperlipidemia are both diagnosable in early life, and both may produce symptoms during the first 10 years. The table on page 103 provides a summary of the major features of these disorders. It is particularly important to look for them when you learn from the history that one of the parents or close relatives of your patient has had a myocardial infarction prior to age 45.

## UNUSUAL ODOR AS A CLUE TO DIAGNOSIS

It is 3:00 A.M. in the nursery, and a call from the nurse informs you that a 2 day old full-term infant, who had been perfectly fine until now, has turned sour. Not recognizing the pun, you sleepily arouse yourself to examine the patient. If you are fortunate, you note that the diaper of the seizing infant smells like sweaty feet. If you are doubly fortunate, you remember that odor long enough to order an amino acid analysis of serum and urine and discontinue all proteins in the patient's diet. That particular baby may have isovalericacidemia. It probably does not, since it is a very rare condition, but the sweaty feet syndrome is just one of several errors of metabolism that may be discovered in the nursery by an alert olfactory organ (see table on page 104).

Some of the above metabolic diseases may be quickly verified by adding 10 per cent ferric chloride drop by drop to 1 ml of the patient's urine (see Poisoning – Ferric Chloride, page 423).

---

Reference: Mace, J.W., Goodman, S.I., Centerwall, W.R., et al.: Clin. Pediatr., *15*:58, 1976.

*Some Features of the Primary Hyperlipoproteinemias*

| TYPE | INCIDENCE | IDENTIFIABLE IN CHILDREN | INHERITANCE | APPEARANCE | CHOLESTEROL | TRIGLYCERIDE | CLINICAL FEATURES IN CHILDHOOD |
|---|---|---|---|---|---|---|---|
| I | Very rare | Yes, in infancy | Autosomal recessive | Cream layer over clear plasma on standing | Normal or increased | Markedly increased | Abdominal pain, pancreatitis, hepatosplenomegaly, eruptive xanthomas, lipemia retinalis |
| II | Common | Yes, in infancy; (?) at birth | Usually autosomal dominant | Clear | Increased | Normal or slightly increased | Rare in heterozygotes; xanthoma, vascular disease, and Achilles tendinitis in homozygotes |
| III | Uncommon | No | (?) | Clear, turbid or milky | Increased | Usually increased | None |
| IV | Common | Occasionally in second decade | Usually autosomal dominant | Turbid or milky with no change on standing | Usually normal | Increased | None |
| V | Uncommon | Occasionally in second decade | (?) autosomal dominant | Cream layer over turbid plasma on standing | Increased or normal | Increased to markedly increased | Same as in Type I |

Reference: Levy, R.I., and Rifkind, B.M.: Am. J. Cardiol., *31*:547, 1973.

*Diseases Associated with Unusual Odors*

| DISEASE | ENZYME DEFECT | ODOR | CLINICAL FEATURES | TREATMENT |
|---|---|---|---|---|
| Diabetes mellitus | Lack of insulin or insulin activity | Acetone on breath | Polyuria, polyphagia, polydipsia, weight loss, acidosis, coma | Insulin administration |
| Phenylketonuria | Phenylalanine hydroxylase | Musty, "mousy," "horsey" | Progressive mental retardation, eczema, decreased pigmentation, seizures, spasticity | Diet low in phenylalanine |
| Maple syrup urine disease | Branched chain decarboxylase | Maple syrup | Marked acidosis, seizures, coma leading to death in first year or two of life or mental subnormality without acidosis or intermittent acidosis without mental retardation | Diet low in branched chain amino acids; protein restriction and/or thiamine in large doses |
| Oasthouse urine disease | Defective transport of methionine, branched chain amino acids, tyrosine, and phenylalanine | Yeast-like Dried-celery-like | Mental retardation, spasticity, hyperpnea, fever, edema | Restrict methionine in diet |
| Odor of sweaty feet, Syndrome I | Isovaleryl CoA dehydrogenase | Sweaty feet | Recurrent bouts of acidosis, vomiting, dehydration, coma, aversion to protein foods | Restrict leucine in diet |
| Odor of sweaty feet, Syndrome II | Green acyldehydrogenase | Sweaty feet | Onset of symptoms in first week of life with acidosis, dehydration, seizures, and death | High CHO diet(?) Low fat diet(?) |

**4**

| | | | | |
|---|---|---|---|---|
| Odor of cats syndrome | Beta-methyl-crotonyl-CoA carboxylase | Cat's urine | Neurologic disorder resembling Werdnig-Hoffmann disease, ketoacidosis, failure to thrive | Leucine restriction(?) Biotin administration |
| Fish odor syndrome | Unknown | Like dead fish | Stigmata of Turner's syndrome, neutropenia, recurrent infections, anemia, splenomegaly | Unknown |
| Fish odor syndrome | Trimethylamine oxidase | Like dead fish | Unusual odor of sweat, skin and urine. Normal development | Elimination of fish from the diet |
| Odor of rancid butter syndrome | Unknown | Rancid butter | Poor feeding, irritability, progressive neurologic deterioration with seizures and death; hepatic dysfunction; possibly same as acute tyrosinosis | Response to decreased phenylalanine and tyrosine intake(?) |

*"The childhood shows the man as morning shows the day."*

Milton

## DISEASES AND POISONINGS ASSOCIATED WITH UNUSUAL BREATH ODOR

The odor of a patient's breath may suggest a particular disease state or ingestion of a toxic substance. The table below lists these suspicious odors and their diagnostic significance.

| ODOR | PRODUCT OR DISEASE STATE TO SUSPECT |
|------|-------------------------------------|
| Acrid (pear-like) | Paraldehyde |
| Alcohol (fruit-like) | Alcohol |
| Ammoniacal | Uremia |
| Bitter almonds | Cyanide (in chokecherry, apricot pits) |
| Coal gas (stove gas) | Carbon monoxide (odorless, but associated with coal gas) |
| Disinfectants | Phenol, creosote |
| Garlic | Phosphorus, tellurium, arsenic (breath and perspiration), parathion, malathion |
| Halitosis | Acute illness, poor oral hygiene |
| Musty fish (raw liver) | Hepatic failure |
| Pungent, aromatic | Ethchlorvynol (Placidyl) |
| Rotten eggs | Hydrogen sulfide mercaptans |
| Shoe polish | Nitrobenzene |
| Sweet acetone (russet apples) | Lacquer, alcohol, ketoacidosis, chloroform |
| Stale tobacco | Nicotine |
| Violets | Turpentine |
| Wintergreen | Methylsalicylate |

Reference: Hospital Physician, March 1976, p. 12.

## CHANGES IN URINE COLOR

Parents as well as children may become alarmed when they note a change in the color of urine. Many drugs and natural substances can produce such alterations. A partial list of such agents and the colors they produce is given below.

4

| URINE COLOR | DRUG OR CHEMICAL |
| --- | --- |
| Blue | Methylene blue<br>Triamterene (Dyrenium) |
| Brown to black | Metronidazole (Flagyl)<br>Nitrites<br>Nitrofurans<br>Phenacetin<br>Rhubarb<br>Senna |
| Green (blue plus yellow) | Amitriptyline (Elavil)<br>Bile pigments<br>Methocarbamol (Robaxin) |
| Purple | Phenolphthalein (urine pH $<$8.0) |
| Orange | Phenazopyridine (Pyridium) |
| Orange to red-brown | Rifampin<br>Warfarin sodium |
| Pink to red to red-brown | Aminopyrine<br>Cascara<br>Deferoxamine (Desferal)<br>Methyldopa (Aldomet)<br>Phenazopyridine hydrochloride<br>    (Pyridium in acid urine)<br>Phenolphthalein (urine pH $>$8.0)<br>Phenothiazines<br>Diphenylhydantoin (Dilantin)<br>Senna (alkaline urine)<br>Urates |
| Yellow or brownish | Aminosalicylic acid<br>Bismuth<br>Mercury<br>Bilirubin<br>Sulfonamides |
| Yellow or green | Methylene blue<br>Carotene-containing foods |
| Pink | Beta-cyanine (beet pigment) in patients<br>    with genetic defect or in children<br>    with iron deficiency |

Reference: Shirkey, H.C. (Ed.): Pediatric Therapy. 5th Ed. St. Louis, C.V. Mosby Company, 1975, p. 226.

## URINARY ELECTROLYTES

The cause of electrolyte abnormalities is usually self-evident, and urinary electrolyte evaluation is unnecessary. In cases where confusion arises, however, 24-hour urinary electrolyte measurement may be helpful. The following table correlates the clinical condition with urinary electrolyte values and the diagnostic possibilities.

| DIAGNOSTIC PROBLEM | URINARY VALUE | PRIMARY DIAGNOSTIC POSSIBILITIES |
|---|---|---|
| Volume depletion | $Na^+$, 0–10 mEq/liter | Extrarenal sodium loss |
| | $Na^+$, >10 mEq/liter | "Renal salt wasting" or adrenal insufficiency |
| Acute oliguria | $Na^+$, 0–10 mEq/liter | Prerenal azotemia |
| | $Na^+$, >30 mEq/liter | Acute tubular necrosis |
| Hyponatremia | $Na^+$, 0–10 mEq/liter | Severe volume depletion; edematous states |
| | $Na^+$, ≥dietary intake | Inappropriate antidiuretic hormone (ADH) secretion; adrenal insufficiency |
| Hypokalemia | $K^+$, 0–10 mEq/liter | Extrarenal potassium loss |
| | $K^+$, >10 mEq/liter | Renal potassium loss |
| Metabolic alkalosis | $Cl^-$, 0–10 mEq/liter | Chloride-responsive alkalosis |
| | $Cl^-$, ≅dietary intake | Chloride-resistant alkalosis |

For purposes of this table, it is assumed the patient is not receiving diuretics.

Reference: Harrington, J.T., and Cohen, J.J.: N. Engl. J. Med., *293*:1241, 1975.

## VITAMIN E ABSORPTION TEST IN THE DIFFERENTIAL DIAGNOSIS OF JAUNDICE IN INFANCY

A variety of diagnostic procedures have been advocated in an attempt to distinguish neonatal hepatitis from biliary atresia. None is correct all the time and some are not readily available. Although the definitive diagnosis ultimately depends on a liver biopsy, operative cholangiogram, and visual inspection of the external biliary duct system, a simple test employing vitamin E can generally predict the operative findings.

Adequate levels of vitamin E are required to prevent the hemolysis of red cells when they are incubated in the presence of dilute solutions of hydrogen peroxide. Vitamin E, a fat-soluble vitamin, requires the presence of bile salts for absorption. In patients with inadequate bile flow, such as occurs in biliary atresia, the absorption of vitamin E will be abnormal and the red cell hydrogen peroxide hemolysis test will be positive.

The vitamin E absorption test is performed as follows:

1. Obtain a fasting serum vitamin E level.
2. Administer 25 mg per kg of vitamin E by mouth (as α-tocopherol acetate — Aquasol E, U.S. Vitamin Corporation).
3. Obtain a second serum specimen 8 hours after the test dose.
4. Calculate the E tolerance index (ETI) as follows:

$$ETI = \frac{\text{8-hr serum E level} - \text{0-hr serum E level}}{25} \times 100$$

| INTERPRETATION DIAGNOSIS | ETI MEAN | RANGE |
|---|---|---|
| Biliary atresia | 0.32 | 0.0 – 1.6 |
| Neonatal hepatitis | 7.00 | 3.1 – 10.6 |
| Normals | 12.40 | 7.2 – 14.9 |

Hydrogen peroxide hemolysis tests may also be performed before and 24 to 48 hours after the administration of vitamin E by mouth. Although patients with hepatitis tend to have normal hydrogen peroxide hemolysis tests and patients with atresia have abnormal results, there is some overlap. After vitamin E, however, the hepatitis patients will demonstrate an improvement in their hemolysis test, whereas the patients with atresia will not.

---

References: Melhorn, D.K., Gross, S., and Izant, R.J., Jr.: J. Pediatr., *81*:1082, 1972. Lubin, B.H., Baehner, R.L., Schwartz, E., et al.: Pediatrics, *48*:562, 1971.

# THE DIFFERENTIAL DIAGNOSIS OF DISORDERS OF CALCIUM AND PHOSPHORUS METABOLISM

| SERUM CALCIUM | SERUM PHOSPHORUS | SERUM ALKALINE PHOSPHATASE | CONSIDER AS DIAGNOSTIC POSSIBILITIES |
|---|---|---|---|
| ↓ | ↓ | ↑ | Rickets<br>  Dietary<br>  Renal disease<br>  Anticonvulsants<br>  Liver disease |
| ↓ | Normal | Normal | Newborn, normal<br>Anticonvulsant therapy<br>Rickets, early<br>Hypoalbuminemia<br>Hypernatremia |
| ↓ | Normal | ↑ | Renal insufficiency<br>Anticonvulsant therapy<br>Rickets |
| ↓ | ↑ | ↑ | Renal insufficiency<br>Pseudohypoparathyroidism |
| ↓ | ↑ | Normal | Normal newborn<br>Hypoparathyroidism |
| Normal | ↓ | Normal | Parenteral alimentation<br>Sepsis (especially gram-negative)<br>Antacid abuse |
| Normal | ↓ | ↑ | Rickets<br>Renal insufficiency |
| Normal | Normal | ↓ | Hypophosphatasia |
| Normal | ↑ | ↑ | Renal insufficiency<br>Pseudohypoparathyroidism |
| ↑ | ↓ | ↑ | Hyperparathyroidism |
| ↑ | Normal | Normal | Vitamin D excess |
| ↑ | ↑ | Normal | Hypoparathyroidism with vitamin D excess |
| ↑ | ↑ | ↑ | Renal insufficiency with vitamin D excess<br>      or<br>Pseudohypoparathyroidism |

Reference: Bergstrom, W.: Personal communication.

# THE THREE-STAGE CHEMICAL EVOLUTION OF RICKETS

4

### Stage 1 (Intestinal Calcium Transport Decreased)

Serum calcium decreased
Serum phosphorus normal
Serum alkaline phosphatase normal
X-ray — normal
Tetany may occur

### Stage 2 (Compensatory Hyperparathyroidism)

Serum calcium normal
Serum phosphorus decreased
Serum alkaline phosphatase increased
Serum bicarbonate decreased
Serum chloride increased
Aminoaciduria
X-ray — active rickets

### Stage 3 (Parathyroid Response No Longer Sustains Normal Serum Calcium)

Serum calcium decreased
Serum phosphorus decreased
Serum alkaline phosphatase increased
Serum bicarbonate decreased
Serum chloride increased
Aminoaciduria
X-ray — florid rickets
Tetany may occur

References: Bergstrom, W.: Personal communication. Fraser, D., and Salter, R.B.: Pediatr. Clin. North Am., 5:417, 1958.

*Rickets*—or avitaminosis D, is named for its discoverer, Dr. Rickets, an "empiric" country practitioner in 17th century England. The term "rachitis," later applied to the same condition, was an apparent attempt by the medical profession to substitute a proper Latinized name for the more plebian rickets.

# 5
# THE
# NEWBORN

# FETAL MONITORING

Pediatricians are working more closely with their obstetrical colleagues in problems focused on the maternal-fetal unit. Pediatricians appear more frequently on the labor floor and the delivery suite. At times you may feel that you have entered a foreign land where an altogether unfamiliar language is spoken. The pediatrician must become familiar with the descriptive terms employed in fetal monitoring and appreciate their significance. Here is a brief guide.

There are three basic patterns of fetal heart rate change that appear in relationship to uterine activity. These patterns are termed either early, variable, or late decelerations and are illustrated in Figure 5–1.

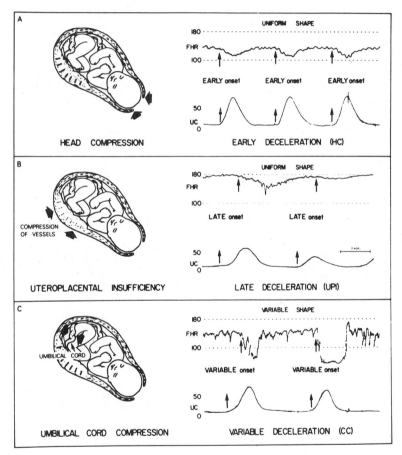

*FIG. 5–1*

FHR = Fetal heart rate;
UC = uterine contraction.

1. *Early decelerations* (Type I Dip) of the fetal heart rate occur early in the uterine contraction cycle. They are seen most frequently when the fetus is descending through the birth canal and are due to compression of the fetal head.

2. *Late decelerations* (Type II Dip) of the fetal heart rate occur 20 or more seconds after the onset of the uterine contraction. They may be observed in cases of prolonged or excessive uterine activity, maternal hypertension, maternal hypotension, or other conditions associated with diminished perfusion of the intervillous space. Late decelerations may be classified in the following fashion:

**115**

|  | DURATION (SEC) | DECREASE IN FETAL HEART RATE |
| --- | --- | --- |
| Mild | <90 | <15 |
| Moderate | <90 | 15–45 |
| Severe | >90 | >45 |

Moderate or severe late decelerations strongly suggest fetal hypoxia or asphyxia.

3. *Variable decelerations* (Type III Dip) of the fetal heart rate may occur at any time during the contraction cycle and are characterized by a very abrupt decrease in the fetal heart rate with an equally abrupt return of the heart rate to baseline values. They are present in 25 to 50 per cent of all monitored labors, and are caused by umbilical cord compression. These are classified as follows:

|  | DURATION (SEC) | FETAL HEART RATE |
| --- | --- | --- |
| Mild | <30 | >80 |
| Moderate | 30–60 | 60–80 |
| Severe | >60 | <60 |

Moderate or severe variable decelerations indicate inadequate fetal blood flow with resultant hypoxia.

References: Hon, E.H.: An Atlas of Fetal Heart Rate Patterns. New Haven, Connecticut, Harty Press, Inc., 1968. Quilligan, E.J., and Collea, J.V.: Adv. Pediatr., *22*:83, 1976.

## PRENATAL CHEMICAL INFLUENCES

Drugs ingested during pregnancy may affect the fetus. It is always useful to review all medications taken by the mother when you assume care of an infant. Drugs that may affect the infant if taken by the mother during pregnancy are listed below.

| DRUG | PRIMARY CLINICAL EFFECT ON INFANT* |
| --- | --- |
| Cigarettes | Low birth weight (?) |
| Alcohol | Fetal alcohol syndrome (see p. 415) |
| Narcotics | Withdrawal signs, prematurity, depression after use in labor |

**5**

| | |
|---|---|
| Lysergic acid diethylamide (LSD) | Chromosomal damage (?), skeletal anomalies (?) |
| General anesthetics (ether, cyclopropane, trichloroethylene) | Respiratory depression or asphyxia |
| Barbiturates | Withdrawal, activation of hepatic microsomal enzymes, respiratory depression after use during labor |
| Dilantin | Cleft palate (?) |
| Corticosteroids | Adrenal suppression |
| Androgens and progestins | Masculinization of female fetuses, enhanced intelligence (?) |
| Estrogens | Adenocarcinoma of vagina (?) |
| Thiocarbamides | Goiter, thyroid suppression |
| Iodides | Goiter, thyroid stimulation or suppression in different dosages |
| Insulin | Fetal death early in pregnancy (?) |
| Tolbutamide | Thrombocytopenia (?), fetal loss (?) |
| Tetracyclines | Staining of teeth and bones |
| Chloramphenicol | Death (gray syndrome) |
| Streptomycin | Hearing loss (?) |
| Sulfonamide | Hyperbilirubinemia, hemolysis in susceptible infants |
| Novobiocin | Hyperbilirubinemia |
| Coumadin | Intrauterine or neonatal bleeding |
| Aspirin (large doses) | Neonatal bleeding |
| Thiazides | Bone marrow depression (?) |
| Reserpine | Transient respiratory symptoms |
| Magnesium sulfate | Respiratory and neuromotor depression |
| Ammonium chloride | Acidosis |
| Methonium compounds | Ileus |
| Naphthalene (as well as certain antimalarials, sulfonamides, nitrofurans, antipyretics) | Erythrocyte hemolysis in susceptible individuals |
| Aminopterin, methotrexate | Fetal death, skeletal anomalies |
| Busulfan | Intrauterine growth retardation, marrow depression, gonadal injury (?) |
| Thalidomide | Skeletal, ear, vascular, and gut anomalies |
| Quinine | Thrombocytopenia, hemolysis in susceptible infants, skeletal anomalies (?), deafness (?) |
| Chloroquine | Deafness (?), hemolysis in susceptible individuals |
| Arsenic | Premature delivery (?) |
| Lead | Growth and mental retardation (?), anemia (?) |

| DRUG | PRIMARY CLINICAL EFFECT ON INFANT* |
|---|---|
| Vitamin D | Hypercalcemia syndrome (?) |
| Vitamin K | Hyperbilirubinemia, hemolysis in susceptible individuals |
| Vaccination | Vaccinia |

*A question mark indicates that the effect is not proved.

Maternal metabolic disease may also affect the unborn child. The list below includes many of these diseases and their effects.

| MATERNAL DISORDER | PRIMARY CLINICAL EFFECTS ON FETUS OR NEWLY BORN INFANT* |
|---|---|
| Endocrine | |
| Diabetes | Excess growth, metabolic instability, respiratory distress syndrome, anomalies, vascular thrombosis |
| Hyperparathyroidism | Hypoparathyroidism and tetany, excess growth (?) |
| Hypoparathyroidism | Hyperparathyroidism, low birth weight |
| Hyperthyroidism | Transient thyrotoxicosis |
| Hypothyroidism | Cretinism in certain instances |
| Cushing's syndrome | Fetal loss |
| Addison's disease | Fetal loss, prolonged gestation (?) |
| Adrenogenital syndrome | None |
| Aldosteronism | Abortion |
| Pheochromocytoma | Fetal loss |
| Herpes gestationis | Transient herpes gestationis |
| Myasthenia gravis | Transient myasthenia |
| Electrolyte and osmolar disturbance | Similar electrolyte or osmolar imbalance |
| Inborn errors of metabolism | |
| Phenylketonuria | Mental retardation, growth failure, microcephaly, anomalies |
| Homocystinuria | CNS damage of offspring (?) |
| Hemoglobinopathies | Low birth weight |
| Cystic fibrosis | Low birth weight (?) |
| Nutritional deprivation | Growth retardation |

*A question mark indicates that the effect is not proved.

Reference: Stevenson, R.E.: Prenatal chemical influences. *In* The Fetus and Newly Born Infant. St. Louis, C.V. Mosby Company, 1973, p. 34.

# CEPHALHEMATOMA
# AND ITS COMPLICATIONS

A cephalhematoma is a subperiosteal hemorrhage. The hematoma is soft and fluctuant, and the outline is well defined with the edge at the bone margin. If the cephalhematoma crosses the midline, a fracture of the skull is present. Cephalhematomas begin to calcify during the first few days of life; a ridge around the hematoma may be felt for as long as six months.

In contrast to the cephalhematoma, a caput succedaneum is soft, but the outline is not well defined. It pits on pressure but is not fluctuant.

Most infants born with cephalhematomas are full term, healthy babies. Cephalhematomas occur in 0.3 to 2.5 per cent of all births, depending largely on the predominant obstetrical techniques employed. It is more common in forceps delivery, vacuum evacuation, prolonged labor, and primiparity. The location of the cephalhematoma depends upon the presentation of the head at birth. The deformity is usually recognized in the nursery, where the pediatrician may observe the child and explain the benignity of the condition to the mother. A small percentage may appear after discharge from the hospital and cause great maternal concern.

Complications with cephalhematoma are unusual, but the pediatrician should be aware of their possibility. In one group of 139 infants with cephalhematoma, a total of 37 showed some complication. The types of difficulty and the number of infants presenting with each complication are listed below.

*Caput succedaneum*—From the Latin. *Caput* means head, and *succedere* means to follow. Refers to the swelling of the head that follows delivery.

| | TYPE OF COMPLICATION | NUMBER OF INFANTS |
|---|---|---|
| Birth to 1 week | Hypoactivity | 5 |
| | Seizures, central nervous system irritation | 5 |
| | Jaundice (>10 mg/100 ml, no Rh, ABO incompatibility) | 9 |
| | Fractures | 6 |
| | Rapidly increasing fronto-occipital circumference | 1 |
| | Localized scalp infection | 1 |
| | Anemia, transfused | 1 |
| 1 week to 2 months | Calcifications | 2 |
| | Large fronto-occipital circumference (>80th percentile) | 3 |
| | Irritability, hyperactivity | 1 |
| | Marked abnormality of fine motor control | 1 |
| | Subdural hematoma | 1 |
| | Erysipelas over cephalhematoma | 1 |
| | Total | 37 |

One of the complications, detectable only by skull roentgenogram, is the linear skull fracture that accompanies the cephalhematoma in about 7 per cent of cases. In most instances, fractures occur in infants who have been delivered by forceps. Since no treatment of the linear fracture is required, skull films are not required unless central nervous symptoms are present, the cephalhematoma is excessively large, or delivery has been extremely difficult.

Reference: Yasunaga, S., and Rivera, R.: Clin. Pediatr., *13*:256, 1974.

# THE JITTERY INFANT

It is frequently necessary to distinguish between the jittery infant and the infant with seizures (see Neonatal Seizures). The movements of the jittery infant are characterized by tremulousness and, occasionally, by clonus. Keeping the following characteristics of jitteriness in mind can help in the distinction between these two conditions.

|  | JITTERINESS | SEIZURE |
|---|---|---|
| Abnormal gaze or eye movement | No | Usually |
| Stimulus-sensitive | Exquisitely | No |
| Predominant movements | Tremor | Clonic jerking |
| On passive flexion | Usually ceases | No change |

The most commonly defined causes of jitteriness:

Hypoxic-ischemic encephalopathy
Hypocalcemia
Hypoglycemia
Drug withdrawal

Reference: Volpe, J.J.: Mead Johnson Symposium on Perinatal and Developmental Medicine, No. 6, 1974, p. 61.

# NEONATAL SEIZURES

Seizures during the neonatal period present special problems. Detection of subtle seizures may be difficult in a neonate. The table below presents the manifestations of such seizures.

*Manifestations of Subtle Seizures*

1. Tonic horizontal deviation ± jerking of eyes
2. Repetitive blinking or fluttering of eyelids
3. Orobuccal movements — drooling, sucking, and the like
4. Tonic posturing of a limb
5. Apnea

Reference: Volpe, J.J.: Mead Johnson Symposium on Perinatal and Developmental Medicine, No. 6, 1974, p. 60.

# PROGNOSIS IN NEONATAL CONVULSIONS

Convulsions occur with relative frequency in the neonatal period, and the physician may be called upon to offer some indication to the parents of the prognosis of the child who seizes. Neonatal convulsions may be divided into two groups: (1) those due to hypocalcemia and occurring after 72 hours of age, and (2) those due to other causes and usually occurring in the first 72 hours of life.

Seizures in the first 72 hours of life are infrequently attributable to hypocalcemia alone. The etiologic factor remains undetermined in many cases, but identifiable causes include cerebral hemorrhage, birth anoxia, congenital cerebral anomaly, hypoglycemia, and meningitis. Mortality and permanent sequelae in this group are high. Approximately 40 per cent of those infants whose seizures are attributed to birth injury or anoxia will die, while 25 per cent will suffer severe mental or developmental handicap. Significant numbers of the infants whose seizures are associated with hypoglycemia (less than 20 mg/100 ml) will demonstrate delayed development, subsequent motor handicap, and seizure activity later in life. Among the group of infants in whom no cause is found for convulsions, approximately 20 per cent will have sequelae in the form of motor or developmental handicap or seizures later in life.

Infants whose seizures are due to hypocalcemia alone are not likely to experience sequelae.

Reference: Keen, J.H., and Lee, D.: Arch. Dis. Child., *48*:542, 1973.

# NEONATAL PHRENIC NERVE PALSY—THE "BELLY DANCER'S SIGN"

Unilateral diaphragmatic paralysis with or without brachial plexus injury may present in neonates as "respiratory distress." The chest roentgenogram may be misleading unless obtained in deep inspiration. Fluoroscopy is required to demonstrate paradoxical motion of the diaphragm on the involved side.

It should be remembered that the existence of diaphragmatic paralysis can be recognized by merely observing the movement of the umbilicus during the respiratory cycle. To perform this maneuver, note the position of the umbilicus at full expiration. Mark this position by placing your pen at the spot. During inspiration, the umbilicus can be seen to shift upward and toward the side of the paralyzed diaphragm. Other suggestive physical findings include unexplained tachypnea without dyspnea, slightly decreased breath sounds on the paralyzed side, fine inspiratory rales on the paralyzed side if atelectasis is present, widening of the subcostal angle on the affected side during inspiration, and flattening of the epigastrium on the side of the paralyzed diaphragm during inspiration. The movement of the umbilicus is the sign most easily identified.

References: Nichols, M.M.: Clin. Pediatr., *15*:342, 1976. Light, J.S.: J. Pediatr., *24*:627, 1944.

5

# A DIAGNOSTIC APPROACH TO NEONATAL JAUNDICE

Determining the cause of jaundice in newborns is a recurrent diagnostic problem. In view of the fact that a variety of disorders may produce elevated bilirubin concentrations, an orderly and systematic evaluation is required in order to minimize unnecessary laboratory studies and most rapidly reach a correct diagnosis. The following guidelines may be employed.

*Which Infants Require Diagnostic Evaluation*

    1. All patients with clinical evidence of jaundice during the first 24 hours of life.

    2. All infants in whom the total serum bilirubin increases by more than 5 mg/dl per day.

    3. All term infants in whom the serum bilirubin exceeds 12 mg/dl.

    4. All premature infants in whom the serum bilirubin exceeds 15 mg/dl.

    5. All infants in whom phototherapy is employed.

    6. All infants in whom the conjugated bilirubin fraction exceeds 2 mg/dl.

    7. All term infants in whom clinical jaundice persists beyond the first week of life, and all premature infants in whom clinical jaundice persists beyond the second week of life.

# DATA COLLECTION SHEET FOR THE EVALUATION OF THE JAUNDICED INFANT

It is easy to forget an important item in the history, physical examination, and laboratory studies of the jaundiced infant. This checklist can help you from "leaving undone those things that ought to have been done."

*Data Collection Sheet for the Jaundiced Infant*

DATA

    *Mother*
      Blood group and blood type
      Maternal serology
      History of previous pregnancies with respect to neonatal jaundice
      Race and/or ethnic origin
      Illness in pregnancy
      Drugs in pregnancy
      History of anemia or jaundice in family

    *Delivery*
      Premature rupture of membranes
      Vacuum extraction
      Oxytocins

Other drugs and anesthetics
Apgar score

*Infant Physical Examination*
General appearance (activity, cry, suck, hydration, plethora, pallor)
Enclosed hemorrhage — cephalhematoma, ecchymoses
Head size, length, weight
Estimate of gestational age
Fundi—chorioretinitis
Liver and spleen size
Umbilical stump
Congenital anomalies

*Infant History*
Age when jaundice first noted
Vomiting
Frequency, volume, and type of feeding
Number of stools noted
Drugs given to infant
Was phototherapy employed prior to diagnostic procedures?
Was hemoglobin followed sequentially?
Was hemoglobin obtained at discharge?

*Laboratory Studies*
Blood type of infant, direct and indirect Coombs' test
Serology of cord blood
Bilirubin — Was conjugated fraction ever determined?
Hemoglobin
Reticulocyte count
Smear morphology
White cell count and differential
Comment regarding platelets
Urine-reducing substance
Any evaluation of sepsis (LP, cultures, IgM, serology)
G-6-PD screen
Hemoglobin electrophoresis
Consultations

## A Schematic Approach to the Diagnosis of Neonatal Jaundice

*Review* maternal history, family history, facts of labor and delivery, infant's caloric intake, and stool history, and perform physical examination.

Initial laboratory studies: Hemoglobin, hematocrit, reticulocyte count, peripheral blood smear, white cell count and differential, urine for reducing substance, direct and indirect Coombs' test, maternal and infant blood groups.

Prolonged Jaundice

Consider: Hepatitis, biliary atresia, Down's syndrome, hypothyroidism, breast milk inhibitors, Crigler-Najjar syndrome, cyanotic heart disease, cystic fibrosis, $alpha_1$-antitrypsin deficiency.

5

*Schematic Approach to the Diagnosis of Neonatal Jaundice*

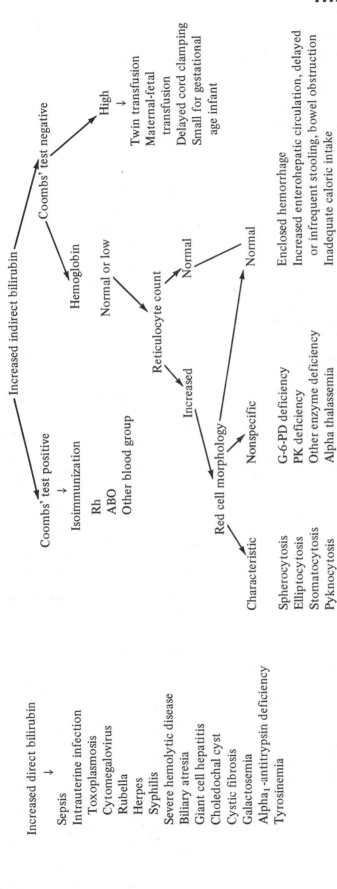

Increased direct bilirubin
→
Sepsis
Intrauterine infection
  Toxoplasmosis
  Cytomegalovirus
  Rubella
  Herpes
  Syphilis
Severe hemolytic disease
Biliary atresia
Giant cell hepatitis
Choledochal cyst
Cystic fibrosis
Galactosemia
Alpha₁-antitrypsin deficiency
Tyrosinemia

Increased indirect bilirubin

Coombs' test positive
→
Isoimmunization
→
Rh
ABO
Other blood group

Coombs' test negative

Hemoglobin

High
→
Twin transfusion
Maternal-fetal
  transfusion
Delayed cord clamping
Small for gestational
  age infant

Normal or low

Reticulocyte count

Normal

Enclosed hemorrhage
Increased enterohepatic circulation, delayed
  or infrequent stooling, bowel obstruction
Inadequate caloric intake
Neonatal asphyxia

Increased

Red cell morphology

Normal

Nonspecific

G-6-PD deficiency
PK deficiency
Other enzyme deficiency
Alpha thalassemia
Disseminated intravascular
  coagulation

Characteristic

Spherocytosis
Elliptocytosis
Stomatocytosis
Pyknocytosis
Frage

# THE USE OF CLINICAL DATA IN DIAGNOSIS OF NEONATAL JAUNDICE

Once a methodical collection of data has taken place, the significance of the information must be appreciated. The tables below indicate what your findings should suggest.

*Clinical Data*

| INFORMATION | SIGNIFICANCE |
|---|---|
| **Family History** | |
| Parent or sibling with history of jaundice or anemia | Suggests hereditary hemolytic anemia, such as hereditary spherocytosis |
| Previous sibling with neonatal jaundice | Suggests hemolytic disease due to ABO or Rh isoimmunization |
| History of liver disease in siblings or disorders such as cystic fibrosis, galactosemia, tyrosinemia, hyper-methioninemia, Crigler-Najjar syndrome, or alpha$_1$-antitrypsin deficiency | All associated with neonatal hyperbilirubinemia |
| **Maternal History** | |
| Unexplained illness during pregnancy | Consider congenital infections such as rubella, cytomegalovirus, toxoplasmosis, herpes, syphilis, or hepatitis |
| Diabetes mellitus | Increased incidence of jaundice among infants of diabetic mothers |
| Drug ingestion during pregnancy | Ingestion of sulfonamides, nitrofurantoins, or antimalarials may initiate hemolysis in G-6-PD deficient infant |
| **History of Labor and Delivery** | |
| Vacuum extraction | Increased incidence of cephalhematoma and jaundice |
| Oxytocin-induced labor | Increased incidence of hyperbilirubinemia |
| Delayed cord clamping | Increased incidence of hyperbilirubinemia among polycythemic infants |
| Apgar score | Increased incidence of jaundice in asphyxiated infants |
| **Infant's History** | |
| Delayed passage of meconium or infrequent stools | Increased enterohepatic circulation of bilirubin. Consider intestinal atresia, annular pancreas, Hirschsprung's disease, meconium plug, drug-induced ileus (hexamethonium) |
| Caloric intake | Inadequate caloric intake results in delay in bilirubin conjugation |
| Vomiting | Suspect sepsis, galactosemia, or pyloric stenosis; all associated with hyperbilirubinemia |
| **Infant's Physical Examination** | |
| Small for gestational age | Infants frequently polycythemic and jaundiced |
| Head size | Microcephaly seen with intrauterine infections associated with jaundice |
| Cephalhematoma | Entrapped hemorrhage associated with hyper-bilirubinemia |
| Pallor | Suspect hemolytic anemia |

| | |
|---|---|
| Petechiae | Suspect congenital infection, overwhelming sepsis, or severe hemolytic disease as cause of jaundice |
| Appearance of umbilical stump | Omphalitis and sepsis may produce jaundice |
| Hepatosplenomegaly | Suspect hemolytic anemia or congenital infection |
| Optic fundi | Chorioretinitis suggests congenital infection as cause of jaundice |
| Umbilical hernia | Consider hypothyroidism |
| Congenital anomalies | Jaundice occurs with increased frequency among infants with trisomic conditions |

## Laboratory Data

| INFORMATION | SIGNIFICANCE |
|---|---|
| *Maternal* | |
| Blood group and indirect Coombs' test | Necessary for evaluation of possible ABO or Rh incompatibility |
| Serology | Rule out congenital syphilis |
| *Infant* | |
| Hemoglobin | Anemia suggests hemolytic disease or large entrapped hemorrhage. Hemoglobin above 22 gm/100 ml associated with increased incidence of jaundice |
| Reticulocyte count | Elevation suggests hemolytic disease |
| Red cell morphology | Spherocytes suggest ABO incompatibility or hereditary spherocytosis. Red cell fragmentation seen in disseminated intravascular coagulation |
| Platelet count | Thrombocytopenia suggests infection |
| White cell count | Total white cell count less than 5000/mm$^3$ or increase in band forms to greater than 2000/mm$^3$ suggests infection |
| Sedimentation rate | Values in excess of 5 during the first 48 hours indicate infection or ABO incompatibility |
| Direct bilirubin | Elevation suggests infection or severe Rh incompatibility |
| Immunoglobulin M | Elevation indicates infection |
| Blood group and direct and indirect Coombs' test | Required to rule out hemolytic disease as a result of isoimmunization |
| Carboxyhemoglobin | Elevated in infants with hemolytic disease or entrapped hemorrhage |
| Urinalysis | Presence of reducing substance suggests diagnosis of galactosemia |

# PROGRESSION OF DERMAL ICTERUS IN THE NEWBORN

The rate of rise of serum bilirubin in the newborn infant who is jaundiced should always be monitored by laboratory determinations. The pediatrician, however, through simple examination of the infant, may make some estimation as to the rate of rise of serum bilirubin.

Dermal icterus has been shown to progress in a cephalopedal fashion; that is, as the infant's bilirubin rises, more of the skin becomes icteric. The icterus begins at the head and neck and progresses caudally to the palms and soles. The following table correlates the level of indirect bilirubin with the area of skin that is icteric in full-term infants whose jaundice is not due to Rh incompatibility.

| AREA OF THE BODY | RANGE OF INDIRECT BILIRUBIN (mg/100 ml) |
|---|:---:|
| Head and neck | 4–8 |
| Upper trunk | 5–12 |
| Lower trunk and thighs | 8–16 |
| Arms and lower legs | 11–18 |
| Palms and soles | >15 |

As icterus progresses, the area that had been jaundiced remains jaundiced, so that the entire body is icteric when the bilirubin rises above 15 mg/100 ml. The fading of the icterus as the bilirubin level falls affects all body areas at the same time, so that the intensity rather than the extent of the staining fades. The staining may progress more rapidly in the low birth weight infant, while the infant with Rh disease may demonstrate a relative lag in dermal staining.

Correct estimation of the extent of icterus involves the examination of the completely undressed infant under blue-white fluorescent light. Icterus may be detected by blanching the skin with pressure of the thumb and noting the color of the underlying skin. This is a more difficult determination to make in deeply pigmented black infants, but the palms and soles, at least, may be easily examined even in these patients.

Reference: Kramer, L.I.: Am. J. Dis. Child., *18*:454, 1969.

## BILIRUBIN LEVELS IN THE TERM INFANT

How frequently will the bilirubin level exceed 12 mg/100 ml in term infants? The figures below demonstrate that this is an unusual event in black and white infants alike. These figures were gathered from the National Collaborative Study. No attempt was made to exclude infants with disease, so it represents realistic expectations in terms of all infants with birth weights in excess of 2500 grams who might be admitted to your nursery.

| BILIRUBIN | PERCENTAGE OF INFANTS | |
|---|---|---|
| (mg/100 ml) | *White* (17,292 infants) | *Black* (18,015 infants) |
| 0 –  7.9 | 73.73 | 74.48 |
| 8 – 12.9 | 20.08 | 21.00 |
| 13 – 15.9 | 3.29 | 2.62 |
| 16 – 19.9 | 1.95 | 1.28 |
| > 20 | 0.95 | 0.62 |

Only 6 out of every 100 term infants will have bilirubin values that exceed 12 mg/100 ml. Never simply ascribe this to a "physiologic" process; do not merely employ phototherapy without trying to determine its cause.

## THE USE OF THE SERUM BILIRUBIN AS THE SOLE CRITERION FOR EXCHANGE TRANSFUSION

In infants with Rh isoimmunization, criteria established many years ago still prove useful in anticipating which infants will require exchange transfusion. Figure 5–2 (for term infants) and Figure 5–3 (for preterm infants) illustrate how the rate of rise in the level of unconjugated bilirubin coupled with the age of the infant can be used as a basis of management.

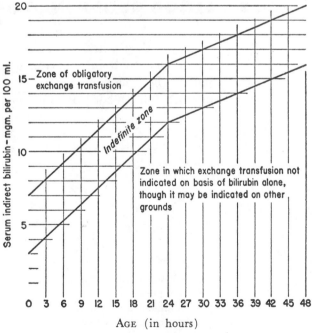

*FIG. 5–2*

Tentative guide to the use of serum indirect bilirubin as the sole criterion for exchange transfusions in term infants.

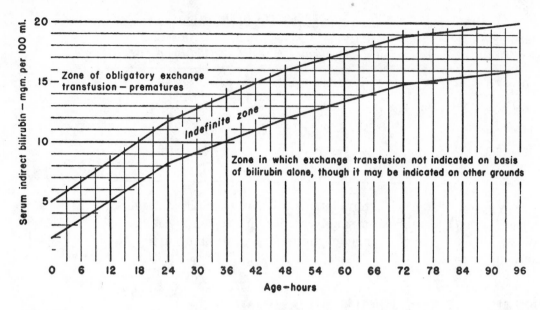

FIG. 5-3

Tentative guide to the use of serum indirect bilirubin as the sole criterion for exchange transfusions in premature infants.

Reference: Allen, F.H., Jr., and Diamond, L.K.: Erythroblastosis Fetalis. Boston, Little, Brown & Company, 1958.

## COMPARISON OF Rh AND ABO BLOOD GROUP INCOMPATIBILITY

If jaundice is noted in an infant at birth or shortly thereafter, blood group incompatibility between mother and infant may well be the cause. The following table compares the findings and recommended treatment in Rh and ABO incompatibility.

|  | Rh | ABO |
|---|---|---|
| *Blood Group Setup* |  |  |
| Mother | Negative | O |
| Infant | Positive | A or B |
| *Type of Antibody* | Incomplete (7S) | Immune (7S) |
| *Clinical Aspects* |  |  |
| Occurrence in first-born | 5% | 40–50% |
| Predictable severity in subsequent pregnancies | Usually | No |
| Stillbirth and/or hydrops | Frequent | Rare |
| Severe anemia | Frequent | Rare |
| Degree of jaundice | +++ | + |
| Hepatosplenomegaly | +++ | + |

*Laboratory Findings*

| | | |
|---|---|---|
| Direct Coombs' test (infant) | + | (+) or 0 |
| Maternal antibodies | Always present | Not clear-cut |
| Spherocytes | 0 | + |

*Treatment*

| | | |
|---|---|---|
| Need for antenatal measures | Yes | No |
| Exchange transfusion | | |
| Frequency | Approx. 2/3 | Approx. 1/10 |
| Donor blood type | Rh-negative | Rh — same as infant |
| | Group specific, when possible | Group O only |
| Incidence of late anemia | Common | Rare |

# THE MULTIPLE CAUSES OF HYDROPS FETALIS

As Rh isoimmunization becomes less common, the other causes of hydrops fetalis take on added diagnostic significance. The following are other recognized causes at birth of a grossly edematous newborn infant.

## Severe Chronic Anemia In Utero

Isoimmunization due to ABO incompatibility or other blood groups
Homozygous alpha thalassemia
Fetal to maternal hemorrhage
G-6-PD deficiency with maternal drug ingestion

## Cardiac Failure

Severe congenital heart disease
Premature closure of foramen ovale
Large arteriovenous malformation
Prolonged supraventricular tachycardia

## Hypoproteinemia

Renal disease (congenital nephrosis, renal vein thrombosis)
Congenital hepatitis

## Intrauterine Infections

Syphilis
Toxoplasmosis
Cytomegalovirus

*Other*

Maternal diabetes mellitus
Umbilical or chorionic vein thrombosis
Fetal neuroblastomatosis
Chagas' disease
Achondroplasia
Cystic adenomatoid malformation of the lung
Pulmonary lymphangiectasia
Choriocarcinoma in situ
Congenital Gaucher's disease
Urethral atresia
Placental chorioangioma

## DETECTION OF ALPHA THALASSEMIA TRAIT IN THE NEWBORN

Heterozygotes for alpha thalassemia compose 2 to 7 per cent of the black population in America. Although this abnormality causes only minor hematologic changes, it may produce a mild microcytic anemia unresponsive to iron therapy.

Alpha thalassemia trait may be detected in the newborn by the identification of greater than 2 per cent hemoglobin Barts (tetramers of gamma chains) on hemoglobin electrophoresis. After the newborn period, the diagnosis is possible only on evaluation of globin chain synthesis.

Evaluation of red cell indices constitutes an efficient screening test for alpha thalassemia. *If the mean corpuscular volume of a black newborn is less than 94 $\mu^3$, a hemoglobin electrophoresis should be performed.* Approximately 67 per cent of these infants will be heterozygotes for alpha thalassemia.

---

Reference: Schmaier, A.H., Maurer, H.M., Johnston, C.L., et al.: J. Pediatr., *83*:794, 1973.

## NORMAL HEMOGLOBIN VALUES IN THE PREMATURE INFANT

How low does the hemoglobin level go in a healthy premature infant during the first 6 to 10 weeks of life? The experience at the Upstate Medical Center is depicted in Figure 5–4. All 50 infants studied had birth weights of less than 1500 grams. None had evidence of isoimmunization. All had hemoglobin values greater than 13.0 gm/dl on the eighth day of life. None were vitamin E deficient or had other nutritional causes for anemia. The solid line represents the mean value, while the shaded area represents all values recorded. It should be noted that the lowest mean hemoglobin value is reached at approximately 6 weeks of age. No infant had a hemoglobin value of less than 8.6 gm/dl at any time. The mean hemoglobin remained above 10.0 gm/dl. When hemoglobin values fall below 8.5 gm/dl during this period of life, something is wrong — a systematic search for an explanation will often be rewarded.

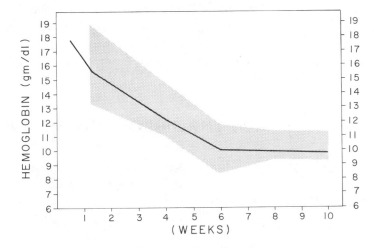

*FIG. 5–4*

# THE NORMAL LEUKOCYTE COUNT IN THE NEWBORN

It is gradually being appreciated that the white blood cell count provides diagnostic information during the first week of life. Variations from normal, either increases or decreases in the total number of polymorphonuclear leukocytes or elevations in the band count, are usually a sign of infection. The following values can be used as a guide to normal values.

| WEIGHT | AGE | ABSOLUTE NEUTROPHIL COUNT (mm³) | ABSOLUTE BAND COUNT (mm³) | B/N RATIO |
|---|---|---|---|---|
| Less than 2500 gm | 0–96 hours | Up to 12,000 | Up to 1,400 | Up to 0.17 |
| | >96 hours | 2,000 – 4.700 | <500 | Up to 0.14 |
| More than 2500 gm | 0–96 hours | Up to 14,000 | Up to 1,400 | Up to 0.17 |
| | >96 hours | 2,400 – 4,500 | <500 | Up to 0.14 |

Elevations in counts were seen in noninfectious disorders, such as infants of diabetic mothers, meconium aspirations, hyaline membrane disease, hypoglycemia, neonatal seizures, and infants with 5-minute Apgar scores of 6 or less. In the absence of these complications, the presence of increased B/N ratios or increases or decreases in the absolute neutrophil count or increases in the absolute band count should be an indication for culturing of the infant and the initiation of antibiotic therapy. Low absolute neutrophil counts are currently most commonly associated with group B streptococcal sepsis.

Reference: Manroe, B., Browne, R., Weinberg, A.G., et al.: Pediatr. Res., *10*:428, 1976.

## THE THROMBOCYTOPENIC NEWBORN

The hallway from the nursery to the obstetric ward is a path too rarely taken by the pediatrician when seeking a diagnosis in a newborn. If an infant's platelet count reveals thrombocytopenia, the mother may well be the source of important information. If her platelet count is normal, the infant's physical examination may provide the answer. (See algorithm on the following page.)

Reference: Oski, F.O., and Naiman, J.L.: Hematologic Problems in the Newborn. Philadelphia, W.B. Saunders Company, 1972, p. 310.

## THE ERYTHROCYTE SEDIMENTATION RATE IN THE NEWBORN

The diagnosis of sepsis in the newborn infant remains a challenging problem. The total neutrophil count and band count (see page 133), buffy coat smears for bacteria, platelet count, alterations in leukocyte morphology (toxic granulations, vacuoles, and Döhle bodies), and the determination of IgM and haptoglobin levels may all be used to facilitate the diagnosis. Another simple test, the "mini-ESR," should also be included in the laboratory investigation.

The test is performed in the following manner.

Fill a standard 75 mm heparinized microhematocrit tube (Fisher Scientific Company, Pittsburgh, Pa., No. 2–668–66) with blood obtained from a heel puncture. Remove all alcohol from the heel before obtaining the blood. Do not allow air bubbles to interrupt the column of blood. Seal one end of the tube with 2 to 3 mm of clay. Collect a similar tube of blood for a microhematocrit determination. Place the microhematocrit tube in an upright, vertical position. The tube may be taped to the isolette or placed in a suitable stand for this purpose. After one hour, measure the distance from the top of the column of blood to the meniscus of the packed red cell column. Express values as mm/one hour. Correct all values to a hematocrit of 40 per cent by reference to Wintrobe correction chart. (See chart on page 136.)

*Diagnostic Approach to the Thrombocytopenic Newborn*

**MOTHER**

1. History
   Previous bleeding (ITP?), drugs, illness, infants with purpura, rubella in pregnancy
2. Placenta – chorioangioma (?)
3. Test for syphilis
4. Platelet count

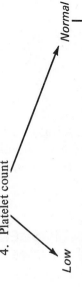

*Low*

1. Maternal ITP, SLE
2. Drug purpura
3. Inherited thrombocytopenia

*Normal*

→ *Examine Infant*

*Congenital Anomalies*

1. Giant hemangioma
2. Rubella syndrome
3. Absent radii
4. Trisomy syndromes

*Hepatosplenomegaly*

1. Infections
   Bacterial sepsis
   Congenital syphilis
   Disseminated herpes
   Cytomegalic inclusion disease
   Rubella syndrome
   Congenital toxoplasmosis
2. Congenital leukemia

*Normal*

1. Isoimmune purpura
2. Thiazides
3. Inherited thrombocytopenia
4. Early congenital aplastic anemia
5. Aminoacidurias

Figure 5–5 depicts the mean value and the 95 per cent confidence limits in normal newborn infants.

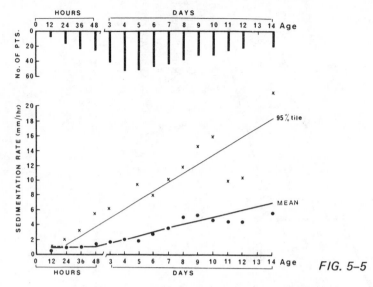

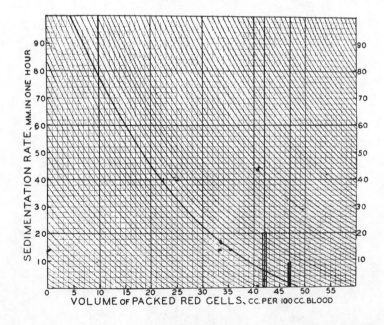

*FIG. 5–5*

Abnormal values may be anticipated in infected infants and in newborns with Coombs'-positive ABO isoimmunization. The ESR is generally elevated within one to two days after the onset of infection. The finding of an elevated "mini-ESR" should be used as presumptive evidence of infection until proved otherwise.

Reference: Adler, S.M., and Denton, R.L.: J. Pediatr., *86*:942, 1975.

## THE WINTROBE AND LANDSBERG CHART FOR CORRECTION OF THE OBSERVED SEDIMENTATION RATE ACCORDING TO THE HEMATOCRIT

*FIG. 5–6*

To use this chart for correction of sedimentation rate for the observed hematocrit, perform the following steps.

1. Find the point on the horizontal axis that corresponds to the patient's hematocrit.
2. Enter the graph, proceeding vertically, until you intercept the line that represents the patient's observed sedimentation rate.
3. Follow the curve that is closest to this point of intercept to the vertical line denoting a hematocrit of 40 per cent. This point of crossing is the patient's corrected sedimentation rate.

### Example

An infant with a hematocrit of 25 per cent is found to have a "mini-ESR" of 28 mm/hr. In this instance, the corrected sedimentation rate would be 4 mm/hr.

---

Wintrobe, M.M., and Landsberg, J.W.: Am. J. Med. Sci., *189*:102, 1935.

# DIFFERENTIAL FEATURES OF HEMORRHAGIC DISEASE OF THE NEWBORN AND DISSEMINATED INTRAVASCULAR COAGULATION

The newborn who is hemorrhaging uncontrollably may have hemorrhagic disease of the newborn due to vitamin K deficiency or disseminated intravascular coagulation. Differential aspects of these two conditions are listed below.

| FEATURES | VITAMIN K DEFICIENCY | DISSEMINATED INTRAVASCULAR COAGULATION |
|---|---|---|
| Uniformity of clotting defect | Constant | Variable |
| Capillary fragility | Normal | Usually abnormal |
| Bleeding time | Normal | Often prolonged |
| Clotting time | Prolonged | Variable |
| One-state prothrombin | Very prolonged (5% or less) | Moderately prolonged |
| Partial thromboplastin time | Prolonged | Prolonged |
| Thrombin time | Normal for age | Usually prolonged |
| Fibrin degradation products | Not present | Present |
| Factor V | Normal | Decreased |

| | | |
|---|---|---|
| Fibrinogen | Normal | Often decreased |
| Platelets | Normal | Often decreased |
| Red cell fragmentation | Not present | Usually present |
| Response to vitamin K | Rapid | Diminished or absent |
| Associated disease | Usually trivial (trauma may be precipitating factor) | Severe. May include sepsis, hypoxia, acidosis, or obstetric accident |
| Previous history | No vitamin K given or mother receiving barbiturates or anticonvulsants | Above illnesses. Vitamin K given |

# MATERNAL ANTICONVULSANTS AND HEMORRHAGE IN THE NEWBORN

The ingestion of anticonvulsants by the pregnant woman increases the risk of serious hemorrhage in the newborn infant. The use of the hydantoins, barbiturates, or primidone, either alone or in combination, produces an exaggerated form of vitamin K deficiency in the newborn infant. The prolonged use of such anticonvulsants during pregnancy is associated with the following:

1. Normal coagulation studies in the mother.
2. Prolongation of the prothrombin time and partial thromboplastin time in the infant with marked depression of the vitamin K dependent factors (II, VII, IX, and X).
3. Neonatal bleeding usually within the first 24 hours of life. Bleeding is frequently intracranial, intrathoracic, or intra-abdominal.

The following precautions should be taken:

1. Discourage the use of metharbital during pregnancy. This barbiturate appears to have the greatest vitamin K antagonism.
2. Avoid all drugs that impair platelet function during the third trimester. Among these are aspirin, thiazides, and indomethacin.
3. If a difficult or traumatic delivery is anticipated, delivery should be by cesarean section.
4. Vitamin K should be given to the mother at least 6 hours prior to delivery, and to the infant immediately at birth. The drug should be administered intravenously to the infant after collection of appropriate cord samples for coagulation studies.
5. Observe the infant carefully for signs of bleeding. Use fresh frozen plasma if the vitamin K has not produced a satisfactory correction of the prothrombin and partial thromboplastin times.

Reference: Bleyer, W.A., and Skinner, A.L.: J.A.M.A., *235*:626, 1976.

# THE CLINICAL DIAGNOSIS OF CONGENITAL HYPOTHYROIDISM

Until routine screening of cord blood specimens for thyroxine ($T_4$) or thyroid-stimulating hormone (TSH) becomes widely available, the diagnosis of congenital hypothyroidism in the nursery will require an alert physician with a high degree of suspicion. The ten warning signs are:

1. Gestation over 42 weeks and/or birth weight greater than 4.0 kg.
2. Large posterior fontanel
3. Respiratory distress
4. Hypothermia, 95° F or less
5. Peripheral cyanosis
6. Hypoactivity, lethargy, poor feeding
7. Lag in stooling beyond 20 hours of age
8. Abdominal distention and/or vomiting
9. Jaundice beyond 3 days of age
10. Edema

The presence of three or more of these signs should make you suspect that the infant may have congenital hypothyroidism ("three or more = $T_4$"). If you miss the diagnosis in the nursery, other clues may manifest themselves within the first 3 months of life. These clues include:

A feeling of coldness to the touch
Mottling of the skin*
Decreased activity
Feeding problems
Enlarged tongue
Hoarse cry
Constipation*
Dry skin
Umbilical hernia*
Unusually large anterior fontanel for age*
Poor growth

*Present in at least 50 per cent of patients.

Reference: Smith, D.W., Klein, A.M., Henderson, J.R., et al.: J. Pediatr., *87*:958, 1975.

# DELAYED URINATION IN THE NEWBORN

One of the kindest acts a neonate can perform for his pediatrician is to urinate early in life. Ninty-nine to 100 per cent of all normal infants urinate at least once by 48 hours of age. Approximately 23 per cent will void first in the delivery room, and the act may not be reported to the nursery.

Failure to urinate by the first 1 to 2 days of life may be due to obstruction of urine flow or to inability to form urine. Causes of obstruction include

> Imperforate prepuce
> Urethral strictures
> Urethral diverticulum
> Hypertrophy of the verumontanum
> Neurogenic bladder
> "Megacystic syndrome"
> Ureterocele
> Renal tumors
> Cystic kidneys

Inability to form urine may result from

> Postnatal intravascular hypovolemia
> Restriction of oral fluids
> Bilateral renal agenesis
> Cortical necrosis
> Tubular necrosis
> Bilateral renal vein thrombosis
> Congenital nephrotic syndrome
> Congenital pyelonephritis
> Congenital nephritis

Nonspecific symptoms or signs such as excessive crying, irritability, poor feeding, pallor, emesis, mottled skin, or weak pulse may suggest the development of uremia.

The physical examination may be more useful in establishing a specific diagnosis.

## Physical Examination

| PALPATION OR PERCUSSION OF DISTENDED BLADDER | NO KIDNEYS PALPABLE | PALPABLE RENAL MASS |
|---|---|---|
| ↓ | ↓ | ↓ |
| Obstruction of urine flow | Bilateral renal agenesis | Renal vein thrombosis |
| ↓ | These infants are usually males and tend to have lowset ears, epicanthal folds, and a flattened nose | Infantile polycystic kidneys |
| Examine meatus for patency and look for epispadias or hypospadias | | |
| | | Hydronephoris |
| | | Cystic dysplasia |
| A urethral diverticulum may give rise to a bulge along the dorsum of the penis | | Neoplasm |

Reference: Moore, E.S., and Galvez, M.D.: J. Pediatr., *80*:867, 1972.

# A TECHNIQUE FOR THE PALPATION OF THE KIDNEYS OF NEONATES

Congenital malformations of the urogenital tract occur in approximately 12 per cent of all newborns. In 0.5 per cent of all newborns, significant renal anomalies are present. These should be detected early in life in order to avoid subsequent complications. Almost all significant anomalies can be detected by careful abdominal palpation. A simple technique that will enable you to palpate the kidneys of 95 per cent of all neonates is as follows:

1. Support the infant in a semireclining position facing you by placing your left hand behind the infant's shoulders, neck, and occiput.
2. Place the fingers of your right hand in the infant's left costovertebral angle posteriorly.
3. Use the thumb of your right hand to search the infant's abdomen systematically, at first superficially and then deeply.
4. Deep palpation is performed by applying gentle, steadily increasing pressure subcostally in a posterior and cephalad direction. The thumb can then be slipped downward without reducing the posteriorly directed pressure. Usually, the upper pole of the kidney can be felt trapped between the descending thumb and the posteriorly placed fingers.
5. Next, change hands and examine the opposite side of the abdomen.

After practice on some two dozen infants, this technique can be mastered and subsequently performed in 30 seconds. Because of its high yield, it deserves your high skill and attention.

Reference: Perlman, M., and Williams, J.: Br. Med. J., 2:347, 1976.

# FIRST STOOL PASSAGE IN THE PREMATURE

When that 1800 gram premie is 18 hours old and has yet to pass the first meconium stool, it might be helpful to have an indication of when to begin thinking of radiologic studies. In the following table, 180 infants of less than 2500 grams at birth were fed at 4 to 6 hours of age or as soon after that as their condition permitted (mean time of first feeding was 18 hours).

Meconium—From the Greek word *mekonion*, which means poppy juice. This juice is thick and greenish and resembles the first stools of the newborn infant.

| AGE (HR) | PRETERM, LOW BIRTH WEIGHT INFANTS | |
|---|---|---|
| | *Number* | *Cumulative Percentage* |
| Delivery room | 11 | 6.1 |
| 0–12 | 92 | 57.2 |
| 12–24 | 40 | 79.4 |
| 24–48 | 36 | 99.4 |
| >48 | 1 | 100.0 |
| Total number of infants | 180 | |

Time of stool passage was not significantly related to weight, gestational age, or time of first feeding. It seems reasonable, then, to expect the first stool in a premature infant in the first 24 hours of life. If the clinical situation is otherwise stable, careful observation and feeding may be appropriate management until a total of 48 hours have passed.

Reference: Mangurten, H.H., and Slade, C.I.: J. Pediatr., *82*:1033, 1973.

## REDUCING SUBSTANCE IN THE STOOL— NECROTIZING ENTEROCOLITIS

The detection of a reducing substance in the stool can provide an early clue to the presence of a gastrointestinal disorder. This is particularly valuable in the newborn infant.

*Procedure:* Mix two parts water with one part stool, mix well, and centrifuge. Place 15 drops of the supernatant in a clean test tube and add a Clinitest tablet. Read the color 15 seconds after the reaction has subsided and compare with a standard urine color chart.

About 5 to 10 per cent of normal term or preterm infants who have begun feedings will demonstrate a 3+ or 4+ reaction. In contrast, 70 per cent of infants with necrotizing enterocolitis will display a 3+ or 4+ reaction from one to four days prior to the onset of abdominal distention, gastrointestinal bleeding, or ileus.

This simple test is also quite useful in older children for the detection of transient or permanent lactase deficiency. Try it — you'll like it.

References: Book, L.S., Herbst, J.J., and Jung, A.L.: Pediatrics, *57*:201, 1976. Kerry, K.R., and Anderson, C.M.: Lancet, *1*:981, 1964.

# THE FIRST STOOL AND HYPERBILIRUBINEMIA

A significant quantity of unconjugated bilirubin accumulates in the intestine of the fetus in utero. Conjugated bilirubin may also be deconjugated in the intestine by the action of the intestinal enzyme beta-glucuronidase. When gut transit time is delayed, this unconjugated bilirubin can be reabsorbed, giving rise to hyperbilirubinemia. This enterohepatic recirculation of bilirubin is often forgotten as a cause of significant jaundice in the otherwise healthy term infant. The relationship of the passage of the first stool to the eventual bilirubin level in term infants can be best appreciated by the following figures.

| TIME OF FIRST STOOL | PERCENTAGE OF INFANTS WITH BILIRUBIN LEVELS IN EXCESS OF 15 mg/100 ml |
|---|---|
| 0 – 6 hours | 1.0 |
| 6 – 9 hours | 6.0 |
| 9 – 12 hours | 7.5 |
| 12 – 15 hours | 9.0 |
| 15 – 18 hours | 10.0 |
| 18 – 21 hours | 8.5 |
| 21 – 24 hours | 12.5 |

Reference: Rosta, J., Makói, J., and Kertész, A.: Lancet, 2:1138, 1968.

# UMBILICAL CATHETER LOCALIZATION

Correct placement of umbilical catheters is often achieved only after one unsuccessful attempt and a trip to the x-ray department. Measurement of the infant from shoulder to umbilicus may allow more accurate estimation of appropriate catheter length prior to placement. Figure 5–7 demonstrates venous catheter lengths required to reach the level of the diaphragm or left atrium.

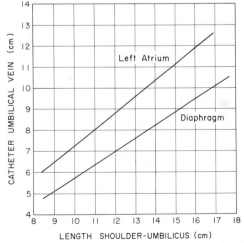

FIG. 5–7

Simply measure the distance from the infant's shoulder vertically to a point lateral to the umbilicus. Correlate this measurement with the umbilical venous catheter length given on the vertical axis of the graph, using the lines drawn.

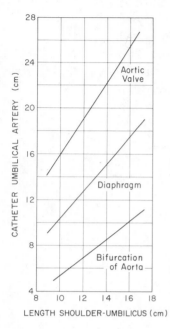

LENGTH SHOULDER-UMBILICUS (cm)    *FIG. 5–8*

The same procedure is used to determine the appropriate umbilical arterial catheter length (Fig. 5–8). In this case, lines are drawn on the graph for estimation of placement of the catheter tip at the aortic valve, the diaphragm, or the bifurcation of the aorta.

Reference: Dunn, P.M.: Arch. Dis. Child., *41*:69, 1966.

## THE STOMACH VOLUME OF THE INFANT

How big is the infant's stomach? How much can it hold? An infant's stomach is about the size of his fist. Unlike a fist, however, it has the capacity to expand. At birth, the stomach of a normal term infant has a 30 to 60 ml capacity. By the tenth day of life it will hold an amount equal to 3 per cent of the infant's weight, so that an infant

*Gavage*—From the French word *gavage*, which means forced feeding; and originally derived from *gaver*, which means to gorge.

of 3.5 kg takes with pleasure a feed of 100 ml over a period of 15 minutes.

The 3 per cent rule holds, with some normal variation, during the first 6 months of life.

Reference: MacKeith, R., and Wood, C.: *In* Infant Feeding and Feeding Difficulties, 4th Ed. London, Churchill Livingstone, 1971, p. 20.

**5**

# BODY POSITION AND GASTRIC EMPTYING IN THE NEONATE

Does the positioning of the infant after feeding influence the rate at which the stomach empties? Most evidence indicates that it does.

The stomach empties fastest when the infant is in the right lateral position. The prone position also produces rapid gastric emptying. The stomach empties much more slowly when the infant is placed supine or in the left lateral position. These latter positions should be avoided in an effort to reduce both gastric distention and regurgitation.

Reference: Yu, V.Y.H.: Arch. Dis. Child., *50*:500, 1975.

# CONGENITAL INFECTION

The signs of congenital infection are varied. Diagnosis often depends upon history and physical examination, since laboratory diagnosis is time-consuming and sometimes unreliable. Use of the following table should facilitate your clinical evaluation.

| DISEASE | TIME OF TRANSMISSION | TERATOGENIC EFFECTS | OTHER MANIFESTATIONS | LABORATORY DIAGNOSIS |
|---|---|---|---|---|
| Rubella | First trimester; early second trimester (problematical) | Cataracts, glaucoma, retinopathy, microphthalmia, microcephaly, congenital heart disease | Thrombocytopenia, hepatosplenomegaly, hepatitis, pneumonia, bone destruction, encephalitis, growth retardation | HI antibody, viral isolation from body fluids |
| Toxoplasmosis | First trimester | Microcephaly, hydrocephaly, cerebral calcifications, chorioretinitis | Encephalitis, myocarditis, hepatosplenomegaly, jaundice, diarrhea, vomiting, convulsions | CF, HI antibody, IgM-FTA specific antibody |
| Cytomegalovirus | Throughout pregnancy | Microcephaly, cerebral calcifications | Same as toxoplasmosis | Neutralizing or CF antibody, isolation of virus from urine, inclusion-bearing cells in urine |
| Herpes simplex | First trimester (transplacental); intrapartum (transplacental); ascending and direct contact | Chorioretinitis, microcephaly, microphthalmia | Cutaneous lesions (vesicles), visceral involvement (granulomas) | Neutralizing or CF antibody, isolation of virus from chorioallantoic membrane tissue culture, growth of virus on rabbit cornea |
| Varicella | First trimester and intrapartum | Chorioretinitis, microcephaly, limb deformities | Skin lesions, encephalomyocarditis, visceral involvement | Growth of virus on tissue culture, CF antibody |

5

| | | | | |
|---|---|---|---|---|
| Group B coxsackie-virus | First trimester and late in pregnancy | Provisional association: genitourinary anomalies, harelip, cleft palate, congenital heart disease, CNS anomalies, pyloric stenosis | Encephalomyocarditis, pneumonia | Neutralization and CF anti-body, growth of virus on tissue culture |
| Syphilis | Second half of pregnancy | Delayed effects on eyes, ears, teeth, joints, CNS | Osteochondritis, jaundice, hepatosplenomegaly, lymphadenopathy, rhagades, anemia | Darkfield examination for spirochetes, FTA-ABS, TPI immobilization |
| Listeria | Intrapartum | Not known | Sepsis, meningitis, hepatitis, diffuse granulomatosis | Isolation of bacteria from blood, urine, or pus. |
| Gonococcus | Last trimester and at delivery | Not known | Sepsis, conjunctivitis, panophthalmitis | Gram stain and culture (Thayer-Martin medium) |
| Tuberculosis | Rarely transplacental; usually following delivery | Not known | Fever, anemia, pulmonary and systemic dissemination | Isolation of organism from gastric washing or maternal lesions, PPD unreliable during neonatal period |

Reference: Evans, H.E., and Glass, L.: Mechanisms of infection. *In* Perinatal Medicine. New York, Harper & Row, 1976, p. 341.

## THE DIAGNOSIS OF CONGENITAL SYPHILIS

The diagnosis of congenital syphilis can be made if:

1. Darkfield examination of the suspicious lesions is positive.
2. Infant's serologic titer is higher than the maternal titer.
3. Infant's titer is sustained during the first months of life.
4. Infant has a confirmed reactive serologic test after an initial negative test.
5. Infant has a confirmed serologic test at 3 months of age.

Remember, if the reagin antibody has been passively transferred, the serologic reaction will be negative in:

90 per cent of infants at 1 month of age
98 per cent of infants at 2 months of age
99 per cent of infants at 3 months of age

If the infant is infected, the serologic reaction will be positive in:

85 per cent of infants at 1 month of age
95 per cent of infants at 2 months of age
100 per cent of infants at 3 months of age

Reference: Solomon, L.M., and Esterly, N.B.: Neonatal Dermatology. Philadelphia, W.B. Saunders Company, 1973, p. 160.

## A DIMPLE ON THE KNEE—A SIGN OF CONGENITAL RUBELLA?

A discrete, deep dimple in the skin overlying the patella is an unusual physical finding. Dimples of this type have been observed in five infants with congenital rubella. This may be a coincidence, but keep the picture on page 149 in mind (Fig. 5–9); it may lead to an unsuspected diagnosis.

*Rubella*—Latin dimunitive of *ruber*, meaning red.

5

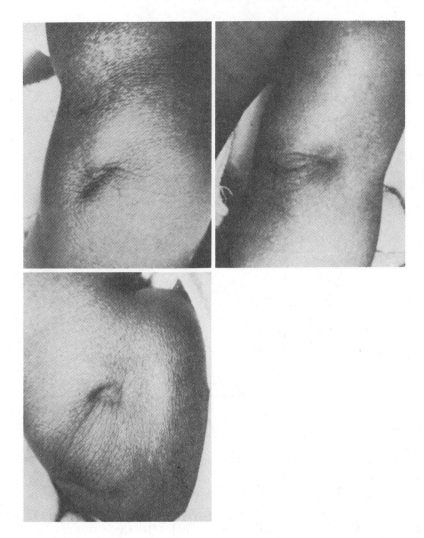

FIG. 5–9

Reference: Hammond, K.: Pediatrics, *39*:292, 1967.

## NORMAL CEREBROSPINAL FLUID VALUES
## IN THE NEONATE

The high-risk neonate who appears to be infected is likely to be subjected to a spinal tap. Frequently, the results of spinal fluid analysis provoke confusion. A CSF white cell count of 10 cells/mm$^3$, while clearly abnormal in an older child, may be within the range of normal for a newborn.

The following table gives the results of CSF analysis in 117 neonates who never developed evidence of viral or bacterial infection.

*Cerebrospinal Fluid Examination in High-Risk Neonates without Meningitis*

| | TERM | PRETERM |
|---|---|---|
| **WBC count (cells/mm³)** | | |
| No. of infants | 87.0 | 30.0 |
| Mean | 8.2 | 9.0 |
| Median | 5.0 | 6.0 |
| SD | 7.1 | 8.2 |
| Range | 0–32.0 | 0–29.0 |
| ± 2 SD | 0–22.4 | 0–25.4 |
| Percentage PMN* | 61.3% | 57.2% |
| **Protein (mg/dl)** | | |
| No. of infants | 35 | 17 |
| Mean | 90 | 115 |
| Range | 20–170 | 65–150 |
| **Glucose (mg/dl)** | | |
| No. of infants | 51 | 23 |
| Mean | 52 | 50 |
| Range | 34–119 | 24–63 |
| **CSF/blood glucose (%)** | | |
| No. of infants | 51 | 23 |
| Mean | 81 | 74 |
| Range | 44–248 | 55–105 |

*PMN = Polymorphonuclear cells.

Though an infected infant may have one or more CSF values that fall within the ranges of normal listed above, only one of 119 infants with meningitis had a totally normal CSF analysis on the first spinal tap.

Reference: Sarff, L.D., Platt, L.H., and McCracken, G.H.: J. Pediatr., *88*:473, 1976.

# CORD IgM AND PERINATAL INFECTION

If a neonate is suspected of having an intrauterine/perinatal infection, a cord serum IgM level determination is in order. Levels above 18 to 20 mg/100 ml are suggestive of such infection, although levels below that arbitrary cutoff value do not rule out infection. In one study of cord sera, the infection rate of infants whose cord IgM was >19.5 mg/100 ml was 42 times the infection rate in those with lower values. Of 192 infants with elevated cord IgM, 69 (36 per cent) had detectable infections. Cord IgM ≥20 to 25 mg/100 ml is a strong indication for further search for perinatal infection by more specific diagnostic methods.

*Infections in 69 Neonates with Elevated Cord IgM*

| AGENTS | PERCENTAGE |
|---|---|
| TORCH (toxoplasmosis, rubella, cytomegalovirus, herpes) | 38 |
| Aseptic meningitis | 17 |
| Urinary tract infections | 14 |
| Bacteremia | 7 |
| Syphilis | 6 |
| Enteropathogenic *E. coli* | 6 |
| Enteroviral | 3 |
| Miscellaneous | 9 |
| | 100% |

Normal IgM levels have been established for infants beyond the immediate newborn period. In addition, the rate of IgM rise in neonates with congenital viral infection exceeds the rate of rise seen in uninfected neonates. For these reasons, an initially normal IgM should be repeated if viral infection is strongly considered.

*Normal IgM Levels During the First Month of Life*

| AGE (DAYS) | MEAN LEVEL (mg/100 ml) | MEAN + 2 SD (mg/100 ml) |
|---|---|---|
| 6–10 | 21 | 38.8 |
| 11–15 | 24 | 44.4 |
| 16–20 | 26 | 49 |
| 21–25 | 27 | 45.8 |
| 26–30 | 24 | 41 |

References: Alford, C.A.: Pediatr. Clin. North Am., *18*:99, 1971. Blankenship, W.J., Cassady, G., Schaefer, J., et al.: J. Pediatr., *75*:1271, 1969.

## GASTRIC ACID FOAM STABILITY TEST AS AN AID IN THE DIAGNOSIS OF THE RESPIRATORY DISTRESS SYNDROME

It is now generally agreed that the respiratory distress syndrome (RDS) is primarily a result of a deficiency in the synthesis and release of surfactant by the Type II cell in the alveoli. Assessment of the lecithin-sphingomyelin ratio in amniotic fluid reflects the level of fetal lung maturity and the potential risk of RDS.

The foam stability test serves as a semiquantitative test of the amount of surface active material in the amniotic fluid. In many clinical circumstances, it may be difficult or impossible to obtain amniotic fluid for the purpose of assessing fetal lung maturity. The foam stability test performed on gastric aspirates has proved to be a useful substitute in such situations. This technique is based on the hypothesis that gastric aspirate collected within 30 minutes of birth represents amniotic fluid swallowed prior to delivery.

### Procedure

1. After appropriate resuscitative care, collect a minimum of 0.5 ml of gastric aspirate via an 8-French nasogastric catheter. Perform procedure within 30 minutes of delivery. Fluid contaminated with blood or meconium cannot be used.

2. Mix the gastric aspirate gently to obtain a uniform suspension.

3. Decreasing amounts of gastric aspirate are pipetted into a series of clean test tubes (length 7.5 cm, diameter 1 cm) and diluted with the appropriate volume of normal saline to produce a final gastric aspirate–normal saline mixture of 1 ml and a dilution of 1:1 to 1:4 as outlined in table below.

### Preparation and Dilution of Gastric Aspirate for the Foam Stability Test

| | TUBE DILUTION | | | |
|---|---|---|---|---|
| Volume (ml) | 1:1 | 1:1.3 | 1:2 | 1:4 |
| Gastric aspirate | 1.00 | 0.75 | 0.50 | 0.25 |
| Normal saline | 0 | 0.25 | 0.50 | 0.75 |
| Ethanol 95% | 1.00 | 1.00 | 1.00 | 1.00 |

One ml gastric aspirate–saline mixture + 1 ml 95 per cent ethanol = 47.5 per cent concentration.

4. One ml of 95 per cent ethanol is added to the gastric aspirate–normal saline mixture to constitute a gastric aspirate–saline-ethanol mixture of 47.5 per cent.

5. The mixture is shaken vigorously for 15 seconds, after which the test tubes are placed on a rack and the results read at the end of 15 minutes following the agitation. The test tubes should not be disturbed during the 15-minute waiting period.

6. Figure 5–10 is used for interpretation of the levels of positivity of the foam stability test. The circle represents the view of the test tube from the top, showing the amount of bubbles formed in the liquid-air interface at the end of 15 minutes. The results are recorded as either positive, intermediate, or negative, depending upon the amount of bubbles present on the liquid surface. When only a minimal amount of gastric fluid is available, the results on the 1:2 dilution (utilizing 0.5 ml gastric aspirate) are used for interpretation. The results obtained by the 1:2 dilution correlate well with those obtained when all four dilutions are performed.

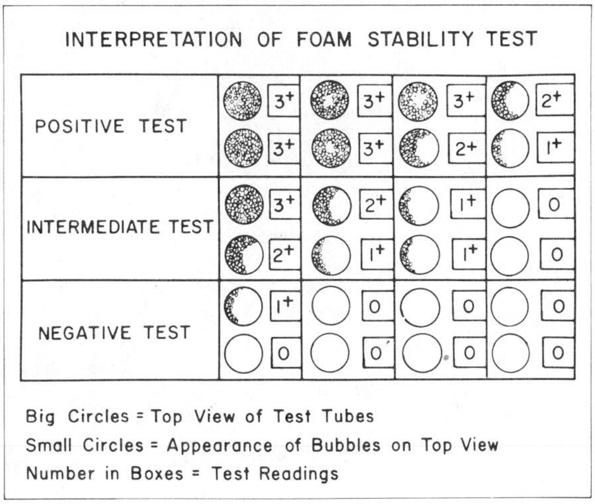

FIG. 5-10

Chart for interpretation of foam stability test; the results in the four columns represent test tubes of various dilutions.

## Interpretation

All infants with negative tests can be expected to develop RDS.

Approximately one-third of infants with intermediate tests may develop RDS.

Less than 10 per cent of infants with a positive test will develop RDS.

Reference: Corwett, R.M., Unsworth, E.J., Hakanson, D.O., et al.: N. Engl. J. Med., 293:413, 1975.

# GROUP B STREPTOCOCCAL SEPSIS OR HYALINE MEMBRANE DISEASE?

Neonatal sepsis with group B beta-hemolytic streptococcus has become a significant problem. Its early onset and associated respiratory distress may mimic classic hyaline membrane disease. The table below describes those features which may be helpful in distinguishing these clinical entities.

| | GROUP B STREPTOCOCCAL SEPSIS | HYALINE MEMBRANE DISEASE |
|---|---|---|
| Gestational age (wks) | 31–38 | 28–36 |
| Prolonged rupture of membranes | Frequent | Infrequent |
| Cocci in gastric aspirate | Frequent | Infrequent |
| Onset of respiratory distress prior to 3 hours of age | Frequent | Frequent |
| Chest roentgenogram consistent with hyaline membrane disease | Frequent | Yes |
| Onset of apnea and/or shock in first 24 hours | Frequent | Infrequent |
| Neutropenia | Frequent | Infrequent |
| Peak inspiratory pressure required on volume cycled respirator is greater than 46 cm of water | Infrequent | Frequent |
| Positive blood culture | Yes | No |

Early recognition, based on these factors, and prompt therapy with penicillin or ampicillin may reduce the reported case fatality rate of 40 to 80 per cent.

References: Ablow, R.C., Driscoll, S.G., Effman, E.L., et al.: N. Engl. J. Med., *294*:65, 1976. Manroe, B., Browne, R., and Weinberg, A.G.: Pediatr. Res., *10*:427, 1976.

*"Better to be driven out from among men than to be disliked of children."*

R. H. Dana

# CARDIAC MURMURS IN THE NEWBORN INFANT

Examination of the heart is an important part of the initial physical examination of the newborn infant. In healthy term infants, one may easily be fooled by the findings on cardiac auscultation. During the first 48 hours of life, as many as 60 per cent of all term infants may have a heart murmur. The types of murmurs and their incidence in the early newborn period are illustrated in Figure 5–11. In some infants, more than one murmur may be audible.

| TYPE | | % BABIES |
|------|------|------|
| Ejection systolic | 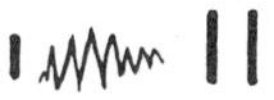 ⌇⋀⋀⋀ ‖ | 56 |
| Continuous | 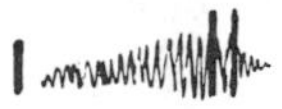 ⌇⋯⋀⋀⋀⋀⋀⋀⋀⋯ | 14 |
| Crescendo | 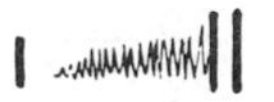 ⌇⋯⋀⋀⋀⋀‖ | 5 |
| Early systolic | 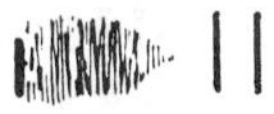 ⫼⫼⫼⋯ ‖ | 4 |
| | Incidence in whole series | 60 |

FIG. 5–11

Some features of these murmurs include the following:

### Ejection Systolic

These are similar in quality to the innocent, vibratory, ejection murmur heard in older children. They are of grade 1/6 to 2/6 in intensity, and are best heard with the bell stethoscope in the pulmonary area or in the fourth left interspace in the parasternal area. This type of murmur is usually present in all infants who also have a continuous murmur.

### Continuous

These murmurs are localized to the pulmonary area and are best heard with the bell stethoscope. They are grade 1/6 to 2/6 in intensity and are not accompanied by a thrill. They may be heard for only a few hours but may persist for several days.

### Crescendo

These are best heard with the bell stethoscope and are of equal intensity in both the pulmonic area and down the left sternal border to the fourth intercostal space. Normally grade 1/6 to 2/6 in intensity.

### Early Systolic

These murmurs can be heard equally well with either bell or diaphragm. They tend to be louder than the other murmurs, with grade 3/6 to 4/6 intensity. They are loudest at the lower left sternal border but are transmitted over the whole precordium and into the axilla. They tend to persist throughout the nursery stay.

The incidence of congenital heart disease is estimated to range from 2 to 7 cases per 1000 births; thus, most infants with murmurs during the first 48 hours of life will prove to be normal. The presence of other anomalies increases the probability that the infant's murmur may be of pathologic significance.

The diagnosis of congenital heart disease requires careful attention to the intensity of the murmur and the color of the patient, and careful monitoring of changes in heart size, heart rate, and other manifestations of cardiac failure. When a murmur is heard during the first 48 hours of life, it should be reevaluated prior to the infant's discharge.

Reference: Braudo, M., and Rowe, R.D.: Am. J. Dis. Child., *101*:575, 1961.

# NEONATAL CYANOTIC CONGENITAL HEART DISEASE

Cyanosis in the newborn may be a manifestation of a variety of disorders. Central nervous system disease, pulmonary disease, and anatomic lesions such as tracheoesophageal fistula and diaphragmatic hernia must be ruled out. If the cyanosis is considered to be of cardiac origin, the most likely anomaly may be deduced from the clinical findings, the chest roentgenogram, and the electrocardiogram.

Figure 5-12 lists the more common congenital defects to be expected with their typical physical and laboratory findings.

| Pulmonary vascular markings | Heart size | ECG | R.V. cavity Small | Systolic murmur | Aorta ant. from R.V. | Two ventricles | Asc. aorta on left | Pulses poor 4 ext. | Pulses poor legs | PA oxygen = Ao oxygen | Aorta from rt. ventricle | Diagnosis |
|---|---|---|---|---|---|---|---|---|---|---|---|---|
| Decreased | Small | LVH | | | | | | | | | | Tricuspid atresia |
| | | RVH | Yes | | | | | | | | | Pulmonary atresia, intact VS (A) |
| | | | No | Yes | Yes | | | | | | | TGA, VSD, PS |
| | | | | | No | Yes | Yes | | | | | "Corrected" TGA, VSD (single V), PS |
| | | | | | | | No | | | | | Tetralogy of Fallot |
| | | | | | | No | | | | | | Single V, PS |
| | | | | No | | | | | | | | Pulmonary atresia, VSD |
| | Large | LVH | | | | | | | | | | Ebstein's anomaly |
| | | RVH | Yes | | | | | | | | | Severe PS |
| | | | No | | | | | | | | | Pulmonic atresia, intact VS (B) |
| Increased | Small Large | LVH | | | | | | | | | | Tricuspid atresia, TGA |
| | | RVH | | Yes | | | | | | | | TGA |
| | | | | No | | | | Yes | | | | Aortic and/or mitral atresia |
| | | | | | | | | No | Yes | | | Preductal coarctation |
| | | | | | | | | | No | Yes | | Total anomalous pulmonary venous return |
| | | | | | | | | | | | Yes | Double outlet RV, subaortic VSD |
| | | BVH | | | | | Yes | | | | | Truncus arteriosus |
| | | | | | | | No | | | | | Single ventricle |

*FIG. 5-12*

Reference: Rashkind, W.J.: Cardiovasc. Clin., *4*:275, 1972.

## CONGENITAL HEART DISEASE IN THE LOW BIRTH WEIGHT INFANT

The small premature infant with a heart murmur is a common inhabitant of the intensive care nursery. Most often the murmur is that of a patent ductus arteriosus. The relative occurrence of PDA and of congenital heart disease other than PDA in one group of 198 premature infants is shown in Figure 5–13.

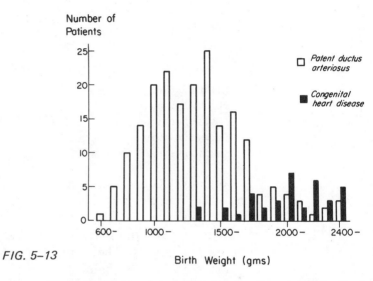

FIG. 5–13

*(Reproduced by permission of The American Heart Association, Inc.)*

The incidence of congenital heart disease other than PDA in the total group of 1150 newborns studied was 3.5/1000 live, low birth weight infants, while the incidence of PDA was 70/1000.

Reference: Leven, D.L., Stanger, P., Kitterman, J.A., et al.: Circulation, *52*:500, 1975.

## DISORDERS ASSOCIATED WITH BREECH PRESENTATION

The pediatrician summoned to be present for the breech delivery of an infant who is subsequently diagnosed as having the trisomy 18 syndrome may question the association of breech presentation and other disorders. A variety of anomalies and syndromes are more frequently present in infants presenting feet first:

Prader-Willi syndrome
Trisomy 13 syndrome
Trisomy 18 syndrome
Trisomy 21 syndrome

Smith-Lemli-Opitz syndrome
Fetal alcohol syndrome
Potter anomaly
Zellweger syndrome
Myotonic dystrophy
Werdnig-Hoffmann syndrome
de Lange syndrome
Familial dysautonomia
Hydrocephalus
Congenital dislocation of the hip
Anencephaly
Meningomyelocele

Breech presentation is also associated with:

Multiple births
Oligohydramnios
Polyhydramnios
Bicornuate or double uterus
Placenta previa

Normally, about 2.5 per cent of term infants are breech presentations. The frequency is two to three times higher in the smaller premature infants. The frequency of major malformations is three times as high as in those born in the vertex position. This difference is not the result of prematurity. The neonatal mortality rate for infants born by breech presentation is about 12 times the mortality rate in nonbreech deliveries. There is a 50 per cent incidence of major malformations in term infants who die after breech delivery. The frequency of neurologic abnormalities and motor retardation at age one year is 63 per cent higher in infants born by breech than by vertex presentation.

Reference: Braun, F.H.T., Jones, K.L., and Smith, D.W.: J. Pediatr., *86*:419, 1975.

## THE ABDOMINAL MASS IN THE NEWBORN

Approximately one-half of the abdominal masses noted in the neonatal period reflect abnormalities of the genitourinary system. The major abnormalities presenting as an abdominal mass during this period of life are:

*Kidney*

Hypoplastic multicystic kidney, unilateral or bilateral
Hydronephrosis secondary to distal obstruction
Mesoblastic nephroma
Solitary cyst
Renal vein thrombosis

5

### Liver and Biliary Tract

Hematoma of the liver
Hemangioma of the liver
Solitary cyst of the liver
Hepatoma
Choledochal cyst
Distended gallbladder secondary to cystic fibrosis

### Gastrointestinal Tract

Duplication of the duodenum, jejunum, or ileum
Mesenteric cyst
Volvulus secondary to meconium ileus
Leiomyosarcoma of the intestine

### Female Genital Tract

Ovarian cyst
Hydro- and hematocolpos

### Retroperitoneal Teratomas

### Adrenal Hemorrhage

### Neuroblastoma

The finding of an abdominal mass in the newborn requires an immediate intravenous pyelogram and ultimate surgical exploration.

It should be noted that malignant tumors are uncommon at birth. Although Wilms' tumor was previously believed to occur with some frequency during this period of life, it is now realized that most of these tumors are mesoblastic nephromas. This tumor is histologically distinct in its fibroblastic appearance and shows only minimal nuclear polymorphism and mitotic activity. Even though these tumors may grow to large size and show evidence of local extension, they do not appear to metastasize, and cure may be achieved with surgery alone.

---

Reference: Arey, J.B.: Pediatr. Clin. North Am., *10*:665, 1963.

## TRACHEOESOPHAGEAL FISTULA

The diagnosis of tracheoesophageal fistula may be suggested by a variety of clinical observations. The five types of fistula are depicted in Figure 5–14 along with the symptoms and signs that typically accompany them.

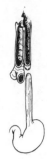

**Type A**
**Symptoms and Signs:**

Excessive mucus, aspiration
    of saliva.
Scaphoid abdomen.
No gas in bowel on x-ray.
Cannot pass catheter into
    stomach.
Gradually increasing respira-
    tory distress.
Polyhydramnios.

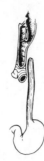

**Type B**
**Symptoms and Signs:**

Polyhydramnios.
Coughing, choking, and
    pneumonia from birth.
Scaphoid abdomen.
No gas in bowel on x-ray.

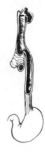

**Type C**
**Symptoms and Signs:**

Most common (80% of
    cases).
Excessive mucus.
Gradually increasing respira-
    tory distress.
Polyhydramnios frequent
    but not severe.
Gas in bowel on x-ray.

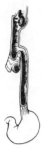

**Type D**
**Symptoms and Signs:**

Coughing, choking, and
    pneumonia from birth.
Gas in bowel on x-ray.

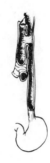

**Type E**
**Symptoms and Signs:**

Difficult to diagnose.
Coughing or cyanosis with
    feeding.
Chronic aspiration pneu-
    monia.

*FIG. 5–14*

The differential diagnosis includes pharyngeal muscle weakness, vascular rings, and esophageal diverticula.

Discovery of a tracheoesophageal fistula should alert the physician to the possibility that other congenital anomalies may be present. Anomalies that have been found to be associated include:

Vertebral
Anal
Cardiac
Renal
Limb

Reference: Brazie, J.V., and Lubchenco, L.O.: *In* Kempe, C.H., Silver, H.K., and O'Brien, D. (Eds.): Current Pediatric Diagnosis and Treatment. Los Altos, California, Lange Medical Publications, 1976, p. 81.

# DIAGNOSIS OF AMBIGUOUS GENITALIA AT BIRTH

The birth of a child is usually heralded by the welcome words "It's a girl," or "It's a boy." It is at that point that parents begin to define their relationship to their child. If sexual identification is impossible at birth, investigation should be undertaken immediately. The following chart will aid in such an investigation.

**5**

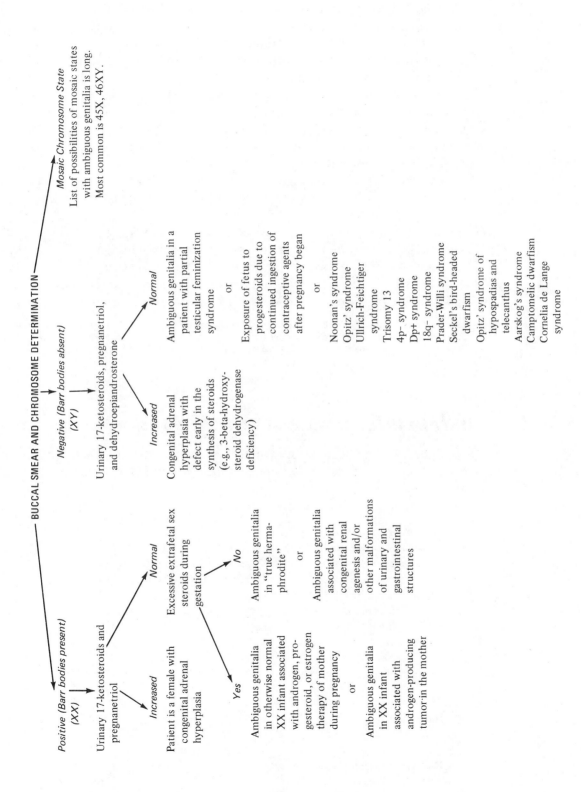

BUCCAL SMEAR AND CHROMOSOME DETERMINATION

*Positive (Barr bodies present) (XX)*

Urinary 17-ketosteroids and pregnanetriol

*Increased*

Patient is a female with congenital adrenal hyperplasia

*Normal*

Excessive extrafetal sex steroids during gestation

*Yes*

Ambiguous genitalia in otherwise normal XX infant associated with androgen, progesteroid, or estrogen therapy of mother during pregnancy

or

Ambiguous genitalia in XX infant associated with androgen-producing tumor in the mother

*No*

Ambiguous genitalia in "true hermaphrodite"

or

Ambiguous genitalia associated with congenital renal agenesis and/or other malformations of urinary and gastrointestinal structures

*Negative (Barr bodies absent) (XY)*

Urinary 17-ketosteroids, pregnanetriol, and dehydroepiandrosterone

*Increased*

Congenital adrenal hyperplasia with defect early in the synthesis of steroids (e.g., 3-beta-hydroxy-steroid dehydrogenase deficiency)

*Normal*

Ambiguous genitalia in a patient with partial testicular feminization syndrome

or

Exposure of fetus to progesteroids due to continued ingestion of contraceptive agents after pregnancy began

or

Noonan's syndrome
Opitz' syndrome
Ullrich-Feichtiger syndrome
Trisomy 13
4p– syndrome
Dp+ syndrome
18q– syndrome
Prader-Willi syndrome
Seckel's bird-headed dwarfism
Opitz' syndrome of hypospadias and telecanthus
Aarskog's syndrome
Camptomelic dwarfism
Cornelia de Lange syndrome

*Mosaic Chromosome State*

List of possibilities of mosaic states with ambiguous genitalia is long. Most common is 45X, 46XY.

Though the buccal smear evaluation is rapid, its interpretation may be difficult without accompanying karyotype analysis. The sex chromatin stains poorly in the newborn, and the diagnosis of certain mosaic states is difficult without chromosome identification. It is recommended that all newborns with ambiguous genitalia have both buccal smear and chromosome evaluation.

While awaiting the results of laboratory tests, daily serum sodium concentration should be ascertained for all newborns in whom genitalia are abnormal, since adrenal hyperplasia of the salt-losing form is a possible diagnosis. The sodium-losing crisis usually occurs at 8 to 10 days of life in these children.

Urinary 17-ketosteroids and pregnanetriol results are accurate in the second week of life. Rarely, the defect in congenital adrenal hyperplasia must be determined by urinary dehydroepiandrosterone or by chromatographic studies (in 3-beta-hydroxysteroid dehydrogenase defect) or by estimation or urinary or serum compound S (11-hydroxylase defect prior to clinically detectable hypertension).

Any male born with bilateral cryptorchidism, even if the genitalia appear otherwise normal, should have a karyotype analysis.

References: Zurbrügg, R.P.: Congenital adrenal hyperplasia; and Schlegel, R.J., and Gardner, L.I.: Ambiguous and abnormal genitalia. *In* Gardner, L.I. (Ed.): Endocrine and Genetic Diseases of Childhood and Adolescence. Philadelphia, W.B. Saunders Company, 1975.

# HYPERTRICHOSIS IN THE NEWBORN

Generalized hypertrichosis can be a normal temporary condition in the newborn or it can be a familial trait. Not all hairy newborns are normal.

Generalized hypertrichosis can be seen in:

Congenital lipodystrophy
Cornelia de Lange syndrome
Craniofacial dysostosis with dental, eye, and cardiac anomalies
Hypertrichosis lanuginosa universalia ("monkey men"); only
    palms, soles, dorsal terminal phalanges, labia minora, prepuce
    and glans penis are spared.
Hypertrichosis with gingival fibromatosis
Leprechaunism

Localized hypertrichosis is observed with:

Congenital hemihypertrophy
Hairy ears
Hairy elbows syndrome
Hairy nevi
Ring chromosome E (low hairline)
Trisomy 18 (back and forehead)
Turner's syndrome (low occipital hairline)

Reference: Solomon, L.M., and Esterly, N.B.: Neonatal Dermatology. Philadelphia, W.B. Saunders Company, 1973, p. 195.

5

# IS IT REALLY ERYTHEMA TOXICUM?

The presence of white papules or pustules in a newborn infant is a common occurrence. They appear with greater frequency in term infants. The eruption is usually termed "erythema toxicum," a disorder of unknown cause. It is now recognized that another vesicopustular eruption may also occur during this period of life. It can be confused with erythema toxicum or a cutaneous skin infection. This eruption has been termed "pustular melanosis." The distinguishing characteristics of these two disorders are described in the table below.

| | PUSTULAR MELANOSIS | ERYTHEMA TOXICUM |
|---|---|---|
| Incidence | More common in black infants | Equal in black and white infants |
| Age of onset | Always present at birth | Rarely present at birth |
| Types of lesions | Vesicopustules with no surrounding erythema; desquamated vesico-pustule with collarette of scale; pigmented macule | White papules with surrounding erythema; vesicopustule; usually with surrounding erythema |
| Sites of involvement | Chin, neck, nape, lower back, and shins; vesicles on palms and soles | Face, forehead, trunk, and extrem-ities; no involvement of palms and soles |
| Duration | Vesicopustules disappear in 24 to 48 hours; pigmented macules fade in 3 weeks to 3 months | Persists for up to 6 days, occasionally longer; no residual pigmentation |
| Smear of lesional contents | Polymorphonuclear leukocytes, cellular debris, sparse eosinophils | Numerous eosinophils |
| Histopathology Pustule | Intracorneal and subcorneal pustules with infiltrate mainly polymorphonuclear leukocytes, variable eosinophils | Intraepidermal or subcorneal pustule involving superficial portion pilo-sebaceous unit, dense infiltrate of eosinophils |
| Pigmented macule | Basketweave hyperkeratosis, focal basilar hyperpigmentation | |

Reference: Ramamurth, R.S., Reveri, M., Esterly, N.B., et al.: J. Pediatr., *88*:831, 1976.

# SCLEREMA NEONATORUM

Sclerema neonatorum is a condition that affects premature or debilitated newborn infants or older infants suffering from severe disease. Infants so affected have smooth, cool, tense, mottled purplish, hard skin that is apparently adherent to the subcutaneous tissues. The skin does not pit, nor can it be pinched into a fold. The process usually begins on the lower extremities and spreads peripherally through the fatty subcutaneous tissues. Sclerema neonatorum is a sign of life-threatening disease, and when it is noted, efforts should be made to identify the disease process.

1. The infant should be assumed to be infected until proved otherwise, and multiple cultures should be taken prior to the institution of antibiotic therapy.

2. Careful investigation should be made for congenital anomalies or signs of trauma so that appropriate treatment may be instituted.

3. Supportive measures, such as maintenance of optimum environmental temperatures, administration of intravenous fluids and blood when indicated, and digitalization if necessary, should be undertaken. Corticosteroids have not been shown to be of value, except when there is evidence of adrenal insufficiency.

Sclerema neonatorum should be distinguished from necrosis of fat that occurs in healthy infants during the first few months of life. Hardened areas attached to the skin but not to the deeper tissue develop over the bony prominences of the infant's body. These areas of fat necrosis disappear gradually, but may soften and become cystic before dissolving completely.

Sclerema neonatorum should also be differentiated from scleredema. Scleredema refers to a pitting edema that is usually generalized and occurs primarily in premature infants. The limbs affected by scleredema are swollen.

In the infant who is already moribund, sclerema neonatorum is a sign of impending death.

---

Reference: Warwick, W.J., Ruttenberg, H.D., and Quie, P.G.: J.A.M.A., *184*:680, 1963.

# DETECTION OF CYSTIC FIBROSIS AT BIRTH

Screening for cystic fibrosis at birth can be rapidly performed based on the detection of albumin in the meconium of affected babies. Unfortunately, false-positive tests may be encountered. The number of false-positives can be reduced by also testing for the presence of lactase in the stool. Lactase activity can be detected in meconium from babies with cystic fibrosis but not in meconium from healthy babies.

The test for lactase in the stool is performed as follows:

1. Add 0.5 ml of 3 per cent lactose solution (prepared in maleate buffer, pH 5.4) to a vial containing meconium.

2. Allow to stand at room temperature for 15 minutes.

3. Test supernatant with a Dextrostix. A blue color denotes the presence of glucose derived from lactose by the lactase in the meconium.

One must be certain that glucose was not already present in the stool. This occurs most commonly in premature babies. To rule this possibility out, the procedure can be repeated with the addition of distilled water rather than a lactose solution. A positive test indicates that glucose was already present.

5

The finding of both albumin and lactase activity in meconium is strong presumptive evidence that the baby has cystic fibrosis.

References: Antonowicz, I., Ishida, S., and Schawachman, H.: Lancet, *1*:746, 1976. Stephan, U., Busch, E.W., Kolberg, H., et al.: Pediatrics, *55*:35, 1975.

# PERSISTENT RHINITIS IN THE NEWBORN

Nasal congestion and rhinorrhea in the newborn may be a difficult problem, since neonates are often obligate nose breathers. The causes of persistent rhinitis in the newborn are listed below along with the treatment of each type.

| ENTITY | CAUSE | TREATMENT |
|---|---|---|
| Transient idiopathic stuffy nose of the newborn | Unknown | Normal saline nosedrops may be instilled and then removed after a few minutes with cotton-tipped applicators or gentle suction on a rubber bulb syringe. If the congestion interferes with feeding, 2 drops of 0.125 per cent phenylephrine (Neo-Synephrine) may be instilled in the nose just before meals for several days. |
| Reserpine side-effects | Caused by mother's taking reserpine | Same as above. |
| Chemical rhinitis | Due to overtreatment of idiopathic stuffy nose with topical nasoconstrictors | Discontinue nosedrops. Use oral decongestants for 2 days. |
| Pyogenic rhinitis | These infants have bacterial infection despite absence of purulent discharge. Diagnose via cultures of discharge | Same as for idiopathic stuffy nose. |
| Congenital syphilis | Maternal syphilis | Penicillin. |
| Hypothyroidism | Congenital hypothyroidism | Thyroid hormone replacement. |
| Choanal atresia | Congenital defect | Place oral airway immediately. Definitive surgery by otolaryngologist. |
| Nasal fracture | Birth trauma | Diagnose by examination for subluxation of the nasal septum causing occlusion of the nasal passages. Refer to otolaryngologist. |

Reference: Schmitt, B.D.: *In* Kempe, C.H., Silver, H.K., and O'Brien, D. (Eds.): Current Pediatric Diagnosis and Treatment. Los Altos, California, Lange Medical Publications, 1976, p. 251.

# INFECTIOUS DISEASE

# CROUP SYNDROMES

Differentiation between epiglottitis, laryngotracheobronchitis (LTB), and spasmodic laryngitis is a common task for the pediatrician. The accompanying table may simplify your efforts. Remember that a foreign body and retropharyngeal abscess may give similar clinical pictures.

| | EPIGLOTTITIS | LTB | SPASMODIC LARYNGITIS |
|---|---|---|---|
| Primary age | 3–8 years | <3 years | 1–3 years |
| Etiology | Usually *Hemophilus influenzae*, occasionally pneumococcus or viral | Viral | Uncertain; viral (?) |
| Onset | Rapid | Gradual | Sudden, usually at night |
| Mean duration of illness before hospitalization | 8.6 hours | 1.9 days | — |
| Presenting complaints | High fever, respiratory distress in younger child, drooling and dysphagia in older child | Cough, hoarseness, fever, inspiratory stridor | No fever |
| Mean temperature | 102.2 F | 102.2 F | Normal |
| Physical examination | Diminished breath sounds, pallor, inspiratory rhonchi | Diminished breath sounds, inspiratory rales | Diminished breath sounds, labored respirations |
| Laryngeal findings | Inflammation of periglottic structures, especially edematous red epiglottis | Edema of vocal cords and subglottic area | Laryngeal spasm |
| Mean white blood count | 24,300 | 13,200 | — |
| Percentage neutrophils | 85% | 63% | — |
| Clinical course | Rapidly progressive, *medical emergency* | Self-limited, may last ≤ 1 week | Self-limited but may be recurrent |
| Bacterial complications | Other organs may be seeded | Rare | None |

**6**

*Croup*—From the Scottish word *croak*, which describes the sound these children make.

| | EPIGLOTTITIS | LTB | SPASMODIC LARYNGITIS |
|---|---|---|---|
| Treatment | Antibiotics and airway maintenance. *Hospitalization is mandatory* | Humidification and support | Humidification, relief of laryngospasm, reassurance |

Reference: Eichenwald, H.P.: Hospital Practice, *11*:81, 1976. Rabe, E.F.: Pediatrics, *2*:255; 415; 559, 1948.

## PHARYNGOTONSILLITIS

Pharyngotonsillitis, the most frequent childhood respiratory infection, is most often viral in origin. Although there is considerable overlap between the viral and streptococcal (strep) forms of this disease, the following table may help differentiate the two forms.

| | STREPTOCOCCAL PHARYNGOTONSILLITIS | | VIRAL PHARYNGOTONSILLITIS |
|---|---|---|---|
| | *<2 Years of Age* | *>2 Years of Age* | *Any Age* |
| Onset | Gradual or sudden | Sudden | Gradual |
| Presenting signs | Nasopharyngitis | Abdominal pain, vomiting, headache | Sore throat (often preceded by malaise and anorexia) |
| Fever | Slight to moderate (rarely, 102° F), often variable | Usually high (103–104° F), but may be moderate | Slight to moderate, sometimes high (reduced by aspirin) |
| Tonsillar involvement | Little or none | May have any or all of: follicular exudate, erythema, petechiae of soft palate | Similar to streptococcal, although petechial mottling is less common and erythema is often less |
| Clinical complaints | Anorexia, runny nose, listlessness, failure to thrive, vomiting | Sore throat | Sore throat, hoarseness, cough, rhinitis, conjunctivitis |
| Laboratory results | Leukocytosis | Leukocytosis | Leukocyte count normal to high |

The following guidelines characterize children who should be cultured for streptococcus:

1. Those with sore throat who have fever, tender anterior cervical nodes, and/or palatal petechiae.
2. Those with oral temperature ≥101° F (38.3° C), even in the absence of a sore throat.
3. Those with any respiratory illness if exposed to a sibling or child with proven streptococcal pharyngitis or if a member of the child's family has a history of rheumatic fever.

4. Those with a scarlatiniform rash.

5. Those with acute onset of nontraumatic hematuria.

Other significant facts to consider when deciding whom to culture and treat:

1. Red throats and tonsillar exudate are nonspecific findings. Most pediatric upper respiratory infections are viral in origin. Those due to streptococcus are no more severe than the others.

2. A 24 to 72 hour delay in therapy will not decrease the antirheumatic fever effect of penicillin.

3. Chronic streptococcal carriers (other than nasal) are usually not contagious; their treatment is indicated only in families with a history of rheumatic fever or in other high-risk situations.

References: Wannamaker, L.W.: J.A.M.A., 235:913, 1976. Eichenwald, H.F.: Hospital Practice, 11:81, 1976. Moffet, H.L.: Pediatric Infectious Diseases. Philadelphia, J.B. Lippincott Company, 1975, p. 26. Townsend, E.H., Jr., and Rodebaugh, J.R.: N. Engl. J. Med., 266:683, 1962.

# DIAGNOSIS OF STREPTOCOCCAL PHARYNGITIS

The diagnosis of streptococcal pharyngitis cannot reliably be made in the absence of a positive throat culture. The following table gives criteria for grouping patients according to high, medium, and low clinical index of suspicion of streptococcal sore throat.

| HIGH | MEDIUM | LOW |
|---|---|---|
| *Symptoms (or history)* | | |
| Close exposure to known streptococcal sore throat | Fever | Minimal fever |
| | Moderately sore throat | Slightly sore or scratchy throat |
| | Abdominal pain | |
| Fever greater than 101.5° F | | |
| Severely sore throat | | |
| *Signs* | | |
| Scarlatiniform rash | Slightly tender, slightly enlarged peritonsillar lymph nodes | Palpebral conjunctivitis |
| Tender, enlarged peritonsillar lymph nodes | | Slightly red or injected pharynx |
| Beefy red pharynx | Moderately red pharynx | Thin, wispy exudate in crypts |
| Moderate exudate | Medium exudate | Hoarseness, cough |
| Petechiae on soft palate or uvula | | |

Reference: Peebles, T.C.: Pediatr. Clin. North Am., 18:145, 1971.

## THE RESPONSE TO PENICILLIN IN STREPTOCOCCAL PHARYNGITIS

If your patient has a streptococcal pharyngitis and you initiate treatment with appropriate doses of penicillin, how soon should you expect to observe a disappearance of the signs and symptoms of the disease?

The following facts should help you in deciding if your diagnosis and treatment were correct.

| SYMPTOM | MEAN DURATION (HOURS) |
| --- | --- |
| Sore throat | 28.8 |
| Headache | 41.1 |
| Abdominal pain | 48.0 |
| Vomiting | 56.0 |

| SIGN | MEAN DURATION (HOURS) |
| --- | --- |
| Fever | 44.0 |
| Pharyngeal injection | 42.0 |
| Pharyngeal petechiae | 40.0 |
| Pharyngeal exudate | 40.0 |

As a general rule, your patient should manifest some evidence of improvement within 48 hours of the start of treatment. The duration of signs and symptoms is somewhat shorter in patients who are treated within 24 hours of the onset of fever.

Reference: Bass, J.W., Crast, F.W., Knowles, C.R., et al.: J.A.M.A., *235*:1112, 1975.

## THE ETIOLOGY OF VIRAL DISEASE

Certain constellations of findings in children should suggest the possibility of viral infections. The table lists the viruses that may be responsible for these findings.

*Roseola*—Latin diminutive of *roseus*, meaning rosy.

*Viral Agents Often Associated with Various Pediatric
Syndromes*

| CLINICAL SYNDROME | VIRUSES |
|---|---|
| Neonatal viral disease | CMV, rubella, HSV, coxsackie |
| Lymphadenopathy | EBV, CMV, cat-scratch disease |
| Pharyngitis | Adenovirus, EBV, HSV, enteroviruses, influenza, parainfluenza |
| Other acute respiratory disease | Adrenovirus, respiratory syncytial virus, influenza, parainfluenza, enteroviruses, rhinovirus, measles (after killed vaccine), EBV |
| Parotitis | Mumps, parainfluenza, LCM, coxsackie B |
| Encephalitis and aseptic meningitis | Mumps, measles, polio, ECHO, coxsackie, HSV, LCM, arboviruses |
| Myocarditis | Measles, mumps, coxsackie B, ECHO, EBV |
| Pericarditis | Coxsackie B, influenza, EBV |
| Hepatitis | Hepatitis A, hepatitis B, EBV, CMV |
| Fever without localizing signs | ECHO, coxsackie, parainfluenza, adenovirus, influenza |
| Rash — petechial | Adenovirus, EBV, measles (after killed vaccine) |
| Rash — maculopapular | Measles, rubella, coxsackie, ECHO |
| Rash — poxlike | Varicella-zoster, HSV, vaccinia, variola |
| Rash — palms/soles | Coxsackie, ECHO, EBV, measles (after killed vaccine) |

CMV = Cytomegalovirus; EBV = Epstein-Barr virus; HSV = herpes simplex virus;
LCM = lymphocytic choriomeningitis.

Although viral diagnostic techniques are relatively slow and
expensive, their use is called for in some situations:

For exclusion of malignancy or treatable nonviral infection (e.g., massive
cervical adenopathy)

To allow discontinuation of antibiotic therapy (e.g., neonatal viral versus
bacterial sepsis)

To justify use of antiviral drug or globulin (e.g., neonatal herpes)

Fatal undiagnosed illness

For early recognition and/or confirmation of outbreak (e.g., measles or
smallpox)

For increased knowledge of epidemiology and transmission of viral agents

To demonstrate susceptibility or immunity of an individual to specific viral
disease (serologic study only)

Serologic studies are almost always indicated as part of viral diagnostic studies. The outstanding major exception is in attempts to document infections caused by the enteroviruses, ECHO and coxsackie, since there are more than three dozen non–cross-reacting serotypes. For these agents, most state or other reference laboratories will perform serologic studies only if a specific enterovirus has been isolated.

An acute (within seven days of onset of illness) serum specimen should be obtained (and saved) from any child with undiagnosed illness for later use in viral or other studies. Convalescent serum, if indicated, can be obtained 14 to 28 days later.

The table on page 175 suggests the timing and sites of additional specimens useful in viral diagnosis.

Viral cultures differ from routine bacteriologic cultures in several important respects. Attention to the following points will improve the possibility of viral isolation.

1. Specimens to be cultured should be bacteriologically sterile whenever possible.

2. Most viruses are destroyed by drying; swabs should be sent to the laboratory in some type of viral "transport medium" (e.g., Hanks solution).

3. Specimens should be packed in dry ice or, if held overnight before culturing, kept in a $-70°C$ freezer.

4. Specimens should be obtained as early in the disease course as possible and should be inoculated immediately.

5. A brief clinical history should accompany all specimens in order to help the virology laboratory decide which viral media, and thus which viruses, are most appropriate to the situation.

---

References: Moffet, H.L.: Pediatric Infectious Diseases. Philadelphia, J.B. Lippincott Company, 1975. Gershon, A.A.: Pediatr. Clin. North Am., *18*:73, 1971.

Specimens in Viral Diagnosis of Specific Clinical Findings

| | THROAT SWAB | STOOL | URINE* | CEREBROSPINAL FLUID | VESICLE FLUID† | OTHER |
|---|---|---|---|---|---|---|
| Optimal time (days) after onset to collect | ≤3 | ≤14 | ≤3 | ≤7 | As soon as possible | |
| *Clinical Findings* | | | | | | |
| Neonatal disease | X | X | X | X | If present | Neonatal and maternal sera, repeat in 3 months |
| Lymphadenopathy | X | | X | | | Urine cytology, rapid mononucleosis slide test |
| Pharyngitis | X | | X | | | Rapid mononucleosis slide test |
| Other acute respiratory disease | X | X | X | | | |
| Parotitis/orchitis | X | X | X | If symptomatic | | |
| Encephalitis/meningitis | X | X | X | X | If present | |
| Myocarditis | X | X | X | | | Rapid mononucleosis slide test |
| Hepatitis | X | X | X | | | Urine cytology |
| Rash | X | X | X | | | |
| Fever without localization | X | X | X | | | |
| Autopsy | | | | | | Cultures of brain, liver, lung |

*Urine for cytomegalovirus may be submitted at any time during the illness.
†Examination of vesicle base scraping stained with Wright or Wright-Giemsa stain (Tzanck prep) may be helpful.

# CLINICAL STAGING IN REYE'S SYNDROME

In order to evaluate therapy, compare your results with those of others, and determine prognosis, it is necessary to utilize a uniform method of classification of the clinical status of patients with Reye's syndrome. The most widely used method of clinical staging is described below.

| STAGE | CLINICAL FINDINGS |
|-------|-------------------|
| 0 | Neurologically normal; chemical evidence of hepatic dysfunction |
| I | Oriented to mildly confused, lethargic, vomiting, amnesic; chemical evidence of hepatic dysfunction |
| II | Agitated delirium, visual unresponsiveness (pupils dilated, react sluggishly to light), hyperactive reflexes, sympathetic hyperactivity, hyperpnea, react to noxious stimuli, decorticate posturing may be present, chemical evidence of liver dysfunction |
| III | Coma, decorticate rigidity, hyperventilation, preservation of sluggish pupillary response to light and oculovestibular reflexes, chemical evidence of liver dysfunction |
| IV | Deep coma, decerebrate rigidity, large fixed pupils, dysconjugate eye movements in response to caloric stimulation of the oculovestibular reflex, loss of corneal reflex, hyperpnea, chemical evidence of mild hepatic dysfunction |
| V | Seizures, loss of deep tendon reflexes, flaccidity, respiratory arrest, circulatory collapse, minimal evidence of hepatic dysfunction |

Remember that the diagnosis and staging of Reye's syndrome are predicated on histologic evidence of liver disease obtained by biopsy at the earliest possible moment in the evaluation process.

References: Lovejoy, F.H., Smith, A.L., Bresnan, M.J., et al.: Am. J. Dis. Child., *128*:36, 1974. Devino, D.C., and Kearing, J.P.: Adv. Pediatr., *22*:175, 1976.

# ATYPICAL MEASLES

Shortly after the introduction of killed measles vaccine in the early 1960s, cases of atypical measles began appearing in vaccine recipients. Although atypical measles differs clinically in many respects from ordinary measles, it can be confirmed by serologic tests. It should be considered in any child whose illness has some of the clinical features described below:

*The History*

> Received killed measles vaccine in past
> Recent exposure to measles-like illness

*The Prodrome*

> High fever that responds poorly to antipyretics
> Headache
> Cough
> Abdominal symptoms, sometimes severe

*The Rash*

> Begins two to three days after onset of illness
> Begins on wrists and feet and usually involves the palms and soles
> Progresses toward the trunk and head
> Is most dense on distal limbs and in skin folds
> Character of rash may be any combination of maculopapular,
>     vesicular, or hemorrhagic lesions
> Is often intensely pruritic

*Respiratory Involvement* is characteristic

> Roentgenogram may show lobar or segmental pneumonia
> Hilar adenopathy is consistently present
> Pleural effusion is common
> Ill-defined nodular lesions may persist on roentgenogram
>     for up to two years
> Arterial hypoxemia may be seen

*Other Symptoms* and signs may be seen. They include:

> Peripheral edema
> Myalgia
> Hypertension
> Strawberry tongue

*Laboratory Findings* often include:

> Elevated WBC with neutrophilia and marked shift to the left
> Appreciable rise in measles HI antibody titers

The illness runs a self-limited course of two to three weeks. No mortality or long-term morbidity has been noted. A few patients have had this illness after having received the live attenuated vaccine now in use.

---

References: Editorial: Br. Med. J., *1*:235, 1971. St. Geme, J.W., and George, B.L.: Pediatrics, *57*:148, 1976.

# INFECTIOUS MONONUCLEOSIS IN YOUNG CHILDREN

Until recently, it has been assumed that infectious mononucleosis was a rare disease in early childhood. This was a consequence of the fact that children under the age of 5 years generally do not produce a heterophile antibody in response to this infection. With the identification of the Epstein-Barr virus as the responsible etiologic agent in this disease and the development of techniques for both viral isolation and the measurement of antibody titers, it is now appreciated that infections with Epstein-Barr virus are very common in early childhood. By the age of 4 years, between 30 and 70 per cent of children have acquired antibodies to this agent.

Symptoms and signs in young children may include fever, diarrhea, pharyngitis, tonsillitis, otitis media, pneumonia, lymphadenopathy, hepatomegaly, and splenomegaly.

The total white count and differential are of little help in suspecting the diagnosis. The presence of 10 per cent or more atypical lymphocytes, however, should alert you to the possibility of infectious mononucleosis. Acute and convalescent titers demonstrating a rise in antibody to Epstein-Barr virus will confirm the diagnosis.

Reference: Tamir, D., Benderly, A., Levy, J., et al.: Pediatrics, *53*:330, 1974.

# COMPLICATIONS OF INFECTIOUS MONONUCLEOSIS

Although most children with infectious mononucleosis experience a typical illness with an uncomplicated course, exceptions do exist. It is important to recognize the many complications of this common disease. They include the following:

*Neurologic*

Guillain-Barré syndrome
Facial nerve palsy
Meningoencephalitis
Aseptic meningitis
Transverse myelitis
Seizures
Peripheral neuritis
Optic neuritis
Acute psychosis
Diplopia
Reye's syndrome
Subacute sclerosing panencephalitis

*Hepatic*

    Hepatitis
    Multiple granulomas

*Cardiac*

    Pericarditis
    Myocarditis

*Hematologic*

    Hemolytic anemia
    Thrombocytopenia
    Aplastic anemia
    Hemolytic-uremic syndrome
    Disseminated intravascular coagulation

*Splenic Rupture*

*Pulmonary Infiltration*

*Airway Obstruction*

*Glomerulonephritis*

Reference: Karzon, D.T.: Adv. Pediatr., *22*:231, 1976.

*"It seems impossible that children should ever grow to be men, and drag the heavy artillery along the dusty road of life."*

H. W. Longfellow

# RUBELLA EXPOSURE DURING PREGNANCY

The dangers of maternal rubella infection during pregnancy are well known. The course to take after an expectant mother has been exposed to rubella is outlined on page 180.

*Management of a Pregnant Female Exposed to Rubella*

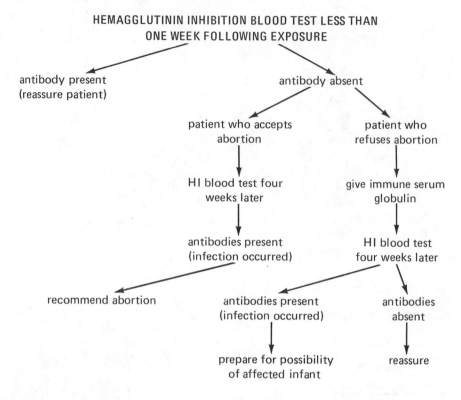

If a blood sample for HI test is obtained more than one week after exposure to rubella, one cannot tell if antibodies present are from a past or the present exposure. Therefore, a second blood specimen taken one or two weeks after the first blood sample is tested for CF, HI, and IgM specific antibody. A rising antibody titer and/or the presence of IgM specific rubella antibody is indicative of current rubella infection.

There is no evidence that immunization of a child whose mother is in the early stages of pregnancy carries any risk of infection to the fetus.

---

Reference: Honig, P.J., and Tunnessen, W.W.: Clinical Diagnostic Quiz, *1*:7, 1976.

## PAPULAR ACRODERMATITIS AND HEPATITIS-B (GIANOTTI'S DISEASE)

Hepatitis-B may manifest itself initially, and sometimes exclusively, as a cutaneous disorder. In children under 3 years of age, papular acrodermatitis appears to be the most common dermatologic sign of hepatitis-B, while in older children and adults the prodromal phase of the illness is accompanied by arthritis, arthralgia, and urticarial or maculopapular eruption that most frequently involves the lower extremities.

The major features of the papular acrodermatitis that is associated with hepatitis-B (Gianotti's disease) are the following:

1. A nonitching, erythematous papular dermatitis, involving the face and extremities, and sparing the major portion of the trunk.
2. Enlargement of lymph nodes in the axillary and inguinal areas.
3. Hepatomegaly.
4. Abnormal liver function tests, including an elevation in the SGOT.

In the absence of obvious jaundice, the diagnosis of hepatitis is frequently not considered. Be suspicious the next time you encounter this characteristic eruption.

6

References: Gianotti, F.: Arch. Dis. Child., *48*:794, 1973. Ishimaru, Y., Ishimaru, H., Toda, T., et al.: Lancet, *1*:707, 1976. Segool, R.A., Lejtenyi, C., and Taussig, L.M.: J. Pediatr., *87*:709, 1975.

# INFLUENZA A$_2$ IN YOUNG CHILDREN

Clinical and laboratory features of influenza infections in young children differ from those found in infected school-age children and adults. The table below presents features of illness found in 75 children with culture-proved influenza A$_2$ infection.

*Principal Features of Influenza in Young Children (n = 75)*

| SYMPTOMS | PER CENT | SIGNS | PER CENT |
|---|---|---|---|
| Cough | 67 | Fever | 87 |
| Anorexia | 56 | Pharyngitis | 72 |
| Rhinorrhea | 53 | Cervical adenopathy | 44 |
| Vomiting | 51 | Otitis media | 44 |
| Diarrhea | 23 | Seizures | 37 |
| | | Lower respiratory signs | 32 |
| LABORATORY DATA | PER CENT | Dehydration | 11 |
| WBC >15,000 | 15 | Generalized adenopathy | 10 |
| WBC <6000 | 1 | Stridor | 10 |
| Neutrophilia | 37 | | |
| Neutropenia | 5 | | |

Certain features seemed particularly age-dependent. For example, 50 per cent of children under 6 months of age had diarrhea. Two-thirds of children under 3 years of age had an associated febrile seizure.

Reference: Price, D.A., Postlethwaite, R.J., and Longson, M.: Clin. Pediatr., *15*:361, 1976.

## VARICELLA AND ZIG

Zoster immune globulin (ZIG), obtained from patients convalescing from varicella or zoster infections, has proved useful in reducing morbidity and mortality from varicella-zoster virus infections in immunocompromised patients. To be effective, ZIG must be given within 72 hours of exposure. Although it does not prevent varicella infection, it does increase the rate of subclinical infection and decrease the rate of disseminated and/or fatal infection in these high-risk patients.

ZIG can be obtained only through a regional ZIG consultant* or the Center for Disease Control (CDC). The table outlines those patient criteria necessary for release of ZIG for varicella prophylaxis.

1. One of the following underlying illnesses or conditions
   Leukemia or lymphoma
   Congenital or acquired immunodeficiency
   Under immunosuppressive medication
   Newly born of mother with varicella
2. One of the following types of exposure to varicella or zoster patient
   Household contact
   Playmate contact (>1 hour play indoors)
   Hospital contact (in same bedroom or adjacent beds in a large ward)
   School contact (same carpool or adjacent desks in classroom)
   Newborn contact (newborn whose mother contacted varicella
       within the 4 days before delivery)
3. Negative or unknown prior disease history
4. Age of less than 15 years
5. Treatment must be initiated within 72 hours of exposure

Adults convalescing from varicella-zoster virus infections should be encouraged to donate plasma (via CDC) to supplement the short supply.

References: *Morbid. Mortal. Weekly Rep., *23*:379, 1974. Gershon, A.A., Sternberg, S., and Brunell, P.A.: N. Engl. J. Med., *290*:243, 1974. Morbid. Mortal. Weekly Rep., *25*:86, 1976.

## COLD AGGLUTININS AND MYCOPLASMA PNEUMONIAE RESPIRATORY ILLNESS

*Mycoplasma pneumoniae* is the etiologic agent that most often comes to mind when the coincidence of respiratory illness and elevated cold agglutinin titer is considered. The titer usually becomes positive at the end of a week of illness and reaches a peak at about four weeks.

Other infectious agents that also produce elevations in the titer of cold agglutinins include:

| Nonviral | Viral |
|---|---|
| Pneumococcus | Influenza A |
| Beta streptococcus | Parainfluenza |
| Psittacosis | Adenovirus |
| | ECHO virus |
| | Cytomegalovirus |
| | Rubella |
| | Respiratory syncytial virus |
| | Epstein-Barr virus |

Most *Mycoplasma* infections in infants and preadolescent children are inapparent. Pneumonia due to this organism, seen in older children, adolescents and adults, may therefore reflect increasing host immune response or repeated exposures to *Mycoplasma*.

References: Murray, H.W., Masur, H., Senterfit, L.B., et al.: Am. J. Med., *58*:229, 1975. Sussman, S.J., Magoffin, R.L., Lenette, E.H., et al.: Pediatrics, *75*:571, 1969. Fernald, G.W., Collier, A.M., and Clyde, W.A., Jr.: Pediatrics, *55*:327, 1975.

## CELLULITIS

Location of a cellulitis may be an important clue to an underlying condition and/or to an etiologic organism. The following table suggests situations associated with cellulitis in specific areas.

| LOCATION | CONDITION OR ORGANISM |
|---|---|
| Periorbital | Ethmoid sinusitis |
| Abdomen | Peritonitis |
| Extremity | Osteomyelitis, septic arthritis |
| Over large node | Adenitis, abscess |
| Perianal | Group A streptococcus (staphylococcus or gram-negative bacteria if abscess) |
| Face (neonate) | Staphylococcus; underlying maxillary osteomyelitis |
| Face (postneonate) | *Hemophilus influenzae;* otitis media |
| Tibia (usually both) | Erythema nodosum (see page 405) |
| Sacrum | Pilonidal cyst or sinus |

Reference: Moffet, H.L.: Pediatric Infectious Diseases. Philadelphia, J.B. Lippincott Company, 1975, p. 295.

# FEVER OF UNKNOWN ORIGIN

Prolonged episodes of fever without an apparent explanation are an uncommon diagnostic problem in pediatrics. Because of their rarity, they represent an exacting challenge and provide the clinician with an unequaled opportunity to demonstrate his skills in both careful history taking and physical examination. At least 50 per cent of "fevers of unknown origin" can be diagnosed by thoughtful attention to details and very simple laboratory studies. Unfortunately, the designation "fever of unknown origin" often prompts a myriad of tests and radiographic procedures in a nonsystematic fashion.

What are the usual causes of obscure, prolonged fevers in children and how do they differ in etiology from those observed in adults? The accompanying table summarizes the findings in two studies involving infants and children and contrasts them with a representative study of adult patients. Fever was defined as the presence of a rectal temperature of 38.5°C (99.8°F) on at least four occasions over a minimum period of two weeks.

## Causes of Fever of Unknown Origin

| INFANTS AND CHILDREN | | ADULTS |
|---|---|---|
| *Pizzo and Associates* | *McClung* | |
| *Infections* (52%) | *Infections* (29%) | *Infections* (40%) |
| Viral syndromes | Respiratory | Tuberculosis |
| Respiratory | Central nervous system | Endocarditis |
| Central nervous system | Salmonella | Localized to peritoneum, |
| Urinary tract | Endocarditis | urinary tract, or liver |
| Osteomyelitis | Histoplasmosis | |
| Endocarditis | Brucellosis | |
| Tuberculosis | Epstein-Barr infection | |
| Herpes simplex, generalized | | |
| Sinusitis | | |
| Salmonella | | |
| *Collagen-Vascular* (20%) | *Collagen-Vascular* (11%) | *Collagen-Vascular* (15%) |
| Rheumatoid arthritis | Rheumatoid arthritis | Rheumatoid arthritis |
| Vasculitis | Lupus | Rheumatic fever |
| Anaphylactoid purpura | Unclassified | Lupus |
| Lupus erythematosus | | Polyarteritis |
| | | Temporal arteritis |
| | | Wegener's granulomatosis |
| *Neoplastic* (6%) | *Neoplastic* (8%) | *Neoplastic* (20%) |
| Leukemia | Leukemia | Leukemia |
| Lymphoma | Lymphoma | Lymphoma |
| | Neuroblastoma | Multiple myeloma |
| | Reticulum cell sarcoma | Colonic, pancreatic, and renal tumors |
| | | Metastatic disease to bone and liver |

| Miscellaneous | (10%) | Miscellaneous | (10%) | Miscellaneous | (20%) |
|---|---|---|---|---|---|
| Agranulocytosis | | Regional enteritis | | Granulomatous disease | |
| Lamellar ichthyosis | | Thyroiditis | |   Sarcoid | |
| Milk allergy | | Salicylate toxicity | |   Hepatitis | |
| Agammaglobulinemia | | Diencephalic syndrome | | Regional enteritis | |
| Behcet's syndrome | | Dehydration fever | | Ulcerative colitis | |
| Anicteric hepatitis | | Immunodeficiency | | Thrombophlebitis | |
| Ruptured appendix | | | | Factitious fever | |
| Central nervous system | | | | Mediterranean fever | |
|   fever | | | | Cirrhosis | |
| Aspiration pneumonia | | | | Whipple's disease | |

*Physically well children* (9%)

| *Undiagnosed* | (12%) | *Undiagnosed* | (32%) | *Undiagnosed* | (5%) |
|---|---|---|---|---|---|

**6**

## The Diagnostic Evaluation

1. *Initial studies* should be determined by clues provided by the history and physical examination. One must particularly search for a history of recent immunizations, transfusions, travel, exposure to animals, or other sick individuals.

2. *Initial diagnostic procedures* should include a complete blood count, urinalysis, erythrocyte sedimentation rate, chest film, and serum protein electrophoresis in addition to more specific studies indicated from the history and physical examination.

3. If sedimentation rate is elevated, if serum electrophoresis reveals a reversed albumin-globulin ratio or increase in the alpha globulin fraction, or if leukocytosis exists, these should all be considered evidence of an active disease process.

4. If initial studies fail to provide a diagnosis, other useful studies might include:

> Blood cultures, urine cultures, stool cultures
> Liver function tests
> Bone marrow biopsy and culture
> Antinuclear antibodies
> Latex fixation test
> Lupus erythematosus preparations
> Upper gastrointestinal films
> Barium enema
> Intravenous pyelogram
> Bone scan
> Sinus films

5. Ultimately, the diagnosis may require a biopsy of skin, muscle, and/or liver.

6. It is useful to establish an orderly timetable for the pursuit of the diagnosis. All too often the investigation proceeds in an aimless fashion without a logical schedule.

References: Pizzo, P.A., Lovejoy, F.H., Jr., and Smith, D.H.: Pediatrics, 55:468, 1975. McClung, J.: Am. J. Dis. Child., *124*:544, 1972. Jacoby, G.A., and Swarts. M.N.: N. Engl. J. Med., *289*:1407, 1972.

## BACTEREMIA AND FEVER

Nature often works against the pediatrician. One of the clear manifestations of that fact is the finding that the children most likely to have positive blood cultures are those under 2 years of age. These infants, their veins hidden under layers of adiposity, may appear only slightly ill. Of 600 febrile children under 24 months of age studied by Teele and coworkers, 19 were found to be bacteremic, but only two were judged to be sufficiently ill to warrant hospitalization before the culture results were known. Other important observations by this group were:

1. No bacteremic child had a rectal temperature less than 38.9° C (102° F).
2. Fifteen of the 19 bacteremic patients had a total WBC of greater than 15,000/mm³.
3. The pathogen in 15 of the 19 children was pneumococcus.
4. Clinical diagnosis of 14 of the 19 bacteremic children was upper respiratory infection/fever of unknown origin or pneumonia.

Conclusion: Suspect bacteremia in febrile infants under 2 years of age. Increase your suspicion if the child has a fever of greater than 38.9° C, a WBC of greater than 15,000/mm³, and symptoms of upper respiratory infection or pneumonia.

---

Reference: Teele, D.W., Pelton, S.I., Grant, M.J.A., et al.: J. Pediatr., *87*:227, 1975.

## PROLONGED AND/OR RECURRENT FEVER IN MENINGITIS

Persistent or recurrent fever in a child under treatment for meningitis is a common yet distressing problem. Data from two large studies provide reassurance as to its significance. Bacteriologic persistence or relapse is an uncommon cause.

The table below displays the first afebrile day (defined as the first day during which a rectal temperature remained below 100° F/38.6° C) for the common pediatric cerebrospinal fluid pathogens.

*First Afebrile Day in Meningitis*

| ORGANISM | PERCENTAGE OF PATIENTS AFEBRILE BY HOSPITAL DAY | | | | | |
|---|---|---|---|---|---|---|
| | *Hospital Day* | | | | | |
| | 1–3 | 4 | 5 | 6–7 | 8–9 | ≥10 |
| Hemophilus influenzae | 40 | 52 | 59 | 73 | 82 | 100 |
| Neisseria meningitidis | 52 | 68 | 78 | 92 | 94 | 100 |
| Streptococcus pneumoniae | 25 | 44 | 62.5 | 81 | 87.5 | 100 |

Prolonged fever (<10 days) was noted in 9 per cent of children with these and other meningitides. *Persistent infection was not a cause in any case.* Drug fever and nosocomial infection were the most common definable causes. No cause was found in the majority of patients.

Recurrence of fever was found in 24 per cent of the children. No recurrence was due to bacteriologic relapse. *Phlebitis was the single most common cause*, as indicated in the table below.

*Cause of Recurrent Fever in Children with Meningitis*

| | PER CENT |
|---|---|
| Phlebitis | 32 |
| Undetermined | 28 |
| Drug | 19 |
| Viral infection | 19 |
| Urinary tract infection | 2 |
| All causes | 100 |

A word of caution: These date were accumulated prior to the emergence of ampicillin-resistant *Hemophilus influenzae* strains. Infection by such a strain should be ruled out by performing a repeat lumbar puncture 18 to 24 hours after initiating therapy with ampicillin.

References: Lipiridon, O., Lozaridon, S., and Manios, S.: Scand. J. Infect. Dis., 5:23, 1973. Bolagtos, R.C., Levin, S., Nelson, K.E., et al.: J. Pediatr., 77:957, 1970.

# SKIN LESIONS AND PROGNOSIS IN MENINGOCOCCAL INFECTIONS

The presence, type, and location of skin lesions in meningococcal infections can serve as a useful, immediate indicator of prognosis.

The skin manifestations may be of three types:

1. No lesions or other abnormalities.
2. Erythematous, macular, and/or petechial lesions in a generalized distribution over the trunk and extremities.
3. Large purpuric or ecchymotic lesions, usually on the extremities, in association with petechiae.

The clinical manifestations of the disease vary little in groups with no lesions or in those with the generalized macular or petechial eruption, although the incidence of meningitis tends to be increased in those with no skin manifestations.

In contrast, patients with ecchymotic and purpuric lesions have a greater incidence of hyperpyrexia, coagulation abnormalities, shock, and death. The table below illustrates these differences.

*Type of Skin Lesions Related to Various Clinical and Laboratory Factors and Mortality*

| CLINICAL AND LABORATORY FACTORS | SKIN MANIFESTATIONS | |
| --- | --- | --- |
| | *No Lesion or Generalized Macular/Petechial Lesion (%)* | *Peripheral Purpuric/ Ecchymotic Lesion (%)* |
| Meningitis | 54 | 21 |
| Leukocytosis | 85 | 53 |
| Hyperpyrexia | 27 | 57 |
| Shock | 8 | 62 |
| Bleeding diathesis | 7 | 62 |
| Mortality | 3 | 44 |

Reference: Toews, W.H., and Bass, J.W.: Am. J. Dis. Child., *127*:173, 1974.

*"Each generation makes its own accounting to its children."*

Robert F. Kennedy

# GINGIVAL LESIONS AND PNEUMOCOCCAL BACTEREMIA

You can make a presumptive diagnosis of pneumococcal bacteremia in a child with fever and leukocytosis if you find a cystic lesion superimposed on a swollen gingiva. Be sure to look carefully in the mouth of your febrile patient. It could prove to be lifesaving.

Reference: Burech, D.L., Koranyi, K., Haynes, R.E., et al.: Am. J. Dis. Child., *129*:1283, 1975.

# PRESENTATION AND TREATMENT OF OSTEOMYELITIS

The patient seems well, the parents are anxious to have their child at home, and the intern swears that there is not another available vein; but parenteral therapy must continue for one more week. This is the situation that tests the resolve of the physician treating a patient with osteomyelitis. Prompt and prolonged treatment of bone infection is essential if chronic disease is to be avoided.

Osteomyelitis occurs more frequently in males, but shows no racial predilection. A history of trauma may be obtained in about one-third of affected patients. Fever with local tenderness, swelling, and heat are the most frequent presentations. White blood cell count is above 15,000/mm$^3$ in only about 30 per cent, and band counts of greater than 5 per cent are found in less than one-third of patients. The erythrocyte sedimentation rate is rarely normal. Bone destruction is frequently evident on radiographic studies, but radiologic diagnosis is unlikely if infection has been present less than 10 days.

Bacteriologic studies of blood or joint fluid or from the bone itself may indicate the specific pathogen responsible. The most frequent pathogen in all age groups is *Staphylococcus aureus*. Streptococci are the next most frequently isolated bacteria, while *Hemophilus influenzae* may be responsible for disease with relative frequency in children under 2 years of age. A variety of other bacterial agents may cause osteomyelitis, and *Salmonella* is an especially frequent pathogen in patients with sickle cell disease.

*Relapse and chronic disease may result in as many as 20 per cent of patients treated with parenteral antibiotics for less than three weeks.*

Reference: Dich, V.Q., Nelson, J.D., and Haltalin, K.C. Am. J. Dis. Child., *129*:1273, 1975.

# SHIGELLOSIS—THE BAND COUNT—A CLUE TO EARLY DIAGNOSIS

It is often difficult to decide whether patients with diarrhea have bacterial or viral gastroenteritis. The table on page 279 should prove of some value in this decision. The white count and differential may also prove to be a helpful diagnostic test.

Approximately 85 per cent of patients with shigellae in their stools will have more band forms than segmented neutrophils in their peripheral blood smears. In contrast, only 17 to 20 per cent of patients with other forms of infectious diarrhea will display this finding.

Lesson — do not rely on the total white count; always request a differential.

Reference: Poh, S.: Pediatrics, *39*:119, 1967.

## FECAL LEUKOCYTES IN DIARRHEA

The presence (or absence) of leukocytes in a methylene blue stain of stool may help delineate the cause of diarrhea. In general, the presence of fecal leukocytes appears to indicate a disruption of distal intestinal mucosa.

The stain is prepared by spreading a small fleck of diarrhea mucus (or stool, if no mucus in specimen) on a clean glass slide. The mucus or stool is then mixed with two drops of methylene blue and covered with a coverslip. A microscopic examination is performed after a two to three minute delay, which allows for good nuclear staining.

*Diarrheas Associated with Fecal Leukocytes*

| ILLNESS | PREDOMINANT LEUKOCYTE | NUMBER OF LEUKOCYTES PER HIGH POWER FIELD |
| --- | --- | --- |
| *E. coli,* enteropathogenic | Polymorphonuclear | >25 in 68% of patients |
| *Shigella* | Polymorphonuclear | |
| *Salmonella* | | |
| Typhoid | Mononuclear | <3 in over 50% of patients |
| Nontyphoid | Polymorphonuclear | |
| Ulcerative colitis | Polymorphonuclear | >25 |

*Diarrheas not Associated with Fecal Leukocytes*

| | |
| --- | --- |
| *E. coli,* enterotoxigenic | *Giardia lamblia* |
| *Vibrio cholerae* | *Entamoeba histolytica* |
| Viral | "Nonspecific" |

Reference: Harris, J.C., Dupont, H.L., and Hornick, R.B.: Ann. Intern. Med., 76:697, 1972.

## THE PARANASAL SINUSES AND THE MASTOID SINUS

Sinusitis is underdiagnosed in infants and children (also frequently misspelled sinisitis, as well). Sinusitis is seen with increased frequency in patients with cyanotic heart disease, in leukemia and aplastic anemia while patients are neutropenic, in cystic fibrosis, and in patients with a history of nasal allergies.

It is useful to remember the ages at which the sinuses are pneumatized. Once a true sinus is present, the possibility of infection exists.

| Sinuses present at birth | Anterior and posterior *ethmoid*. Maxillary antra. |
| Two to four years | Pneumatization of *frontal* sinuses begins — complete by 5 to 9 years of age. *Sphenoid* sinus becomes visible by age 3. |

The *mastoid antrum* is present at birth, and pneumatization of the temporal bone starts in early infancy. The *mastoid process* is not present at birth, but begins to grow during the first year. Pneumatization is a slow, irregular process, but is generally complete prior to adolescence.

**6**

# BACTERIAL INFECTION AND THE WBC

Elevated total white counts frequently provide evidence for bacterial infection. Data now show that the absolute number of neutrophils or neutrophil precursors/mm$^3$ (percentage neutrophils or bands X total WBC/mm$^3$) may more accurately predict infection. Eighty per cent of patients presenting with an absolute band count greater than 500/mm$^3$ or an absolute neutrophil count greater than 10,000/mm$^3$, or both, will have a bacterial infection. The nature of the bacterial infection may also be inferred from analysis of neutrophil values.

| NEUTROPHIL COUNT | BAND COUNT | |
| --- | --- | --- |
| | >500 | <500 |
| >10,000 | Either gram-positive or gram-negative | Gram-positive |
| <10,000 | Gram-negative | Infection less likely |

The absence of the above values should not be used to exclude infection in a child whose clinical picture indicates its presence, and treatment should not be based on these criteria alone. Commonly, children with osteomyelitis, septic arthritis, or lymphangitis due to streptococcal or staphylococcal infections will have total neutrophil counts that fall within the normal range.

*Pertussis*—From the Latin *per*, meaning intensive, and *tussis*, or cough.

The blood smear may also provide evidence for bacterial infection. Toxic granules and Döhle bodies are often seen, but vacuolization of the neutrophils is most specific for bacterial infection.

Some bacterial infections present with unusual WBC pictures:

| DISEASE | CHARACTERISTIC WBC PICTURE | COMMENTS |
| --- | --- | --- |
| Tuberculosis, typhoid fever, and para-typhoid fever | Absence of leukocytosis and neutrophilia | Presence of neutrophilia is suggestive of complications or localization, such as tuberculous meningitis |
| Scarlet fever and brucellosis | Eosinophilia | |
| Pertussis | Absolute lymphocytosis; 75 per cent of children will have absolute lymphocyte count $> 10,000/mm^3$ | Total WBC count may vary from leukocytosis and is not very helpful; adenovirus infections, which mimic pertussis, can also produce high WBC counts with absolute lymphocytosis |
| Shigellosis | 85 per cent of children with shigellosis will have more band forms than neutrophils | Stool examination for leukocytes is helpful; children with *Shigella, Salmonella,* and invasive *Escherichia coli* gastroenteritis often exhibit fecal neutrophils, whereas children with viral diarrhea, noninvasive toxigenic *E. coli* diarrhea, and diarrhea secondary to parasites rarely exhibit fecal leukocytes |

The WBC count and differential may be less useful when it is altered by drugs or noninfectious conditions.

| CONDITION | EFFECT ON PERIPHERAL WBC PICTURE | COMMENTS |
| --- | --- | --- |
| Epinephrine adminis-tration, stress, or strenuous activity | Leukocytosis and increased absolute number of neutro-phils; no shift to left | Changes in WBC picture occur within minutes |
| Corticosteroid administration, Cushing's syndrome | Leukocytosis and increased absolute number of neutro-phils; shift to left occurs with eosinopenia | Changes in WBC picture occur within 4 hours of oral corti-costeroid administration and return to normal within 24 hours of administration of last dose |
| Addison's disease or panhypopituitarism | Neutropenia, eosinophilia, lymphocytosis | |
| Diabetic ketoacidosis | Leukocytosis as high as $25,000/mm^3$ with increased absolute neutrophil count and shift to left | |
| Burns, operation, crush injuries, fractures, neoplasms | Leukocytosis, increased absolute neutrophil count, and shift to left | |

| Acute hemorrhage | Leukocytosis, increased absolute neutrophil count, and shift to left | Leukocytosis and shift to left are greater if bleeding is against serous membrane than if it is external |
| --- | --- | --- |
| Acute hemolysis | Leukocytosis, increased absolute neutrophil count, and shift to left | Children with sickle cell anemia, erythroblastosis fetalis, auto-immune hemolytic anemia, or any other hemolytic process often exhibit profound leukocytosis and shift to left in absence of infection |

Reference: Weitzman, M.: Am. J. Dis. Child., *129*:1183, 1975.

**6**

# THE ATYPICAL LYMPHOCYTE

Atypical lymphocytes do not always mean that the patient has infectious mononucleosis. Do not forget to consider some of the other diseases listed below.

More than 20 per cent of the white blood cells may be atypical lymphocytes in:
Infectious mononucleosis
Viral hepatitis
The "post-transfusion" syndrome
PAS hypersensitivity
Dilantin and Mesantoin hypersensitivity
Cytomegalovirus

Less than 20 per cent of the white blood cells are atypical lymphocytes in:
Infections
Mumps
Varicella
Rubeola
Rubella
"Primary atypical pneumonia"
Herpes simplex
Herpes zoster
Roseola infantum
Influenza
Mycoplasma
Nonspecific upper respiratory infection
Many other viral illnesses
Tuberculosis
Rickettsialpox
Radiation
Other
Letterer-Siwe disease
Agranulocytosis
Lead intoxication
Stress

Uncommon causes of atypical lymphocytosis:
    Tertiary syphilis
    Congenital syphilis
    Smallpox
    Bullis fever
    Tetrachlorethane poisoning
    TNT poisoning
    Organic arsenical hypersensitivity
    Severe dermatitis herpetiformis

Reference: Modified from Wood, T.A., and Frenkel, E.P.: Am. J. Med., *42*:929, 1967.

## USE OF THE SINGLE SEROLOGIC TEST

There are only a few inflammatory or infectious illnesses in which the physician may escape the incessant plea of the infectious disease consultants for "convalescent serum." These are conditions in which a single antibody titer may be so high as to be virtually diagnostic or in which the presence of any antibody is abnormal.

*Serologic Tests in which Testing a Single Serum May be Useful*

VDRL
Histoplasmosis titer (by complement fixation)
Heterophil/rapid mononucleosis slide test
Toxoplasmosis dye titer
Rubella titer (by hemagglutination inhibition)
Antinuclear antibody (abnormal if present)
Hepatitis-B antigen
Rheumatoid factor (abnormal if present)
Aspergillus precipitin titer
Trichina bentonite flocculation

Reference: Modified from Moffett, H.L.: Pediatric Infectious Diseases. Philadelphia, J.B. Lippincott Company, 1975, p. 379.

## PARASITES

"Stool for ova and parasites" is often ordered with little thought given to the possible parasitic pathogen in a given clinical situation. Parasitic disease is much less frequent in the United States than in most of the rest of the world, but the pediatrician should be familiar with parasites that may be encountered here and abroad.

The table on the following pages lists parasites that are likely to be encountered in the United States. Some, such as the plasmodia and the tapeworms, are included because of the frequency with which they are found in U.S. citizens who travel abroad or in immigrants from other countries. Treatment regimens are not listed because of the frequency with which treatment recommendations change.

6

| NAME OF PARASITE | ROUTE OF ENTRY INTO HUMAN BODY | MECHANISM OF INFECTION | CLINICAL MANIFESTATIONS | METHOD OF DIAGNOSIS |
|---|---|---|---|---|
| *Enterobius vermicularis* (pinworm) | Patient acquires eggs from skin during scratching and transfers them to mouth. Eggs may also be swallowed when inhaled while handling clothes and bedclothes of infected individuals. | Worm inhabits the rectum or colon and emerges onto perianal skin during sleep, causing intense itching. | No systemic manifestations. | Application of transparent adhesive tape to perianal skin and inspection of tape under microscope. |
| *Ascaris lumbricoides* (roundworm) | Acquired through ingestion of eggs found in soil contaminated with human feces. | Inhabits the small intestine. Larvae penetrate intestinal villi, enter portal circulation, proceed to lungs. They ascend to oropharynx where they are swallowed, and they inhabit the small intestine and mature to adult worms. | May be asymptomatic. May have fever, malaise, eosinophilia. Large number of worms may cause intestinal obstruction. May migrate to appendix, perforate, and cause peritonitis. | Detection of ova in the stool. |
| *Toxocara canis* (dog roundworm) | Acquired through ingestion of eggs found in soil contaminated with dog feces. | Larvae hatched in small intestine, migrate aimlessly through tissue (thus the disease is called visceral larva migrans). | Eosinophilia to 50 per cent of the white blood count. Larvae may enter central nervous system, eye, lung, liver, and so on. | Detection of larvae in liver biopsy and/or high titers of human isohemagglutinins. |
| *Necator americanus* and *Ancylostoma duodenale* (hookworm) | Eggs are deposited with stool and become larvae, which penetrate human skin and enter the blood stream. They pass through the lungs to the pharynx where they are swallowed. | Adult worms inhabit small intestine and feed on the villi. | Anemia, hypoproteinemia, malnutrition. | Detection of ova in the stool. |

| NAME OF PARASITE | ROUTE OF ENTRY INTO HUMAN BODY | MECHANISM OF INFECTION | CLINICAL MANIFESTATIONS | METHOD OF DIAGNOSIS |
|---|---|---|---|---|
| *Giardia lamblia* | Cyst is ingested in water contaminated by human feces. | Inhabit the duodenum. | May be asymptomatic. May cause protracted, severe diarrhea with fever and weight loss. | Detection of trophozoite or cysts in the stool. Stool examination should be done multiply. Examination of duodenal fluid may be required. |
| *Taenia saginata* and *Taenia solium* (tapeworm) | Ingested head (scolex) from poorly cooked beef or pork establishes itself in the small intestine. | Generated segments (proglottids) increase length of worm. The proglottid is regurgitated into the stomach and may lead to migration and formation of cysts in the brain or eye. | Cramps, pain. | Detection of proglottids or ova in the stool. |
| *Echinococcus granulosus* (dog tapeworm) | Ingestion of eggs contained in dog feces. | Cysts form in liver, lung, and elsewhere. | Cysts act as space-occupying lesions and, if ruptured, may lead to metastatic cysts. | Casoni skin test. Serologic tests. |
| *Entamoeba histolytica* | Cysts contained in human feces are ingested in contaminated food or water. | Excystation allows deposit of trophozoites in the colonic mucosa. | May be asymptomatic. May cause protracted colitis. Infrequently leads to hepatic abscess, lung or skin infections. | Detection of trophozoites or cysts in stool. Serologic tests. |
| *Strongyloides stercoralis* | Larvae enter the human skin from contaminated soil. Larvae hatched in patient's intestine may reinfect the same patient via penetration of the intestinal wall and travel through the blood stream. | Inhabits the small intestinal mucosa. | May be asymptomatic. May cause protracted mucoid diarrhea and malabsorption. | Detection of larvae in stool. |

**6**

| Organism | Life cycle / Transmission | Pathology | Clinical features | Diagnosis |
|---|---|---|---|---|
| *Trichuris trichiura* | Eggs deposited in soil are ingested. Larvae hatch in the small intestine and migrate to the cecum and large intestine. | Inhabits large intestine. The anterior end is buried in the mucosa. | Usually asymptomatic. No eosinophilia. With heavy infection there may be diarrhea and tenesmus. | Detection of ova in stool. |
| *Trichinella spiralis* | Larvae encysted in skeletal muscle of pork or bear. They mature in the small intestine. Larvae pass to the lungs, are shunted to the left side of the heart and the systemic circulation. | Migrating larvae lodge in muscle and sometimes in central nervous system. | Gastroenteritis, periorbital edema, myositis, petechial hemorrhages, fever, eosinophilia. | Skin test, serology, appropriate history. |
| *Schistosoma mansoni* | Larvae emerge into water from infected snail. The larvae penetrate human skin and proceed to liver sinusoids. They grow there and migrate to venules throughout the body. | Larvae obstruct the portal circulation. Granulomas are formed in any tissue in which worms are embedded. | Fibrosis of liver, lung; circulatory obstruction, cor pulmonale, pseudopolyps of bladder, neurologic manifestations. | Detection of ova in stool or urine. May have to be done often, since relatively few eggs reach intestinal lumen. |
| *Plasmodium falciparum,* *Plasmodium malariae* | Parasite enters human blood stream via bite of a female anopheline mosquito. Parasite may also be transferred to a patient who receives blood from an infected donor. | Parasites mature in the liver for up to two weeks. They are then able to infect erythrocytes and additional hepatocytes. | Fever during erythrocyte infection. Musculoskeletal pain, headache, diarrhea, anemia. *P. falciparum* may cause hemoglobinuria, coma, convulsions, death. "Induced" malaria contracted from infected blood donor has no erythrocyte phase. Fever is only manifestation. | Detection of parasites in erythrocytes on usual blood smear or "thick smear." |

| NAME OF PARASITE | ROUTE OF ENTRY INTO HUMAN BODY | MECHANISM OF INFECTION | CLINICAL MANIFESTATIONS | METHOD OF DIAGNOSIS |
|---|---|---|---|---|
| *Pneumocystis carinii* | Person to person contact (?). Asymptomatic carriers (?). | Patients affected are immuno-suppressed, have primary immune deficiency or malignancy. | Dyspnea, fever, unproductive cough, tachycardia, tachypnea, mild anemia. Chest roentgenogram shows bilateral diffuse or patchy interstitial infiltrates. | Lung biopsy, bronchial washings, tracheal aspirate. |
| *Toxoplasma gondii* | Acquired: ingestion of raw or poorly cooked meat. Contact with oocysts via cat feces. | Parasite invades host tissues. Usually localized to lymph nodes, but may invade brain, heart, lung, liver, and muscle in immuno-suppressed host. | Clinically evident infection is rare. Lymphadenopathy is usually the only symptom. Immunosuppressed patient may have generalized involvement with hepatitis, pneumonitis, pericarditis, myocarditis, meningo-encephalitis. | Serologic tests. |
| | Congenital: infection acquired trans-placentally. | Congenital infection is generalized. Infant is more severely affected with acquisition in late gestation. | Hepatosplenomegaly, enlarged lymph nodes, myocarditis, anemia, edema, exudates in the body cavities. The eye is usually involved with white scars visible on the fundus. There may be intracerebral calcifications, hydro-cephalus, convulsions. | |

References: Katz, M.: J. Pediatr., *87:*165, 1975. Beverley, J.K.A.: Bri. Med. J., *2:*475, 1973. Walzer, P.D., Perl, D.P., Krogstad, D.J., et al.: Ann. Intern. Med., *80:*83, 1974.

# ANIMALS AS DISEASE SOURCE

It is 4:00 A.M. You are just completing an admission note on a child with a confusing constellation of signs and symptoms. Suddenly, the third year student announces that he has learned that the child recently returned from a summer at a grandmother's goat farm and that several of the goats were ill.

The accompanying table may help you to handle such situations constructively by suggesting or ruling out various zoonoses once a careful environmental history has been obtained.

*Potential Host Distribution of Selected Zoonoses*

6

Column groups: **DOMESTIC ANIMALS** = Horses, Cattle, Sheep, Goats, Swine, Dogs, Cats, Lab rodents, Poultry. **WILD ANIMALS** = Invertebrates, Fish, Amphibians, Reptiles, Birds, and **MAMMALS** = Rodents, Primates, Carnivores, Ungulates, Other.

| Disease | Horses | Cattle | Sheep | Goats | Swine | Dogs | Cats | Lab rodents | Poultry | Invertebrates | Fish | Amphibians | Reptiles | Birds | Rodents | Primates | Carnivores | Ungulates | Other |
|---|---|---|---|---|---|---|---|---|---|---|---|---|---|---|---|---|---|---|---|
| **VIRUS DISEASES** | | | | | | | | | | | | | | | | | | | |
| Arbovirus encephalitis | X | X | X | X | X | | | | | X | X | | X | X | X | | X | X | |
| Cat-scratch disease (virus suspected) | | | | | | | X | | | | | | | | | | X | | |
| Lymphocytic choriomeningitis | | | | | | | | X | X | | | | | | X | | | | |
| Newcastle | | | | | | | | | X | | | | | X | | | | | |
| Rabies | X | X | X | X | X | X | X | X | X | | | | | | X | X | X | X | X |
| Vesicular stomatitis | X | X | | | X | | | | | X | | | | | | | | | |
| Yellow Fever | | | | | | | | | | X | | | | | X | X | | | X |
| **RICKETTSIAL DISEASES** | | | | | | | | | | | | | | | | | | | |
| Q fever | | X | X | X | | | | | | | | | | | X | X | | | |
| Rocky Mountain spotted fever | | X | X | | | | | | | X | | X | | | X | | | | |
| **SPIROCHETAL DISEASES** | | | | | | | | | | | | | | | | | | | |
| Leptospirosis | X | X | X | X | X | X | X | X | | | | | | | X | X | X | X | X |
| Rat-bite fever | | | | | | X | X | | | | | | | | X | X | | | |
| **BACTERIAL DISEASE** | | | | | | | | | | | | | | | | | | | |
| Anthrax | X | X | X | X | X | X | X | X | X | | | | | | X | X | X | X | X |
| Brucellosis | X | X | X | X | X | X | X | X | X | | | | | | | X | X | X | X |
| Erysipelas | | | | | | | X | | X | X | | X | | | X | X | | | |
| Hemorrhagic septicemia | X | X | X | X | X | X | X | X | X | X | | | | | | | | | |
| Listeriosis | X | X | X | X | X | X | | | | X | | | | | X | X | X | | |
| Melioidosis | X | X | X | X | X | X | X | X | | | | | | | X | | | | |
| Plague | | | X | X | | X | X | X | | | | | | | X | X | X | | X |
| Pseudotuberculosis | | | X | X | X | X | | | | X | X | | | | | | | | |
| Psittacosis | | | | | | | | | | X | | | | | X | | | | |
| Salmonellosis | X | X | X | X | X | X | X | X | X | X | X | X | X | X | X | X | X | X | X |
| Scarlet fever | | X | | | | X | | | | | | | | | | | | | |
| Septic sore throat | | X | | | | | | | | | | | | | | | | | |
| Staphylococcosis | | X | | | | | | | | | | | | | | | | | |
| Tetanus | X | | | | | | | | | | | X | | | | | X | | |
| Tuberculosis | X | X | X | X | X | X | X | X | X | X | | X | | | X | | X | X | X |
| Tularemia | | X | X | X | X | X | X | | | | | | | | X | X | X | X | X |
| Vibriosis | | X | X | X | | | | | | | | | | | | | | | |
| **FUNGUS DISEASES** | | | | | | | | | | | | | | | | | | | |
| Actinomycosis | X | X | X | X | X | X | X | | | | | | | | X | | X | X | X |
| Aspergillosis | X | X | X | X | X | | X | X | | | | | | | X | | | | |

| | DOMESTIC ANIMALS | | | | | | | | | WILD ANIMALS | | | | | MAMMALS | | | | |
|---|---|---|---|---|---|---|---|---|---|---|---|---|---|---|---|---|---|---|---|
| | Horses | Cattle | Sheep | Goats | Swine | Dogs | Cats | Lab rodents | Poultry | Invertebrates | Fish | Amphibians | Reptiles | Birds | Rodents | Primates | Carnivores | Ungulates | Other |
| Coccidioidomycosis | X | X | X | X | X | X | | | | | | | | | X | X | X | X | |
| Cryptococcosis | X | X | X | X | X | X | X | | | X | | | | X | | X | X | X | |
| Epizootic lymphangitis | X | | | | | | | | | | | | | | | | | | |
| Histoplasmosis | X | X | X | X | X | X | X | X | X | X | | | | | X | X | X | | X |
| Nocardiosis | X | X | X | X | X | X | X | | | | | | | | | X | | | X |
| North American blastomycosis | X | | | | | X | | | | | | | | | | | | | |
| Rhinosporidiosis | X | X | | | | | | | | | | | | | | | | | |
| Ringworm | X | X | X | X | X | X | X | X | X | X | | | | | X | X | X | X | X |
| Sporotrichosis | X | X | | | | X | | X | | | | | | | | | | | |
| Streptothricosis | X | X | X | X | | X | | | | | | | | | | | | X | |
| **PROTOZOAN** | | | | | | | | | | | | | | | | | | | |
| Amebiasis | | | | | | | | | | | | | | | | X | | | |
| Balantidiasis | | | | | X | | | | | | | | | | | X | | | |
| Leishmaniasis | | | | | | X | | | | | | | | | X | | X | | |
| Plasmodium (malaria) | | | | | | | | | | | | | | | | X | | | |
| Sarcocystis | X | X | X | X | | X | | | | | | | | | X | | | | X |
| Toxoplasmosis | | X | | | | X | X | X | | | | | | | X | X | | X | X |
| Trypanosomiasis | X | X | X | X | X | X | X | X | | X | | | | | | | | X | X |

Reference: Fowler, M.E.: Curr. Probl. Pediatr., *4*:3, 1974.

# RABIES: PROPHYLAXIS OR NOT

The question of rabies prophylaxis for animal bite victims involves balancing the risk of treatment complications against the risk of rabies in the exposed individual.

Initial management of a patient bitten by an animal should include:

1. Flushing the wound with copious amounts of a quaternary ammonium compound such as Zephiran (after rinsing off soap).
2. Appropriate surgical wound care.
3. Capture of the animal for observation or for sacrifice and fluorescent antibody study of brain.

Figure 6–1 provides an algorithmic approach to the prophylaxis question; the subsequent table suggests specifics of prophylaxis should this appear necessary.

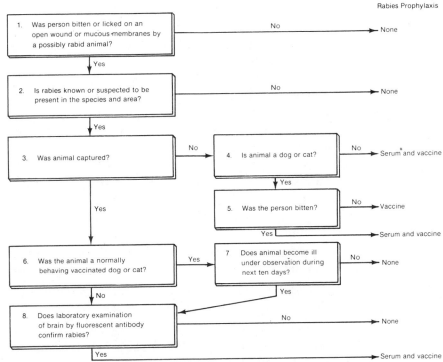

Rabies Prophylaxis

1. Was person bitten or licked on an open wound or mucous membranes by a possibly rabid animal? — No → None

2. Is rabies known or suspected to be present in the species and area? — No → None

3. Was animal captured? — No → 4. Is animal a dog or cat? — No → Serum and vaccine

4. Is animal a dog or cat? — Yes → 5. Was the person bitten? — No → Vaccine; Yes → Serum and vaccine

6. Was the animal a normally behaving vaccinated dog or cat? — Yes → 7. Does animal become ill under observation during next ten days? — No → None; Yes →

8. Does laboratory examination of brain by fluorescent antibody confirm rabies? — No → None; Yes → Serum and vaccine

*FIG. 6–1*

Postexposure rabies prophylaxis algorithm.

## *Postexposure Antirabies Guide*

| SPECIES | CONDITION | TREATMENT AND EXPOSURE | |
| --- | --- | --- | --- |
| | | *For Bite* | *For Nonbite* |
| *Wild* | | | |
| Skunk | Regard as rabid | S-V-1 | S-V-1 |
| Fox | Regard as rabid | S-V-1 | S-V-1 |
| Raccoon | Regard as rabid | S-V-1 | S-V-1 |
| Bat | Regard as rabid | S-V-1 | S-V-1 |
| *Domestic* | | | |
| Dog | Healthy | None-2 | None-2 |
| | Escaped (unknown) | S-V | V-3 |
| Cat | Rabid | S-V-1 | S-V-1 |
| *Other* | Consider individually | | |

S = antirabies serum; V = rabies vaccine.

1. Discontinue vaccine if fluorescent antibody tests of animal killed at time of attack are negative.

2. Begin S and V at first sign of rabies in biting dog or cat during 10-day observation period.

3. Fourteen doses of duck embryo vaccine.

Reference: Corey, L., and Hattwick, M.A.W.: J.A.M.A., *232*:272, 1975.

# BONE MARROW BIOPSY IN DIAGNOSIS OF GRANULOMATOUS DISORDERS

Needle biopsy of the bone marrow employing either the Vim-Silverman or Westerman-Jensen needle makes it possible to obtain a core of bone and its enclosed marrow. A bone marrow aspirate can be obtained through the biopsy needle before performing the marrow biopsy. This procedure has virtually eliminated the need for open surgical trephine biopsy.

The needle biopsy is particularly useful for the rapid diagnosis of a variety of granulomatous disorders. A granuloma consists of a nodule of macrophages that have enlarged to form epithelioid cells, surrounded by a rim of lymphocytes. In some instances they also may be surrounded by eosinophils and plasma cells. Granulomas may be observed in the bone marrow in miliary tuberculosis, disseminated histoplasmosis, infectious mononucleosis, sarcoidosis, brucellosis, and lymphomas. Unless a specific organism can be identified by special stains or by bacteriologic culture, there are no diagnostic features of a granuloma characteristic of a specific disorder. Prominent caseous necrosis does favor the diagnosis of tuberculosis or histoplasmosis. The following facts may help you in deciding to request this procedure:

Bone marrow biopsies and cultures are diagnostic in *miliary tuberculosis* in 15 to 40 per cent of patients. Only liver biopsy provides a higher yield in this disease.

Bone marrow cultures are positive in 60 to 75 per cent of patients with *disseminated histoplasmosis*. This is a higher yield than is obtained with blood and sputum cultures. Organisms may be quickly identified with special stains.

In approximately 20 per cent of patients with *sarcoidosis*, the bone marrow contains granuloma.

Reference: Ellman, L.: Am. J. Med., *60*:1, 1976.

# INFECTION FROM PERIPHERAL INTRAVENOUS CATHETERS

An indwelling intravenous (IV) cannula always carries the risk of infection. As judged by positive cannula-tip cultures, infection risk is similar for "scalp vein" and plastic or Teflon cannulae after 48 hours "in situ." Scalp vein needles are somewhat less infection prone within the first 48 hours. Patients with malignant diseases are at a greater risk of catheter-associated infection.

Observance of the following guidelines will help minimize the risk of cannula-associated infections in your patients.

1. Prepare the IV site as if for a blood culture.
2. Use scalp vein needles when possible.
3. Inspect site for phlebitis daily.
4. If local inflammation, unexplained fever, or signs of sepsis appear, change IV site and culture tip of cannula as well as performing other clinically indicated cultures.
5. Change to new site at least every 48 hours.

References: Collin, J., Constable, F.L., Collin, C., et al.: Lancet, *2*:150, 1975. Feld, R., Leers, W.D., Curtis, J.E., et al.: Med. Pediatr. Oncol., *1*:175, 1975. Maki, D.G., Drink, P.J., and Davis, T.E.: N. Engl. J. Med., *292*:1116, 1975.

# 7

# ALLERGY/ IMMUNOLOGY

# APPROACH TO IMMUNODEFICIENCY

Initial evaluation of the child with frequent or unusual infections is within the capability of any pediatrician and almost any hospital laboratory. Your approach may be streamlined by the use of the following guidelines.

A. Frequent mild respiratory infections without complications (up to 14 per year may be normal) are usually *not* suggestive of immunologic deficit. These are especially common in the preschool child and tend to decrease with age. Similarly, pneumonias that recur (or persist) at a single anatomic site are not likely to be due to immunodeficiency.

B. Several patterns of illness *are* suggestive of immune defect:
   1. Family history positive for immunologic problems, lymphoproliferative disorders, or autoimmune disease.
   2. Recurrent infections caused by bacteria of high-grade virulence.
   3. Those caused by bacteria that are ordinarily nonpathogens.
   4. Those caused by fungi.
   5. Unusual reaction to live vaccine or to ordinarily mild viral illnesses.
   6. Infections at unusual sites.
   7. Infections that persist or that resolve unusually slowly.

C. Many patterns of infection that initially appear to suggest immunodeficiency may be explainable on a nonimmunologic basis, such as:
   1. Mechanical or other host factors:
      a. CNS: e.g., cranial or dermal sinuses, neurenteric cysts, posttraumatic skull defect.
      b. Respiratory tract: e.g.,, tracheoesophageal fistula, foreign body, cystic fibrosis.
      c. Urinary tract: e.g., neurogenic bladder, posterior urethral valves, urethral stenosis.
      d. Secondary immunodeficiencies: e.g., malnutrition, malignant diseases, drugs.
      e. Miscellaneous conditions favoring infection, e.g., diabetes mellitus, congenital heart disease, burns, indwelling catheters, eczema, sickle cell anemia, trisomy-21.

   *or by*

   2. Microbiologic factors:
      a. Inadequately treated infections: e.g., incorrect drug, incorrect dose, occult abscess.
      b. Repeated exposure to pathogens: e.g., streptococcal carrier in family.
      c. Unusual resistance of common organism: e.g., ampicillin-resistant *Hemophilus influenzae.*
      d. Presence of unidentified (and therefore untreated) organism.

D. If the preceding points have been considered and an immunodeficiency is still being sought, the following table provides clinical clues and suggestions for *screening* tests in each area of host defense.

7

| TYPE OF DEFICIT (AND RELATIVE FREQUENCY) | LIKELY PATHOGENS OR PROBLEMS | HISTORY AND PHYSICAL EXAMINATION CLUES | SCREENING TESTS AND EXPECTED RESULTS |
|---|---|---|---|
| T cell (5%) | Viruses, fungi, protozoans, autoimmunity, surveillance against malignancy | Growth failure, vaccinial scar, ataxia-telangiectasia, absence of lymph nodes | 1. Lymphocyte count low ($<1200$) 2. Lymphocyte morphology may be abnormal 3. Absence of thymic shadow on infant roentgenogram 4. No response to standard anergy tests |
| Combined T and B cell (25%) | | Features of T cell (above) and B cell (below) both occur in the combined immunodeficiency | |
| B cell (50–75%) | Severe bacterial infections | Usually well until 5 to 6 months, then: growth failure, eczema, petechiae, arthritis, absence of lymph nodes | 1. Decrease in hemoglobin common 2. Decrease in level of one or more immunoglobulins 3. Absence of expected specific antibodies, e.g., ASO, isohemagglutinins 4. Decreased platelet count in Wiskott-Aldrich 5. Plasma cells in bone marrow or periphery, if present, suggest *some* B cell function |
| Phagocytes (1%) | Recurrent bacterial infections and/or abscesses | Mouth ulcers, impalpable spleen, abscesses, draining sinuses | 1. Abnormal appearance and/or low number of neutrophils. Repeat weekly for one month if cyclic neutropenia is considered 2. Howell-Jolly bodies 3. Low NBT in some defects |
| Complement (1%) | Recurrent bacterial infections and/or abscesses; auto-immune disease | Mouth ulcers, abscesses, impalpable spleen, draining sinuses | 1. Low $C_3$ 2. Low $CH_{50}$ |

References: Norman, M.E., and South, M.A.: Clin. Pediatr., *13*:644, 1974. Ammann, A.J., and Wara, D.W.: Curr. Probl. Pediatr., Vol. 5, 1975.

# CHRONIC GRANULOMATOUS DISEASE (CGD) OF CHILDHOOD

What are its manifestations and what are the organisms that produce most of the problems?

## Signs and Symptoms

| FINDING | PER CENT OF PATIENTS |
|---|---|
| Marked lymphadenopathy | 92 |
| Pneumonitis | 87 |
| Male sex | 87 |
| Suppuration of nodes | 86 |
| Hepatomegaly | 84 |
| Dermatitis | 84 |
| Onset of signs by 1 year of age | 78 |
| Splenomegaly | 74 |
| Hepatic-perihepatic abscess | 45 |
| Death before age 7 years | 37 |
| Osteomyelitis | 33 |
| Onset with dermatitis | 30 |
| Onset with lymphadenitis | 30 |
| Persistent rhinitis | 25 |
| Conjunctivitis | 23 |
| Persistent diarrhea | 22 |
| Perianal abscess | 18 |
| Ulcerative stomatitis | 16 |

## Infecting Organisms

Most organisms that produce infections in patients with CGD are catalase-positive and are capable of destroying their own hydrogen peroxide, thus protecting themselves.

Common bacterial infecting agents, in order of frequency, include:

*Staphylococcus aureus*
*Klebsiella-Aerobacter* organisms
*Escherichia coli*
*Staphylococcus albus*
*Serratia marcesans*
*Pseudomonas* and *Proteus* species
*Salmonella* organisms
*Paracolobactrum* organisms

Fungal agents that also produce disease include:

*Candida albicans*
*Aspergillus* organisms
*Nocardia* organisms
*Actinomyces*

Note that pneumococci, beta-hemolytic streptococci, and *Hemophilus influenzae* do not cause infections in these patients with increased frequency.

Reference: Johnston, R.B., Jr., and Baehner, R.L.: Pediatrics, *48*:733, 1971.

# TESTING FOR DELAYED HYPERSENSITIVITY

Skin testing for delayed hypersensitivity is becoming more and more common as patients are evaluated for possible immunologic defects. Interpretation of such tests has been hampered by the fact that many apparently normal children are anergic. The table below provides some figures on the percentage of positive reactions, of varying sizes, in patients of different ages, employing four different skin testing agents.

| | No. | CANDIDA ALBICANS | | | | | DIPHTHERIA-TETANUS | | | | | MUMPS | | | | | SK/SD | | | | |
| --- | --- | --- | --- | --- | --- | --- | --- | --- | --- | --- | --- | --- | --- | --- | --- | --- | --- | --- | --- | --- | --- |
| | | Induration† | | | Erythema† | | Induration | | | Erythema | | Induration | | | Erythema | | Induration | | | Erythema | |
| | | ≥2 | ≥5 | ≥10 | ≥10 | ≥15 | ≥2 | ≥5 | ≥10 | ≥10 | ≥15 | ≥2 | ≥5 | ≥10 | ≥10 | ≥15 | ≥2 | ≥5 | ≥10 | ≥10 | ≥15 |
| Newborn infant | 2 | 0 | 0 | 0 | 0 | 0 | 0 | 0 | 0 | 0 | 0 | 0 | 0 | 0 | 0 | 0 | 0 | 0 | 0 | 0 | 0 |
| 0–6 mo | 18 | 27 | 5 | 0 | 0 | 0 | 53* | 7 | 0 | 15 | 0 | 100 | 61 | 0 | 44 | 16 | 8 | 0 | 0 | 0 | 0 |
| 7–12 mo | 14 | 50 | 42 | 7 | 21 | 7 | 100 | 50 | 0 | 28 | 7 | 100 | 84 | 0 | 76 | 53 | 7 | 0 | 0 | 0 | 0 |
| 1–5 yr | 26 | 65 | 46 | 3 | 23 | 3 | 88* | 73 | 3 | 42 | 19 | 100 | 92 | 7 | 88 | 53 | 20 | 16 | 7 | 20 | 16 |
| 6–10 yr | 18 | 66 | 50 | 22 | 44 | 16 | 100 | 88 | 16 | 50 | 16 | 100 | 100 | 50 | 100 | 94 | 51 | 55 | 33 | 50 | 44 |
| 11–15 yr | 19 | 63 | 47 | 15 | 36 | 15 | 100 | 73 | 21 | 68 | 36 | 100 | 100 | 31 | 84 | 74 | 73 | 73 | 63 | 73 | 68 |
| 16–20 yr | 17 | 88 | 76 | 23 | 70 | 35 | 88* | 82 | 23 | 58 | 41 | 100 | 94 | 11 | 82 | 82 | 82 | 76 | 76 | 82 | 64 |

*Includes patients not receiving DPT immunization.
†Induration and erythema expressed in millimeters.

The following reagents were used:

1. Oidiomycin (*Candida albicans*) 1/100 (Hollister-Stier).
2. Mumps skin test antigen – undiluted (Eli Lilly).
3. Streptokinase/streptodornase – diluted with buffered saline to 40 units SK and 10 units SD/ml (Lederle).
4. Diphtheria and tetanus toxoids, adsorbed (pediatric DT) – diluted 1/100 with buffered saline (Dow).

Reference: Franz, M.L., Carella, J.A., and Galant, S.P.: J. Pediatr., *88*:975, 1976.

# THE FUNGAL SKIN TEST— A DIAGNOSTIC HINDRANCE

7

A common error of clinical practice is the reliance on a fungal skin test to make a diagnosis of an acute fungal infection. Test results are misleading. The following points should be remembered.

1. *Cross reactions* can occur because of shared antigens.
2. *Elevations of antibody titers* may be produced by the introduction of small amounts of antigen via the intradermal route.
3. *False-negative skin test* reactions are very common during the acute phase of fungal infections.

Measuring changes in complement-fixing antibodies is of far greater significance in establishing a diagnosis in patients suspected of having coccidioidomycosis, histoplasmosis, or blastomycosis. A titer of 1:16 or greater should be considered as presumptive evidence of a recent infection with one of these agents and should result in intensive efforts to isolate the organism by culture of sputum, urine, bone marrow, or other body fluids.

*Blastomycin*, as a skin test antigen, may elevate histoplasmosis antibodies and usually produces a negative result in patients with active blastomycosis.

*Histoplasmin* can elevate the complement-fixing antibody titer to histoplasmin, and will produce elevations of antibody titer to blastomycin as well.

*Coccidioidin* is the most specific of the skin test antigens but frequently may be negative during the acute phase of the illness.

These three skin tests should not be applied in the evaluation of patients with fevers of undetermined origin. These skin tests can be of more value as prognostic indicators in patients with culture-proved fungal disease, as epidemiologic tools in community studies, as antigens for in vivo determination of cellular immunity, and as indicators of past fungal exposure in patients in whom immunosuppressive therapy is to be instituted.

Reference: Levin, S.J.: J. Infect. Dis., *122*:343, 1970.

# THE NASAL TURBINATES AS AN INDICATOR OF ALLERGY

The pediatrician spends a great deal of time looking up a child's nose. What can you learn from the appearance of the nasal turbinates? Unfortunately, as with many physical signs, no one change in the nasal turbinates appears to be diagnostic of any one condition, but their appearance can provide a clue. The findings described in the table below can serve as a provisional guide.

| TURBINATE | MOST LIKELY DIAGNOSIS |
| --- | --- |
| *Pale and/or violaceous* | |
| Nasal turbinates should be compared with other mucous membranes, and the mucous membrane of the lower lip in particular. | Adenoidal hypertrophy<br>Bacterial infection |
| *Swollen* | |
| The turbinates may be judged to be swollen if one or more touches the nasal septum. | Allergic rhinitis |
| *Wet* | |
| The turbinates may be judged to be wet if several broad strands of clear mucous adhere to them or if there is a pool of fluid. | Allergic rhinitis |

Reference: Murray, A.B.: Ann. Allergy, *30*:245, 1972.

*"If your basic attitude is one of loving kindness, you may yell at children and even cuff them around a bit without doing any real harm."*

Dr. Smiley Blanton

# ALLERGIC RHINITIS

The diagnosis of allergic rhinitis in the pediatric patient is particularly important because of the need to differentiate it from chronic infectious rhinitis. The following table differentiates allergic rhinitis, infectious rhinitis, and vasomotor rhinitis.

| | ALLERGIC RHINITIS | INFECTIOUS RHINITIS | VASOMOTOR RHINITIS |
|---|---|---|---|
| Etiology | IgE-mediated immunologic reaction | Respiratory infection | Autonomic nervous system disorder |
| Precipitating factors | Air-borne allergens: pollen, mold, dust, animal dander, wool, feathers, and so on | Viruses, bacteria | Temperature changes, alcohol ingestion, non-antigenic irritants: tobacco smoke, perfume, strong odors, and the like |
| Symptoms | Appear suddenly, disappear slowly | Appear and disappear slowly | Appear and disappear suddenly |
| Environmental factors | Symptoms may lessen indoors, especially with air conditioning or air purifier | No effect | Varies, symptoms may lessen or worsen indoors |
| Seasonal | Often | No | No |
| Fever | No | Often | No |
| Pruritus | Yes | No | Mild or absent |
| Conjunctivitis | Yes | No | No |
| Discharge | Watery, colorless | Mucopurulent | Watery, colorless |
| Nasal smear | Eosinophils | Neutrophils | Normal |
| Skin tests | Positive | Negative | Negative |
| Antibiotics | No effect | Sometimes helpful | No effect |

The physical examination can provide additional clues to the diagnosis of allergic rhinitis. The allergic child may have "allergic shiners." This bluish cast under the eyes is a result of venous congestion from sinusitis. The patient may also demonstrate a "nasal crease"; this is a transverse line extending across the nose at the junction of the lower and middle thirds. It is a result of chronic manipulation of the nose by the palm of the hand in an up and down fashion. This maneuver has been termed the "allergic salute." Most patients with colds, in contrast, rub their nose, under the nostrils, in a horizontal fashion.

Reference: O'Loughlin, J.M.: Drug Ther., *4*:52, 1974.

# COW'S MILK ALLERGY

Many physicians still remain skeptical about the diseases that may be produced by allergy or sensitivity to whole cow milk protein.

Careful observations do indicate, however, that from 7 to 25 per cent of infants may manifest symptoms upon exposure to whole cow milk. As a general rule, the earlier the introduction of the whole cow milk into the diet, the more likely the adverse symptoms are likely to develop. Diseases that may be produced by whole cow milk include:

### Gastrointestinal Bleeding

Approximately one-half of all infants and children found to have iron deficiency anemia have associated whole cow milk–induced gastrointestinal bleeding. Removal of whole cow milk from the diet results in the disappearance of occult fecal blood loss within 48 hours.

### Malabsorption Syndrome

In its most severe form, these children demonstrate diarrhea and failure to thrive. Vomiting, recurrent respiratory infections, and eczema are also commonly present. Serum IgA levels are increased; milk antibodies are present. Jejunal mucosa shows alterations and may be flat. Elimination of cow milk produces improvement in days to several months. Reintroduction of cow milk reproduces symptoms in hours or may take three to four weeks. Some of these infants also manifest sensitivity to soy and wheat as well.

### Exudative Enteropathy

Patients manifest edema, hypoproteinemia, and anemia. Symptoms frequently are first observed when cow milk has been fed during a diarrheal disease. Some, but not all, children will have diarrhea. Many will have eosinophilia and eosinophils in the stool. Stool often contains milk antibodies.

### Recurrent Serous Otitis Media, Bronchiolitis, Bronchitis, Skin Rashes and Vomiting

These may occur as individual illnesses, or the child may manifest multiple symptoms. Because of the common nature of such symptoms, strict criteria must be applied before allergy to cow milk can be claimed to be the cause. Clinical criteria should include the following:
1.  Symptoms subside after dietary elimination of milk.
2.  Symptoms recur within 48 hours after milk challenge.
3.  Reactions to three such challenges must be positive and have a similar onset, duration, and clinical features.
It is important to remember that about 20 per cent of children allergic to cow milk protein will also be allergic to soy protein.

Other diseases in which cow milk protein allergy may play a role include idiopathic pulmonary hemosiderosis, enuresis, steroid-dependent nephrosis, and the "tension-fatigue" syndrome. This latter entity is probably on the shakiest ground in terms of its relationship to cow milk. Its symptoms and signs include:

| Tension | overactivity, restlessness |
| --- | --- |
| | clumsiness |
| | inability to relax |
| | irritability |
| | oversensitivity |
| | insomnia |
| | hypersensitivity to pain |

| Fatigue | tiredness |
| --- | --- |
| | achiness |
| | sluggishness |
| | torpor |

and

pallor
nasal stuffiness
infraorbital circles
infraorbital edema
abdominal pain
headache
enuresis
arthralgias

Only a scrupulously administered elimination diet with careful observation of symptoms can establish this constellation of signs and symptoms as a manifestation of milk allergy.

---

References: Walker-Smith, J.: Arch. Dis. Child., *50*:347, 1975. Crook, W.C.: Pediatr. Clin. North Am., *22*:227, 1975.

# PRIMARY IMMUNIZATIONS OF CHILDREN NOT IMMUNIZED IN INFANCY

Not infrequently, the pediatrician is faced with a child who is over 1 year of age and who has not been immunized. The following schedules should be used to accomplish immunization as rapidly as possible.

If the child is 1 to 5 years of age:

First visit — DPT, TOPV, tuberculin test
1 month later — measles, rubella, mumps
2 months later — DPT, TOPV
4 months later — DPT, TOPV
6 to 12 months later or preschool — DPT, TOPV
Age 14–16 years — Td; continue every 10 years

If the child is 6 years of age and over:

First visit — Td, TOPV, tuberculin test
1 month later — measles, rubella, mumps
2 months later — Td, TOPV
6 to 12 months later — Td, TOPV
Age 14–16 years — Td; continue every 10 years

DPT = Diphtheria, Pertussis, Tetanus; TOPV = Trivalent Oral Polio Vaccine; Td = adult type diphtheria tetanus toxoid.

Reference: American Academy of Pediatrics: Report of the Committee on Infectious Diseases. 1974, p. 9.

# 8

# THE BLOOD

# ANEMIA—A DIAGNOSTIC APPROACH

The child with anemia is either overlooked or overstudied on many occasions. The accompanying flow diagram suggests a means of arriving at a probable diagnosis with a minimum of laboratory studies. The evaluation begins with a careful history that should include information regarding age, sex, color, ethnic background, birth weight and neonatal course, diet, drugs, diarrhea, infections, history of other family members with anemia, and a statement about the presence or absence of pica. The initial laboratory studies should include a calculation of *red cell indices, a reticulocyte count,* and *examination of a well-prepared peripheral blood smear.* With these facts in hand, proceed to determine if your patient has a hypochromic-microcytic anemia, a normocytic anemia, or a macrocytic anemia. Follow the logical steps to diagnosis.

8

*A Diagnostic Approach to Anemia*

## MICROCYTIC–HYPOCHROMIC

6 mos — 2 yrs — MCV <70
2 yrs — 5 yrs — MCV <73
5 yrs — 12 yrs — MCV <76

Iron deficiency
Thalassemia syndromes
  alpha
  beta
Lead poisoning
Chronic infection
Severe protein deficiency
Siderocrestic
  pyridoxine–responsive

Studies:
  Serum iron, TIBC, FEP,
    Hb electrophoresis
  Brilliant cresyl blue prep
  Fetal hemoglobin
  Marrow iron stain

**HISTORY**

| | | |
|---|---|---|
| Age | | *Drugs* |
| Sex | | Diarrhea |
| Color | and | *I*nfection |
| *E*thnic | | Inheritance |
| *N*eonatal | | *P*ica |
| Diet | | |

## MACROCYTIC

(MCV >96 $\mu^3$)

Macrocytosis
Reticulocytosis
Liver disease
Hypothyroidism
Down's syndrome
Normal newborn

Macro-ovalocytosis with anemia
Bone marrow

**MEGALOBLASTIC**

*Folic Acid*
Dietary
Malabsorption
Dilantin

*B₁₂ Deficiency*
Pernicious anemia
  Juvenile
  Adult
Grasbock
Ileal disease

OROTIC ACIDURIA

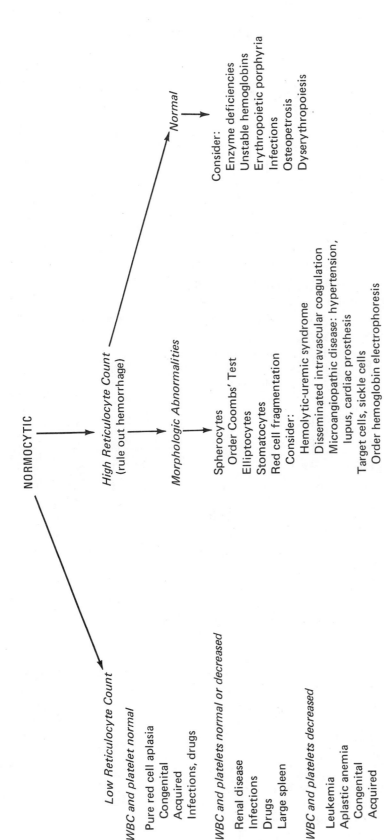

NORMOCYTIC

*High Reticulocyte Count*
(rule out hemorrhage)

*Morphologic Abnormalities*

Spherocytes
    Order Coombs' Test
Elliptocytes
Stomatocytes
Red cell fragmentation
    Consider:
    Hemolytic-uremic syndrome
    Disseminated intravascular coagulation
    Microangiopathic disease: hypertension,
        lupus, cardiac prosthesis
Target cells, sickle cells
    Order hemoglobin electrophoresis

*Normal*

Consider:
    Enzyme deficiencies
    Unstable hemoglobins
    Erythropoietic porphyria
    Infections
    Osteopetrosis
    Dyserythropoiesis

*Low Reticulocyte Count*

*WBC and platelet normal*

Pure red cell aplasia
    Congenital
    Acquired
    Infections, drugs

*WBC and platelets normal or decreased*

Renal disease
Infections
Drugs
Large spleen

*WBC and platelets decreased*

Leukemia
Aplastic anemia
    Congenital
    Acquired

8

# THE RISE IN HEMOGLOBIN WITH IRON THERAPY

How fast should the hemoglobin rise when you start treating your iron deficient patient with oral iron?

Two important factors must be considered when judging the adequacy of the hematologic response. They are the initial hemoglobin value and the duration of the period of observation. The lower the initial hemoglobin, the greater is the hemoglobin rise per day. The shorter the observation period, the greater is the calculated hemoglobin rise per day. As one gets closer to a normal hemoglobin value, the daily rise in hemoglobin is much less. In our own experience in treating patients with hemoglobin values of less than 8.0 gm/100 ml, one may anticipate a hemoglobin rise of 0.2 to 0.3 gm per day during the first 7 to 10 days of therapy. During the period of 10 to 24 days, the hemoglobin rises at a rate of 0.15 gm per day and slows after that point to a rate of 0.10 per day until a normal level is achieved. Normally, the reticulocyte count begins to increase in 48 to 72 hours and reaches a peak 7 to 10 days after the initiation of therapy.

Listed below is another guide to the expected response as a function of the initial hemoglobin level.

| INITIAL HEMOGLOBIN (gm/dl) | HEMOGLOBIN RISE IN ONE WEEK (gm/dl) |
|---|---|
| 2.0 – 5.0 | 1.61 |
| 5.1 – 6.0 | 1.53 |
| 6.1 – 7.0 | 1.17 |
| 7.1 – 8.0 | 1.11 |
| 8.1 – 9.0 | 0.98 |
| 9.1 – 10.0 | 0.57 |
| 10.1 – 11.0 | 0.72 |
| 11.1 – 12.0 | 0.40 |

Optimal responses to oral iron therapy are achieved by treating the patient with ferrous sulfate. A patient should receive 2 to 3 mg of elemental iron per kg three times per day. The iron should be given between meals and never administered with milk.

The major reasons for failing to achieve a satisfactory response include:

1. Patient did not receive the iron.
2. Iron given improperly.
3. The presence of an intercurrent infection.
4. The presence of associated lead poisoning.

5. You made the wrong diagnosis.

6. Patient is continually bleeding, possibly as a result of cow milk sensitivity.

---

Reference: Mehta, B.C., Lotliker, K.S., and Patel, J.C.: Indian J. Med. Res., *61*:1818, 1973.

# ANEMIA IN EARLY INFANCY

During the first months of life there are many causes of anemia. Anemia during the first three months of life is rarely a result of nutritional iron deficiency. The accompanying table is intended to call your attention to the more likely causes of anemia that occur at birth and at two or three months of age as well as provide you with leads to establishing the diagnosis.

*Common Causes of Anemia in Early Infancy*

| AGE | DIAGNOSIS | SUPPORTING DATA |
|---|---|---|
| At birth | Hemorrhage | |
| | *Obstetric accidents* (placenta previa, abruptio placentae, incision of placenta, rupture of cord, rupture of anomalous placental vessel | History and visual inspection of placenta and cord |
| | *Occult hemorrhage* | |
| | Fetomaternal | Demonstration of fetal cells in maternal circulation |
| | Twin-to-twin | Demonstration of significant difference in hemoglobin values of identical twins |
| | *Internal hemorrhage* (intracranial, retroperitoneal, intrahepatic, intrasplenic, cephalhematoma) | Physical examination |
| | Isoimmunization | Blood groups of mother and infant; evidence of antibody on infant's red cells |
| | Inherited defect of red cell (includes G-6-PD deficiency, pyruvate kinase deficiency, hereditary spherocytosis, elliptocytosis, stomatocytosis, etc.) | Red cell morphology, family history, and appropriate screening tests |
| | Acquired defect (generally in association with hypoxemia, acidosis, or infection) | Physical findings, red cell morphology, coagulation disturbance, blood and urine cultures, and serologic studies and gamma-M determination |
| | Red cell hypoplasia (Blackfan-Diamond syndrome, congenital leukemia, osteopetrosis) | Rare disorders; bone marrow aspirate |
| 2–3 months | Iron deficiency as a consequence of previous hemorrhage | Obstetric history when available |
| | Late manifestation of previous isoimmunization | Blood types of mother and infant; maternal antibody titers |

| AGE | DIAGNOSIS | SUPPORTING DATA |
|---|---|---|
| 2–3 months | Hereditary defects of the red cell | Persistence of hemolytic anemia; red cell morphology and laboratory tests |
| | Thalassemia major | Red cell morphology, splenomegaly, persistence of fetal hemoglobin elevation, family studies |
| | Sickle cell anemia | Red cell morphology, hemoglobin electrophoresis |
| | Vitamin E deficiency | Infant of low birth weight; red cell morphology, low serum E level, positive hydrogen peroxide hemolysis test |
| | Folic acid deficiency | Premature infant, history of infections or diarrhea, red cell and marrow morphology, response to folic acid |
| | Persistent infection | Elevated titers to rubella, cytomegalovirus, toxoplasmosis |
| | Renal tubular acidosis | Acidosis, hypochloremia, mild azotemia, urine pH of 6.0 or greater in presence of acidosis |

# IRON DEFICIENCY OR THALASSEMIA TRAIT?

Children with mild microcytic anemias are commonly encountered in the practice of pediatrics. Most of these patients have either iron deficiency or thalassemia trait. The use of red cell indices can provide a simple means of making a presumptive diagnosis without requiring serum iron determinations or hemoglobin electrophoresis.

Two formulas employing these indices have been proposed. They are as follows:

1. The Mentzer Formula $= \dfrac{\text{MCV}}{\text{Red Cell Count}}$

*Interpretation:* Values in excess of 13.5 strongly suggest that the patient has iron deficiency anemia, while values below 11.5 indicate that thalassemia trait is the most likely diagnosis.

2. The Discriminant Function = MCV - RBC - (5 × Hb) - 3.4

*Thalassemia*—From the Greek *thalassa*, meaning sea, and *haima*, meaning blood. So named because the originally recognized patients all lived around the Mediterranean Sea.

*Interpretation:* Positive values suggest a diagnosis of iron deficiency, while negative values indicate that thalassemia trait is the cause of the microcytic anemia.

*Caution:* These formulas are useful only in uncomplicated situations. Confusing answers may be obtained in patients with associated hemolytic anemias or in patients with thalassemia minor who have hemorrhage or are pregnant, or in patients who are polycythemic secondary to chronic hypoxemia.

These formulas are useful in initial evaluation of patients. If iron deficiency is suggested by the formula and the patient does not respond to iron therapy, then further evaluation is indicated. A diagnosis of thalassemia trait should be confirmed in at least one family member.

References: Mentzer, W.C., Jr.: Lancet, *1*:882, 1973. England, J.M., and Fraser, P.: Lancet, *1*:449, 1973.

**8**

*"Children, blessings seem, but torments are."*

Otway

# FREE ERYTHROCYTE PROTOPORPHYRIN AS A DIAGNOSTIC AID

With the development of a simple, rapid, and inexpensive method for the measurement of free erythrocyte protoporphyrin (FEP), screening for both iron deficiency and lead poisoning has become simplified and can be performed on capillary samples of blood.

Normal values for FEP may vary from laboratory to laboratory, but in general the following values can be applied:

> Upper limit of normal:
> 90 micrograms/100 ml RBCs
> or
> 30 micrograms/100 ml whole blood

Modest elevations of the FEP (30 to 190 micrograms/100 ml of whole blood) may be observed in iron deficiency, while values in excess of 190 signify lead poisoning or the rare patient with erythropoietic protoporphyria.

> *Pica*—From the Latin *pica*, meaning magpie. The magpie picks up and eats and hoards odd objects. A scavenger bird of prey.

*Iron Deficiency and Thalassemia Minor*

When the FEP is used in conjunction with the measurement of erythrocyte mean corpuscular volume (MCV), a very accurate means of distinguishing iron deficiency from thalassemia minor is provided. The FEP is normal in patients with thalassemia minor unless they have associated iron deficiency anemia. The accompanying diagram illustrates a suggested approach to the initial diagnosis of these disorders employing the MCV, derived from the Coulter Counter, and the FEP.

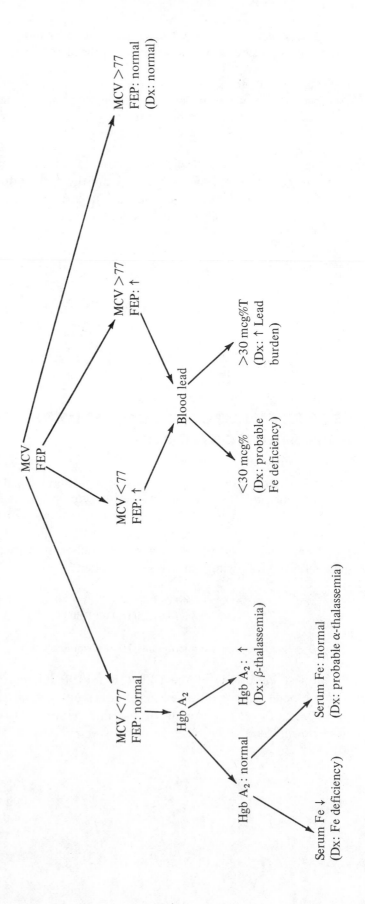

*Lead Poisoning*

The Center for Disease Control has provided the following guidelines for the use of the FEP in the diagnosis and management of patients with lead poisoning:

1. The FEP should be used for the initial screening for lead poisoning.
2. Children with an elevated FEP should have a blood lead determination performed.
3. With the results of the FEP and blood lead, the patients may be classified into four major categories:

| TEST | CLASS I<br>Normal | CLASS II<br>Minimally<br>Elevated | CLASS III<br>Moderately<br>Elevated | CLASS IV<br>Extremely<br>Elevated |
|---|---|---|---|---|
| Pb (mcg/100 ml) | 29 | 30–49 | 50–79 | 80 |
| FEP (mcg/100 ml<br>whole blood) | 59 | 60–109 | 110–189 | 190 |

4. In situations where there is a discrepancy between the blood lead and the FEP, the FEP is more likely to reflect the true status of the patient.
5. Some Class I children may be placed into two additional categories. Class Ia would include those children with iron deficiency anemia. Class Ib children appear, on the basis of present experience, to have transient or declining blood lead elevations. The anticipated combinations of blood lead and FEP as a suggested guideline to estimate the most likely degree of risk are:

| TEST<br>RESULTS | FEP<br>≤59 | FEP<br>60–109 | FEP<br>110–189 | FEP<br>≥190 |
|---|---|---|---|---|
| Pb ≤29 | I | Ia | Ia | EEP+ |
| Pb 30–49 | ↓Ib | II | ↑III | ↑IV |
| Pb 50–79 | * | ↓II | III | ↑IV |
| Pb ≥80 | * | * | * | IV |

EEP+ = Erythropoietic protoporphyria.
  * = Combination of results is not generally observed in practice; when blood lead is repeated, the results will generally indicate contamination of the first specimen.
  ↓ = Downgrading of the estimate of risk of lead intoxication suggested by blood lead is altered on the basis of the FEP results.
  ↑ = Upgrading of the estimate of risk of lead intoxication suggested by blood lead is altered on the basis of the FEP results.

6. Guidelines for management are as follows:

Class I    Routine rescreening until age 6 years.

Class Ia    Diagnosis and treatment of iron deficiency anemia.

Class Ib    Reevaluation at monthly intervals until it is certain that the child does not have undue body lead burden.

Class II      Should be considered to have increased lead absorption if there is no iron deficiency. Both conditions may exist. Look for other evidence of lead poisoning (long bone films, urinary coproporphyrin, EDTA mobilization test). If mobilization is abnormal, perform chelation. If no evidence of lead poisoning, evaluate at three-month intervals after it is determined that patient is no longer exposed to lead. If lead exposure continues, evaluate at monthly intervals.

Class III      If asymptomatic, perform EDTA mobilization test. If test is positive, then chelate. If patient is symptomatic, then hospitalize immediately and begin chelation therapy. If chelation is unnecessary, follow at monthly intervals.

Class IV      These children, regardless of lack of symptoms, should be hospitalized for evaluation and chelation therapy.

---

References: Piomelli, S.: Pediatrics, *51*:254, 1973. Stockman, J.A., Weiner, L.S., Simon, G.E., et al.: J. Lab. Clin. Med., *85*:113, 1975. Center for Disease Control: J. Pediatr., *87*:824, 1975.

# THE SLOW SEDIMENTATION RATE

All of the factors responsible for determining the rate at which erythrocytes sediment have not been identified. Factors that are known to influence the sedimentation rate include the quantity of fibrinogen, alpha$_1$-globulin, the gamma-M globulin, and the serum cholesterol, with the quantity of fibrinogen perhaps playing the most important role. In addition, alterations in the morphologic characteristics of the red cell or in cell surface charge that hinder rouleau formation will affect the erythrocyte sedimentation rate.

Everyone is familiar with the long and nondescript list of diseases that produce an increase in the erythrocyte sedimentation rate. It is generally not appreciated that certain disorders or drugs characteristically produce a slow sedimentation rate or a rate that is slower than would be anticipated. Disorders that produce a slow sedimentation rate include:

Anorexia nervosa
Hypofibrinogenemia, congenital or acquired
Abetalipoproteinemia (acanthocytosis)
Sickle cell anemia (if many sickled forms are present)
Pyruvate kinase deficiency (usually postsplenectomy if associated with
   marked morphologic alterations of the erythrocytes)
Hereditary spherocytosis
Congestive heart failure
Nephrotic syndrome
Steroid therapy
Aspirin administration
Serum sickness

In patients with the nephrotic syndrome in whom an infection is suspected, the measurement of the C-reactive protein provides a useful alternate screening test.

# SCREENING FOR RED CELL G-6-PD DEFICIENCY—INTERPRETATION

In view of the fact that red cell glucose-6-phosphate dehydrogenase deficiency is presently recognized to be the most common inborn error of metabolism in the world (it affects over 100 million individuals), a simple means of detection should always be available. A variety of screening tests have been developed. A test that is performed easily in both the ward and office setting is one employing dye reduction. It can be performed as follows:

*Reagents*

1. 0.001M brilliant cresyl blue (National Aniline Division of Allied Chemical Corporation, distributed by Eastman Kodak), mol wt 320; 32 mg are dissolved in 100 ml of water.

2. 0.2M Tris buffer (trishydroxymethylaminomethane), mol wt 121.4; 2.43 gm are dissolved in 60 ml of water. The pH is adjusted to 8 with 0.2M hydrochloric acid (0.5 ml concentrated hydrochloric acid in 30 ml of water). After the pH is adjusted, sufficient water is added to make 100 ml.

3. 0.002M triphosphopyridine nucleotide (TPN), mol wt 757; 25 mg are dissolved in 16.5 ml of water.

4. 0.05M disodium glucose-6-phosphate, mol wt 331; 250 mg are dissolved in 15.7 ml of water.

*Procedure*

Reagent mixture (sufficient for 60 tests):

| | |
|---|---:|
| 0.001M brilliant cresyl blue | 25 ml |
| 0.2M Tris buffer, pH 8.0 | 20 ml |
| 0.002M TPN | 7 ml |
| 0.05M disodium glucose-6-phosphate | 5 ml |

Stored at 4 to 10°C, this mixture generally is stable for four months. When adult control samples do not cause decoloration of the dye within 60 minutes, the reagent mixture should be discarded.

Hemolyze 0.02 ml of fresh or anticoagulated blood with 1 ml of water. When the hematocrit of the patient is between 15 and 25 per cent, twice the amount of blood is used. Within 30 minutes, 0.6 ml of the reagent mixture is added to the hemolysate. Mix and cover with approximately 0.5 ml of mineral oil. Incubate at 37°C and observe at 40, 60, 90, and 120 minutes for a color change. The blood of normals will decolor the dye within 60 minutes. Since reduced brilliant cresyl blue is colorless, the blue color will disappear, leaving only the red color of hemoglobin.

The common form of G-6-PD deficiency results only in anemia when patients are stressed by a variety of oxidant drugs or by metabolic products that are generated during the course of a variety of illnesses. During a hemolytic episode, the diagnosis of G-6-PD deficiency may be missed when employing a screening test. This is particularly true when the patient has the $Gd^{A-}$ form of the enzyme mutant. This enzyme mutant is seen primarily among black individuals. The decreased level of the enzyme in the red cells of $Gd^{A-}$ individuals does not result from a defect in synthesis but rather from the in vivo instability of the enzyme. A similar mechanism underlies the other common type of deficiency, $Gd^{Mediterranean}$. This mutant is seen primarily among Greeks, Italians, and other racial groups in the Middle East. The rate of decline of G-6-PD activity in vivo in these two mutants is contrasted with the normal rate of enzyme decay observed in $Gd^{B+}$ individuals in Figure 8–1.

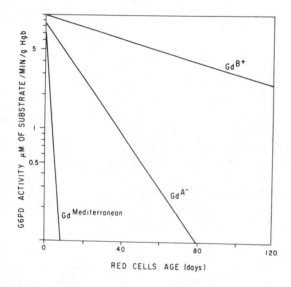

FIG. 8–1

In normal red cells, the activity of G-6-PD falls approximately 50 per cent as cells age from time of bone marrow release to senility at 120 days. In normal blood, a fourfold reduction in mean red cell age from 60 to 15 days increases the enzyme activity from 5.0 to 8.3 units. In the blood of $Gd^{A-}$ individuals, a comparable reduction in mean cell age, from 50 to 12 days, would raise the enzyme level from 0.6 to 5.0 units and would bring it into the normal range. Thus, in $Gd^{A-}$ individuals with acute or chronic hemolysis, the enzyme deficiency might not be apparent. In these circumstances, the oldest enzyme-deficient cells are destroyed and, at the same time, bone marrow compensation produces a large number of enzyme-sufficient reticulocytes. The net result is a market reduction in the mean cell age of the erythrocyte population. If the mean cell age becomes less than 12 days, the enzyme activity of the circulating red cells may even appear higher than normal. It is for this reason that the diagnosis may be missed if reliance is placed on simple screening techniques. In patients with the Gd^Mediterranean mutant, the liability of the enzyme is so great that normal activity is never reached even in the midst of a hemolytic episode.

If one suspects G-6-PD deficiency as the cause of a hemolytic anemia in a patient with Gd^A⁻ mutant, the following procedures might be followed in an attempt to establish the diagnosis:

1. Separation of oldest cells and enzyme assay of this fraction.
2. Cytochemical study of individual cells for G-6-PD activity.
3. Electrophoresis of enzyme to demonstrate presence of mutant.
4. G-6-PD enzyme assay. If enzyme value is not substantially increased above normal in presence of reticulocytosis, one should strongly suspect G-6-PD deficiency.
5. Restudy patient when hemolytic episode has resolved.

The clinical differences between Gd^A⁻ and Gd^Mediterranean males are outlined in the table below.

|  | Gd^A⁻ | Gd^Mediterranean |
|---|---|---|
| **Steady State** | | |
| Activity of RBCs | 5–15% | 0–5% |
| Activity of WBCs | 100% | 20% |
| Life span of RBCs | 100 days | 100 days |
| **Hemolytic Crisis** | | |
| Interval after exposure to hemolytic agent | 24–36 hours | 3–24 hours |
| Hemoglobinuria | Common | Constant |
| Jaundice | Common | Constant |
| Anemia | Moderate (rarely <6 gm Hgb) | Severe (often <6 gm Hgb) |
| Duration of hemolysis | Self-limited | May be fatal |

Reference: Piomelli, S.: *In* Nathan, D.G., and Oski, F.A. (Eds.): Hematology of Infancy and Childhood. Philadelphia, W.B. Saunders Company, 1974, p. 363.

# RECOGNIZING A HEMOLYTIC ANEMIA

The physician is often confronted with the question, "Does my patient have a hemolytic anemia?" In most instances, this question can be answered without recourse to elaborate diagnostic procedures.

Hemolysis refers to the premature destruction of erythrocytes. It can result from a finite reduction in red cell life span, such as that seen in many hereditary hemolytic anemias, or from superimposed random destruction of red cells, such as occurs in burns, incompatible blood transfusions, or microangiopathic processes. It can occur extravascularly in liver, spleen, and bone marrow, or intravascularly.

Patients may have a shortened red cell life span without being anemic. The normal individual can increase the rate of red cell production some sixfold in an attempt to compensate for accelerated red cell destruction.

As a general rule, a hemolytic anemia should be suspected in all patients in whom the absolute number of reticulocytes is increased (100,000/mm$^3$) in association with a stable or falling hemoglobin level. This general rule assumes that the patient is not actively bleeding.

The readily available laboratory tests that are useful in confirming the presence of a hemolytic anemia are listed in the accompanying table.

*Laboratory Findings in Hemolytic Anemias*

| LABORATORY TEST | INTERPRETATION |
|---|---|
| Peripheral blood smear | The presence of polychromasia, nucleated red blood cells, and alterations in red cell morphology all suggest the presence of a hemolytic anemia. Hemolysis is always present when spherocytes or red cell fragments are observed in the peripheral blood. |
| Plasma haptoglobin | Haptoglobin is decreased in patients with hemolytic anemias of both the intravascular and extravascular types. Haptoglobin is an alpha-2 globulin of plasma that rises rapidly in inflammatory states. It specifically binds hemoglobin dimers. The hemoglobin-haptoglobin complex is rapidly cleared by the reticuloendothelial system. In situations accompanied by intravascular hemolysis, the haptoglobin generally becomes quickly saturated, and free hemoglobin appears in the plasma. The measurement of haptoglobin is of limited diagnostic value in neonates because values are normally low. |
| Plasma hemopexin | Hemopexin is a plasma beta globulin that binds heme. It is not generally measured in most laboratories. When free hemoglobin appears in the circulation, it is readily oxidized to methemoglobin and its disassociated heme groups are bound to hemopexin. This heme-hemopexin complex is rapidly removed from the circulation and the concentration of hemopexin falls. Hemopexin levels are also too variable in newborns to be used for diagnostic purposes. |
| Hemoglobinemia, hemoglobinuria, and hemosiderinuria | When plasma haptoglobin is depleted by excessive hemolysis, the hemoglobin dimers pass through the glomerulus and into the glomerular filtrate. Some of the dimers are taken up by the tubular cells, and the iron of the heme is converted into hemosiderin. The remaining hemoglobin dimers appear in the urine, where they can be detected by a variety of reagents designed to indicate the presence of occult blood. With chronic hemolysis, the urinary sediment will contain tubular cells laden with hemosiderin. This hemosiderin can be easily recognized in the unstained sediment or precisely identified by staining of the sediment with the Prussian blue reaction. |
| Serum lactic dehydrogenase | Serum LDH rises in patients with intravascular hemolysis, with marked extravascular hemolysis, and with ineffective erythropoiesis — particularly of the megaloblastic type. |
| Carboxyhemoglobin | One mole of carbon monoxide is formed for each mole of heme catabolized. Excessive hemoglobin catabolism — be it intravascular, extravascular, or in entrapped hemorrhages — will result in elevations in blood carboxyhemoglobin levels. Measurement of blood carboxyhemoglobin level, where available, is the best and most sensitive test of hemolysis. Accurate measurements can be made only by gas chromatography and not by spectrophotometry. Smoking or environmental contamination will also produce elevations in blood carboxyhemoglobin values. Normal COHb levels in newborns should not exceed 0.9 per cent, while normal values in older, nonsmoking subjects, should not exceed 0.6 per cent. |

8

Outlined below are the sequences that occur when free hemoglobin enters the plasma.

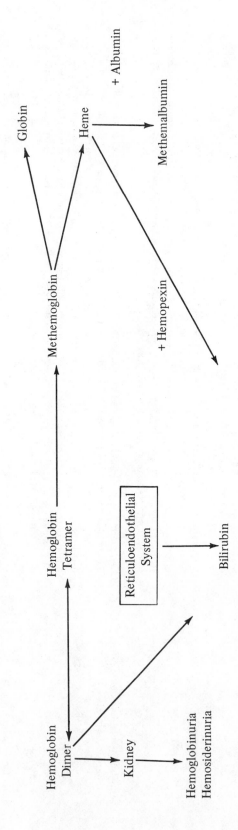

# VOLUMES FOR SUCCESSFUL EXCHANGE TRANSFUSION

How much blood needs to be removed and replaced to achieve a successful exchange transfusion? This obviously varies as a function of the weight of the infant. The nomogram depicted in Figure 8–2 has proved useful in determining the effectiveness of an exchange transfusion. It indicates the volume of donor's blood necessary to replace from 60 to 90 per cent of the infant's blood. To use it, one locates the diagonal line corresponding to the body weight of the patient and notes where it intersects the horizontal line representing the percentage of blood desired to be removed. The vertical projection of this point of intersection on the bottom scale shows the volume of donor's blood to be used.

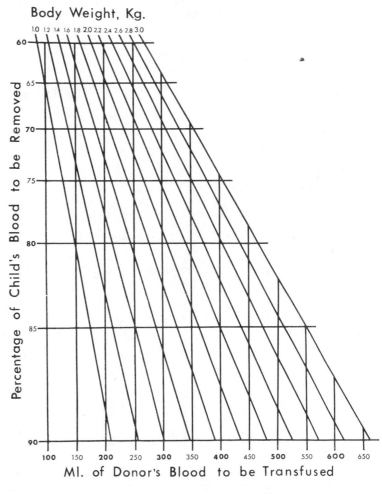

FIG. 8–2

For patients weighing more than 3 kg, the nomogram can still be employed by dividing the patient's weight by a factor that brings it on scale and then multiplying the volume of donor blood to be employed by the number used in the division. For example, in a patient weighing 22 kg in whom you wish to achieve 90 per cent exchange, divide the patient's weight by 11 and use the diagonal line originating from the 2 kg mark. This will indicate the need for a 440 ml exchange. This figure should then be multiplied by 11, and the answer will indicate that your 22 kg patient requires an exchange transfusion of 4840 ml of blood to remove 90 per cent of his blood volume.

---

Reference: Huerga, J., Smetters, G.W. and Sherrick, J.C.: *In* Sunderman, F.W., and Sunderman, F.W., Jr. (Eds.): The Clinical Pathology of Infancy. Springfield, Illinois, Charles C Thomas, 1967, p. 360.

## THE RATIONAL USE OF BLOOD PRODUCTS

Transfusion of blood or blood products is a frequent need on a busy pediatric service. The most scientific use of this procedure requires an estimation of the blood product requirement of the patient. The following pages outline methods for such estimations.

### Simple Transfusion (With Packed Red Cells)

Assuming a packed cell hemoglobin (Hgb) content of 22 gm/100 ml and a postneonatal blood volume of 75 ml/kg, this formula states:

$$\frac{\text{Volume of packed}}{\text{cell transfusion (ml)}} = \frac{\text{Wt (in kg)} \times 75 \text{ ml/kg} \times \text{desired rise in Hgb (gm/100 ml)}}{22 \text{ gm/100 ml}}$$

*Example:* To raise the Hgb of an 11 kg child from 4 gm/100 ml to 10 gm/100 ml, one would calculate:

$$\frac{\text{Transfusion}}{\text{volume (ml)}} = \frac{11 \text{ kg} \times 75 \text{ ml/kg} \times 6 \text{ gm/100 ml}}{22 \text{ gm/100 ml}} = 225 \text{ ml}$$

If for some reason whole blood must be used, or if packed cell Hgb differs from that assumed, substitution of the correct value in the denominator will still provide an accurate estimate of transfusion needs.

---

Reference: Oski, F.A., and Naiman, J.L.: Hematologic Problems in the Newborn. Philadelphia, W.B. Saunders Company, 1972.

### Partial Exchange Transfusion

In situations when time or volume considerations suggest use of partial exchange transfusion (e.g., anemia with heart failure), a modification of the previous formula may be useful:

$$\frac{\text{Exchange}}{\text{volume (ml)}} = \frac{\text{Wt (in kg)} \times 75 \text{ ml/kg} \times \text{desired rise in Hgb}}{22 \text{ gm/100 ml} - \text{Hgb}_R}$$

$Hgb_R$ = mean of the initial and final hemoglobin. This represents the Hgb content of blood *removed* during the exchange.

$$\frac{(Hgb \text{ initial} + Hgb \text{ desired})}{2}$$

*Example:* To raise the Hgb of a 17 kg child from 3.0 gm/100 ml to 7.0 gm/100 ml using a partial exchange transfusion with packed cells, one could calculate:

$$\frac{\text{Exchange}}{\text{volume (ml)}} = \frac{17 \text{ kg} \times 75 \text{ ml/kg} \times 4 \text{ gm/100 ml}}{22 \text{ gm/100 ml} - \frac{(3 \text{ gm/100 ml} + 7 \text{ gm/100 ml})}{2}} = 300 \text{ ml}$$

---

Reference: Nieburg, P.I., and Stockman, J.A.: Am. J. Dis. Child. (in press).

## Exchange Transfusion with Plasma

Neonates or older children with significant polycythemia may benefit from a partial exchange transfusion designed to reduce their hemoglobin.

This can be accomplished by using plasma in the exchange transfusion as indicated in the following formula:

$$\frac{\text{Exchange}}{\text{volume (ml)}} = \frac{\text{Wt (kg)} \times 100 \text{ ml/kg}* \times \text{ desired fall in Hgb (gm/100 ml)}}{Hgb_R}$$

$Hgb_R$ = mean of initial and desired hemoglobin = $\frac{(Hgb \text{ initial} + Hgb \text{ desired})}{2}$

*Example:* To lower the Hgb of a 4 kg neonate from 24 gm/100 ml to 16 gm/100 ml, one would calculate:

$$\frac{\text{Exchange}}{\text{volume}} = \frac{4 \text{ kg} \times 100 \text{ ml/kg} \times 8 \text{ gm/100 ml}}{20 \text{ gm/100 ml}} = 160 \text{ ml}$$

*Neonatal blood volume.

---

Reference: Oski, F.A., and Naiman, J.L.: Hematologic Problems in the Newborn. Philadelphia, W.B. Saunders Company, 1972.

## Platelet Transfusion

Infusion of 0.2 units/kg of fresh platelets will provide a post-infusion rise in platelet count of approximately 60,000 to 90,000 platelets/mm$^3$.

*Example:* To raise the platelet count by 60,000 to 90,000/mm$^3$ in a 15 kg child, the following calculation would be made:

$$\text{Platelet units} = 0.2 \text{ units/kg} \times 15 \text{ kg} = 3 \text{ units}$$

# NEUTROPENIA

The total polymorphonuclear count is below 1500/mm³. What are the causes of this neutropenia? The accompanying table can provide a guide to sorting out this complex and heterogenous group of disorders. In general, it can be stated that an increased risk of infection does not occur in these patients unless the total polymorphonuclear count decreases to less than 500/mm³, and reaches alarming proportions only when the count remains below 200/mm³.

*The Clinical and Laboratory Features of the Neutropenias*

| DIAGNOSIS | CLINICAL FEATURES | LABORATORY FINDINGS |
|---|---|---|
| Neutropenia secondary to infection | Infant ill with septicemia, pneumonia, meningitis, or profound diarrhea. | Total white count frequently less than 5000/mm³ with neutrophils of less than 1000/mm³. *E. coli*, *Streptococcus*, and *Shigella* recognized causes. Toxic granulation often prominent. Blast forms may be present. |
| Neutropenia associated with maternal neutropenia | Infant usually asymptomatic. | Neutropenia present in both mother and infant. Mother may have lupus erythematosus. A leukocyte agglutinin may be present in maternal sera. |
| Neutropenia associated with maternal isoimmunization to fetal leukocytes | Infant generally asymptomatic, but serious infection has been described. | Bone marrow aspirate generally reveals a paucity of myeloid forms beyond the myelocyte stage of maturation. Leukocyte agglutinin present in maternal sera directed against infant's white cells. |
| Genetic agranulocytosis | Infections include otitis media, pneumonia, meningitis, multiple furuncles, deep abscesses, and omphalitis. May involve more than one family member. | Bone marrow may be hypocellular or of normal cellularity with virtual absence of white cell precursors or maturation arrest at myelocyte stage. |
| Chronic benign granulo-cytopenia of childhood | Infant usually asymptomatic. May have furuncles, paronychia, ulcerations in genital area, or gingivitis. | Marrow cellular with all but the most mature myeloid forms present in normal numbers. Spontaneous cure may occur in later childhood. |
| Neutropenia and pancreatic insufficiency | Infants usually asymptomatic in neonatal period. Steatorrhea and growth failure may be observed early in life. | Bone marrow hypocellular. Mild thrombocytopenia may also be present. Absence of pancreatic enzymes with normal sweat electrolytes. Epiphyseal stippling may be observed. More than one family member may be involved. |

8

| Reticular dysgenesis | Infants profoundly ill with overwhelming septicemia. Total white count 0 to 600 600/mm$^3$. | No granulocytes or granulocyte precursors present in bone marrow. Spleen and thymus devoid or virtually devoid of lymphocytes. |
|---|---|---|
| Drug-induced neutropenia | Cutaneous infections may be present. More severe infections uncommon. | Maternal ingestion of thiazides, Dilantin, amidopyrine, thiouracil, propylthiouracil, phenothiazines, trimethadione, sulfonamides, and others. Marrow reveals either a maturation arrest or depletion of myeloid precursors. |
| Cyclic neutropenia | Symptoms not reported in neonatal period. By 6 weeks of age, infant may have recurrent attacks of stomatitis, otitis media, furunculosis, and pneumonia. | Neutropenia intermittent. Cycles frequently of 21 days. Neutropenia generally associated with maturation arrest of myeloid elements. More than one family member involved. |
| Lazy leukocyte syndrome | Symptoms uncommon in newborn. Clinical features include unexplained fever, stomatitis, otitis media, furunculosis, and pneumonia. | Marrow appears normal. Leukocytes have impaired chemotaxis and random mobility. |
| Neutropenia associated with inborn errors of metabolism | Symptoms are those of underlying metabolic error. Lethargy, vomiting, and ketosis common. | Neutropenia observed in hyperglycinemia, methylmalonic acidemia, and isovalericacidemia. |

## EOSINOPHILIA

The presence of more than 700 eosinophils per mm³ is defined as eosinophilia. A heterogeneous group of disorders may be associated with eosinophilia. The mnemonic NAACP may help you to categorize them (Neoplasia, Allergy, Addison's disease, Collagen-vascular disease, Parasites). More specific causes include the following.

### Neoplasms

Hodgkin's disease*
Any neoplasm
Eosinophilic leukemia*
Myeloproliferative disorders

### Allergy

Asthma
Hay fever
Urticaria
Eczema
Drug sensitivity*

### Adrenal insufficiency

### Collagen-vascular diseases

Periarteritis nodosa*
Rheumatic fever

### Parasites

Helminthic: Trichinosis, ascariasis, hookworm, strongyloidiasis*
Toxocara (visceral larva migrans)*
Malaria

### Miscellaneous

Fanconi's aplastic anemia
Cirrhosis
Dermatitis herpetiformis
Radiation therapy
Peritoneal dialysis
Congenital heart disease
Hereditary familial eosinophilia
Idiopathic hypereosinophilic syndrome*

*Marked eosinophilia

---

References: Lukens, J.N.: Pediatr. Clin. North Am., *19*:969, 1972. Muido, L.: Supplied the mnemonic.

## THROMBOCYTOSIS

Often the report of a peripheral blood smear contains the observation "platelets appear increased." Often this is disregarded.

Elevations in platelet count frequently have diagnostic significance. Just recently it provided the clue to the fact that one patient had a neuroblastoma. The causes of thrombocytosis (platelet count in excess of 400,000/mm³) are listed below. Those in italics are the most common.

Hereditary
   *Asplenia*
   Myeloproliferative disorder in Down's syndrome

Nutritional deficiency
   *Iron deficiency*
   Megaloblastic anemia
   *Vitamin E deficiency*

Metabolic
   Hyperadrenalism

Immume
   Graft vs. host reaction
   Nephrotic syndrome

Infectious
   Virus
   Bacteria
   Mycobacteria

Drug response
   *Vinca alkaloids*
   Citrovorum factor
   Corticosteroid therapy

Neoplastic
   *Chronic myelogenous leukemia*
   Histiocytosis
   Carcinoma
   Lymphoma
   Megakaryocytic leukemia
   Neuroblastoma

Traumatic
   *Surgery*
   Fractures
   *Hemorrhage*

Miscellaneous
   *Splenectomy*
   Caffey's disease
   Inflammatory bowel disease
   Pulmonary embolism
   Thrombophlebitis
   Cerebrovascular accident
   Sarcoidosis
   Idiopathic

8

Reference: Addiego, J.E., Jr., Mentzer, W.E., Jr., and Dallman, P.R.: J. Pediatr., *85*:805, 1974.

## EASY BRUISING—A COAGULATION DEFECT OR PLATELET DISORDER?

Easy bruising is a common complaint. Certain simple features of the history and physical examination allow you to distinguish bleeding as a result of defect in the fluid phase of coagulation from a platelet or capillary defect.

| CLINICAL FEATURES | COAGULATION DEFECTS | PLATELET AND CAPILLARY DEFECTS |
|---|---|---|
| Bleeding from superficial cuts and abrasions | Usually not excessive | Often profuse and prolonged |
| Spontaneous bruises and hematomas | Often deep and spreading hematoma; only a few at any one time | Usually small; superficial, and multiple |
| Hemarthroses | Common in severe cases | Very rare |
| Bleeding from deep cuts and tooth extractions | Onset often delayed for minutes or hours; not permanently controlled by local pressure | Onset usually immediate; frequently permanently arrested by local pressure |
| Most common bleeding manifestations | Deep tissue hemorrhages, often involves joints and muscle; prolonged bleeding after injury | Epistaxis, menorrhagia, and gastrointestinal bleeding |
| Petechiae | Rare | Common |

Reference: Hardisty, R.M., and Ingram, G.I.C.: Bleeding Disorders. Philadelphia, F.A. Davis Company, 1965, p. 9.

## DIAGNOSTIC APPROACH TO THE BLEEDING PATIENT

The patient admitted for surgery who has a history of prolonged bleeding following dental extractions, the very ill patient who suddenly begins leaking blood from IV sites, and the child with a history of easy bruisability should each have immediate screening tests to determine if a coagulation defect exists. The results of the prothrombin time (PT), partial thromboplastin time (PTT), and platelet count are telephoned from the lab, and the most logical next step must be chosen. Logical steps are not always easy to come by, but reference to the chart below may provide the appropriate one.

*A Diagnostic Approach to the Bleeding Patients*

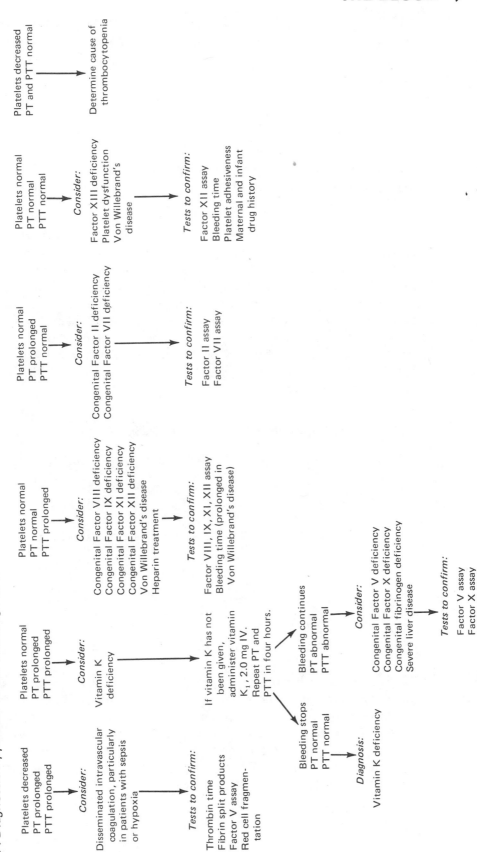

Platelets decreased
PT prolonged
PTT prolonged

*Consider:*

Disseminated intravascular
coagulation, particularly
in patients with sepsis
or hypoxia

*Tests to confirm:*

Thrombin time
Fibrin split products
Factor V assay
Red cell fragmen-
tation

Platelets normal
PT prolonged
PTT prolonged

*Consider:*

Vitamin K
deficiency

If vitamin K has not
been given,
administer vitamin
K₁, 2.0 mg IV.
Repeat PT and
PTT in four hours.

Bleeding continues
PT abnormal
PTT abnormal

Bleeding stops
PT normal
PTT normal

*Diagnosis:*

Vitamin K deficiency

*Consider:*

Congenital Factor V deficiency
Congenital Factor X deficiency
Congenital fibrinogen deficiency
Severe liver disease

*Tests to confirm:*

Factor V assay
Factor X assay
Fibrinogen assay

Platelets normal
PT normal
PTT prolonged

*Consider:*

Congenital Factor VIII deficiency
Congenital Factor IX deficiency
Congenital Factor XI deficiency
Congenital Factor XII deficiency
Von Willebrand's disease
Heparin treatment

*Tests to confirm:*

Factor VIII, IX, XI, XII assay
Bleeding time (prolonged in
Von Willebrand's disease)

Platelets normal
PT prolonged
PTT normal

*Consider:*

Congenital Factor II deficiency
Congenital Factor VII deficiency

*Tests to confirm:*

Factor II assay
Factor VII assay

Platelets normal
PT normal
PTT normal

*Consider:*

Factor XIII deficiency
Platelet dysfunction
Von Willebrand's
disease

*Tests to confirm:*

Factor XII assay
Bleeding time
Platelet adhesiveness
Maternal and infant
drug history

Platelets decreased
PT and PTT normal

Determine cause of
thrombocytopenia

Along with the information included in the chart, it may be helpful to remember that the most common cause of congenital coagulation abnormality is von Willebrand's disease, inherited in an autosomal dominant pattern.

## STEROID-INDUCED PLATELET RESPONSE IN ITP

Should a child with acute idiopathic thrombocytopenic purpura be treated with steroids? Hematologists appear to have differences of opinion. Most agree, however, that the ultimate prognosis of children under 10 years of age presenting with ITP will be unaffected by the use of steroids, with approximately 90 per cent demonstrating complete recovery within a year of onset of their disease. When steroids are employed in the acute phase of the illness, in a dose of 2 mg of prednisone/kg/day, how fast should you anticipate observing a rise in the platelet count? This table should prove to be a useful guide for the child less than age 10 years.

*Per Cent of Patients with a Platelet Count >25,000/mm³*

| DAY OF TREATMENT | WITH STEROIDS | NO STEROIDS |
|:---:|:---:|:---:|
| 1 | 0 | 0 |
| 3 | 10 | 0 |
| 5 | 30 | 4 |
| 7 | 35 | 14 |
| 9 | 52 | 14 |
| 11 | 58 | 19 |
| 13 | 72 | 30 |
| 15 | 75 | 42 |
| 21 | 83 | 55 |
| 180 | 93 | 100 |

In patients with chronic ITP, about 50 per cent will show a rise in platelet count following steroid therapy. In almost none of these patients will the response be sustained.

Patients with acute ITP who are treated with steroids should have the drug discontinued after three weeks of therapy. After this time, the side-effects outweigh the benefits, and prolonged therapy may actually induce thrombocytopenia.

---

Reference: Simons, S.M., Main C.A., Yaish, H.M., et al.: J. Pediatr., *87*:16, 1975.

# EFFECTS OF DRUGS ON PROTHROMBIN TIME

The prothrombin time that is unexpectedly high or low may be a manifestation of the effect of any number of drugs. The following table lists drugs that increase or decrease the prothrombin time. The mechanism of prothrombin time increase is listed, while the mechanism for a shortened test is not known.

*Drugs that Increase Prothrombin Time*

By causing a decrease in vitamin K synthesis or absorption:

| | |
|---|---|
| Cathartics | Neomycin |
| Chlortetracycline | Streptomycin |
| Cholestyramine | Succinylsulfathiazole |
| Kanamycin | Sulfamethoxazole |
| Mineral oil | |

By decreasing clotting factor synthesis:

| | |
|---|---|
| Acetaminophen | L-Asparaginase |
| Acetylsalicylic acid | 6-Mercaptopurine |
| (large doses) | Quinidine |
| Aminosalicylic acid | Quinine |

By altering liver function (bile salt excretion, cholestasis, hepatotoxicity):

| | | |
|---|---|---|
| Acetohexamide | Methotrexate | Sulfisoxazole |
| Chlordiazepoxide | Methyltestosterone | Tetracycline |
| Chlorpromazine | Niacin | Thiazides |
| Chlorpropamide | Oral contraceptives | Tolazamide |
| Halothane | Prochlorperazine | Tolbutamide |
| Mepazine | Promazine | Trifluoperazine |

By decreasing prothrombin concentration or activity:

| | |
|---|---|
| Chloramphenicol | Doxycycline |
| Cremomycin | Pyrazinamide |
| Cyclophosphamide | Sulfachlorpyridazine |
| Demeclocycline | |

*Drugs that Shorten the Prothrombin Time*

Acetylsalicylic acid (small doses)
Anabolic steroids
Azathioprine
Edetic acid (early in therapy)
Kanamycin (early in therapy)
Vitamin K

# MORPHOLOGIC ABNORMALITIES OF THE LEUKOCYTES

There are a number of hereditary morphologic abnormalities of the leukocytes that have diagnostic significance. For example, appreciation of this fact may enable you to make a presumptive diagnosis of trisomy 13–15 (D group) before the chromosome analysis is completed.

The Chédiak-Higashi syndrome can be presumptively diagnosed by inspection of a peripheral blood smear. Suspect it in patients with a history of multiple pyogenic infections in association with partial albinism, hepatosplenomegaly, and mild mental retardation.

A list of some of these morphologic abnormalities and their diagnostic significance appears below.

### Anomalies of the Leukocytes

| ANOMALY | APPEARANCE | ASSOCIATED FINDINGS |
|---|---|---|
| Increased numbers of nuclear projections of the neutrophils | 15 percent or more of the neutrophils contain two or more nuclear projections | Trisomy for one of chromosomes of the D group |
| The Pelger-Huët anomaly | Virtual absence of leukocytes containing more than two lobes | Autosomal dominant inheritance; no associated disease |
| The May-Hegglin anomaly | Leukocytes containing Döhle bodies; giant platelets | Thrombocytopenia may be present; autosomal dominant inheritance |
| Hereditary hyper-segmentation of the neutrophils | Most neutrophilic leukocytes contain four or more lobes | Autosomal dominant inheritance (Undritz, 1939); must be distinguished from the hypersegmentation of the leukocytes observed in pernicious anemia |
| The Chédiak-Higashi anomaly | Multiple refractile gray-green inclusions in the leukocytes; large red or blue inclusions in the lymphocytes | Multiple pyogenic infections, albinism, hepatosplenomegaly, mental retardation, increased incidence of lymphoma |
| Jordan's anomaly | Vacuoles in cytoplasm of granulocytes | One family with muscular dystrophy, another with icthyosis |
| Adler's anomaly | Increased numbers of coarse dark azurophilic granules in the cytoplasm of the neutrophils | No pathologic significance; must be distinguished from toxic granulation; inherited as an autosomal recessive |
| Reilly bodies | Same as Adler's anomaly | Observed in patients with gargoylism; in these patients, lymphocytic inclusions and bone marrow granules of acid mucopolysaccharide may also be seen |

## PROGNOSTIC FACTORS IN LEUKEMIA

More and more children with acute lymphoblastic leukemia are surviving for at least five years from the time of diagnosis without experiencing an initial relapse. In some studies, at least 50 per cent of children can anticipate such a course. It is now recognized that certain factors occur with increased frequency in those patients who do not do well. The major unfavorable prognostic factors include:

1. Initial white blood cell count above 20,000/mm$^3$.
2. Age less than 2 years or greater than 10 years.
3. Central nervous system involvement at the time of diagnosis.
4. The presence of a mediastinal mass.
5. The presence of significant organomegaly or renal involvement at the time of diagnosis.
6. Being black.

## NONHEMATOLOGIC ABNORMALITIES IN FANCONI'S SYNDROME (CONSTITUTIONAL APLASTIC ANEMIA)

When should you suspect that a child who has aplastic anemia has the disease on a congenital basis rather than as a result of an acquired process? The distinction is important because patients with the congenital form of the disturbance generally respond well to androgen therapy. The presence of abnormalities in the physical examination should make you suspect the diagnosis. The most common abnormalities include:

| ABNORMALITY | PER CENT OF PATIENTS |
|---|---|
| Increased pigmentation | 68 |
| Skeletal deformities | 59 |
| Stunted growth | 56 |
| Small head | 43 |
| Renal anomalies | 26 |
| Strabismus | 26 |
| Mental deficiency | 21 |
| Microphthalmia | 13 |
| Hypogonadism | 22 |

The most common of the skeletal abnormalities are those of the thumb. Many patients also display a reduced number of ossification centers at the wrist.

Most patients develop their hematologic abnormalities between 4 and 10 years of age. When patients with the abnormalities described above are seen early in life, they should be followed carefully for the development of aplastic anemia.

Reference: Nelsson, L.B.: Acta Paediatr., *49*:518, 1960.

# 9

# HEART, VESSELS, LUNGS

# CEREBROVASCULAR ACCIDENTS AND CYANOTIC CONGENITAL HEART DISEASE

Cerebrovascular accidents (CVAs), unrelated to surgery, brain abscess, or subacute bacterial endocarditis, still remain a serious complication in patients with cyanotic congenital heart disease.

Frequently, they are attributed to the presence of the associated polycythemia. CVAs, however, are far more common in those children with iron deficiency anemia.

*Virtually all children under 2 years of age with a stroke will have hypochromic microcytic red cell indices.* These children are functionally anemic for their level of hypoxia.

When caring for patients with cyanotic congenital heart disease, do not rely on hemoglobin or hematocrit values alone in evaluating hematologic normality. Always determine the patient's red cell indices. All patients with low MCVs (below 70 $\mu^3$ until 2 years of age) should be evaluated for iron deficiency. If it is present, *these children should be treated regardless of their hemoglobin or hematocrit level.*

Phlebotomy may be considered to maintain the hematocrit at less than 70 per cent once iron deficiency has been corrected.

References: Cottrell, C.M., and Kaplan, S.: Am. J. Dis. Child., *125*:484, 1973. Phornphutkel, C., Rosenthal, A., Berenberg, W., et al.: Pediatr. Res., *6*:329, 1972.

# CONGENITAL HEART DISEASE— THE PRIMARY MANIFESTATION

Different forms of congenital heart disease present in different ways. The primary manifestation may be cyanosis, congestive heart failure, tachycardia or bradycardia, or a heart murmur. Which primary finding suggests which defect? This table should serve as a useful guide.

## Marked Cyanosis

Transposition of the great arteries
Pulmonary atresia and stenosis with intact ventricular septum
Tetralogy of Fallot with severe pulmonary stenosis
Complex pulmonary atresias
Tricuspid atresia
Ebstein's malformation of the tricuspid valve

## Congestive Heart Failure

Aortic atresia
Coarctation of the aorta
Double outlet right ventricle syndrome
Patent ductus arteriosus
Truncus arteriosus
Ventricular septal defect
Arteriovenous fistulas

### Abnormal Heart Rate

Supraventricular tachycardia
Heart block

### Heart Murmur

Patent ductus arteriosus
Pulmonary stenosis
Aortic stenosis
Pulmonary artery stenosis
Ventricular septal defect
Arteriovenous fistulas
Atrioventricular valve regurgitations

---

Reference: Rowe, R., and Mehrizi, A.: The Neonate with Congenital Heart Disease. Philadelphia, W.B. Saunders Company, 1968, p. 105.

# EXTRACARDIAC ANOMALIES IN INFANTS WITH CONGENITAL HEART DISEASE

Approximately 25 per cent of infants with congenital heart disease are found to have extracardiac anomalies. It is often possible to associate particular extracardiac anomalies with a specific type of cardiac defect. The following table lists the frequency of these associations.

Frequency of ECA in the Most Common Cardiac Diagnostic Categories in Infancy

| CARDIAC MALFORMATION* | TOTAL NUMBER | EXTRA-CARDIAC ANOMALY (NUMBER) | PER CENT | NUMBER AND PER CENT WITH ANOMALIES IN BODY SYSTEM | | | | |
|---|---|---|---|---|---|---|---|---|
| | | | | Musculoskeletal | Respiratory | Central Nervous | Genitourinary | Gastrointestinal |
| VSD–Simple | 159 | 44 | 27.6 | 20 (12.6) | 7 ( 4.4) | 14 ( 8.8) | 6 ( 3.8) | 4 (2.5) |
| HLV | 122 | 15 | 12.3 | 6 ( 4.6) | — | 2 ( 1.6) | 4 ( 3.3) | — |
| PDA | 116 | 42 | 36.2 | 12 (10.3) | 5 ( 4.3) | 13 (11.2) | 9 ( 7.8) | 5 (3.1) |
| TOF | 104 | 31 | 29.8 | 13 (12.5) | 4 ( 3.8) | 9 ( 8.7) | 4 ( 3.8) | 10 (9.6) |
| TGA–Simple | 103 | 8 | 7.8 | 3 ( 3.0) | — | 3 ( 2.9) | 1 ( 1.0) | 1 (1.0) |
| CoAo–Complex | 86 | 22 | 25.6 | 7 ( 8.1) | 2 ( 2.3) | 5 ( 5.8) | 8 ( 9.3) | 4 (4.7) |
| ECD | 75 | 38 | 51.0 | 6 ( 8.0) | 1 ( 1.3) | 2 ( 2.7) | 3 ( 4.0) | 7 (9.3) |
| VSD–Complex | 74 | 23 | 31.1 | 9 (12.1) | — | 8 (10.8) | 4 ( 5.4) | 3 (4.1) |
| TGA–Complex | 65 | 7 | 10.8 | 4 ( 6.2) | — | 1 ( 1.5) | 2 ( 3.1) | 1 (1.5) |
| Mal | 58 | 20 | 34.5 | 4 ( 6.9) | 6 (10.3) | 5 ( 8.6) | 8 (13.8) | 5 (8.6) |
| SV | 49 | 10 | 20.4 | 5 (10.4) | 1 ( 2.0) | 5 (10.4) | 2 ( 4.1) | 1 (2.0) |
| PA | 48 | 2 | 4.2 | 1 ( 2.1) | — | 1 ( 2.1) | 1 ( 2.1) | — |
| PS | 48 | 9 | 18.7 | 4 ( 8.4) | 1 ( 2.1) | 5 (10.4) | 1 ( 2.1) | 3 (6.3) |
| Myo | 37 | 7 | 18.9 | — | 2 ( 5.4) | 3 ( 8.1) | 2 ( 5.4) | 2 (5.4) |
| Truncus | 37 | 5 | 13.5 | — | — | 2 ( 5.4) | 2 ( 5.4) | 1 (2.7) |
| TAPVR | 37 | 5 | 13.5 | — | 2 ( 5.4) | 1 ( 2.7) | 1 ( 2.7) | 2 (5.4) |
| ASD | 36 | 13 | 36.1 | 8 (22.2) | 2 ( 5.6) | 4 (11.1) | 2 ( 5.6) | 3 (8.4) |
| PA, VSD | 33 | 6 | 18.2 | 1 ( 3.0) | 2 ( 6.1) | 1 ( 3.0) | 1 ( 3.0) | — |
| CoAo–Simple | 25 | 5 | 20.0 | 2 ( 8.0) | 2 ( 8.0) | 1 ( 4.0) | — | 1 (4.0) |
| DORV | 18 | 3 | 16.7 | 3 (16.7) | 1 ( 5.6) | — | 1 ( 5.6) | 1 (5.6) |
| CTGA | 17 | 2 | 11.8 | 2 (11.8) | — | — | 1 ( 5.9) | — |
| Other lesions | 219 | 78 | 35.6 | | | | | |
| Total | 1566 | 395 | 25.2 | | | | | |

*VSD = ventricular septal defect; HLV = hypoplastic left ventricle; PDA = patent ductus arteriosus; TOF = tetralogy of Fallot; TGA = transposition of the great arteries; CoAo = coarctation of the aorta; ECD = endocardial cushion defect; Mal = malposition; SV = single ventricle; PA = pulmonary atresia; PS = pulmonary stenosis; Myo = myocardial disease; Truncus = truncus arteriosus; TAPVR = total anomalous pulmonary venous return; ASD = atrial septal defect; PA, VSD = pulmonary atresia and ventricular septal defect; DORV = double outlet right ventricle; CTGA = corrected transposition of the great arteries.

9

Chromosomal and nonchromosomal syndromes may also be associated with certain cardiac anomalies. The following tables list the cardiovascular defects found in association with the syndrome listed.

*Chromosomal Syndromes Associated with Cardiovascular Malformations in Infants*

| SYNDROME | NUMBER OF PATIENTS | NUMBER AND DIAGNOSIS OF CHD* |
|---|---|---|
| 21 Trisomy (Down) | 63 | 32 ECD; 6 VSD; 6 TOF; 4 PDA; 2 ASD; 2 VSD and ASD; 2 Cor Pul; 2 TAPVR; 1 TA; 1 MA; 1 NSHD; 1 SV; 1 MR; 1 VSD and PDA; 1 ASD primum |
| E Trisomy (Edwards) | 7 | 3 VSD and PDA, 2 Dextro and CHD, 1 VSD, 1 VSD and ASD |
| D Trisomy (Patau) | 5 | 1 TOF; 1 AoAtres; 1 PDA; 1 CoAo and PDA; 1 ASD secundum |
| Turner (XO) | 5 | 1 severe CoAo; 1 AoAtres; 1 Levoc-Asplen; 1 TGA and IVS; 1 Truncus |
| Klinefelter (XXY) | 1 | 1 VSD |
| Cat Eye (Trisomy extra small chromosome) | 1 | 1 TA and TAPVR |
| XYY | 1 | 1 TGA and IVS |
| A Translocation | 1 | 1 PDA |
| C Translocation | 2 | 1 TOF; 1 systemic hypertension |
| D Deletion | 2 | 1 VSD; 1 VSD and ASD |
| G Translocation | 1 | 1 TAPVR |

*ECD = endocardial cushion defect; VSD = ventricular septal defect; TOF = tetralogy of Fallot; PDA = patent ductus arteriosus; ASD = atrial septal defect; Cor Pul = cor pulmonale; TAPVR = total anomalous pulmonary venous return; TA = tricuspid atresia; MA = mitral atresia; NSHD = no significant heart disease; SV = single ventricle; MR = mitral regurgitation; Dextro, CHD = dextrocardia with heart disease; AoAtres = aortic atresia; CoAo = coarctation of the aorta; Levoc-Asplen = levocardia, asplenia syndrome; TGA = transposition of the great arteries; IVS = intact ventricular septum; Truncus = truncus arteriosus.

*Nonchromosomal Syndromes in Infants with CHD*

| SYNDROME | NUMBER | CARDIAC LESIONS AND NUMBER* |
|---|---|---|
| Congenital rubella | 25 | 13 PDA; 2 PS and IVS; 2 CoAo, PDA and VSD; 1 CoAo and VSD; 1 TGA with VSD; 1 ASD secundum; 1 Truncus; 1 VSD; 1 TAPVR; 2 NSHD |
| Pierre Robin | 5 | 2 TOF; 1 VSD; 1 ECD; 1 CoAo and PDA |
| DiGeorge | 3 | 2 AoAtres; 1 Interr Ao and HLV |
| Beckwith | 3 | 1 ASD secundum; 1 VSD; 1 AoAtres |
| Cornelia de Lange | 2 | 1 TOF; 1 CoAo, Complex |
| Holt-Oram | 1 | 1 TGA, PS and VSD |
| Goldenhar | 1 | 1 TOF |
| Rubinstein-Taybi | 1 | 1 Mesocardia, asplenia, CoAo and VSD |
| Marfan | 1 | 1 VSD |
| Noonan | 1 | 1 TGA and IVS |

*PDA = patent ductus arteriosus; PS = pulmonary stenosis; IVS = intact ventricular septum; CoAo = coarctation of the aorta; VSD = ventricular septal defect; TGA = transposition of the great arteries; ASD = atrial septal defect; Truncus = truncus arteriosus; TAPVR = total anomalous pulmonary venous return; NSHD = no significant heart disease; TOF = tetralogy of Fallot; ECD = endocardial cushion defect; AoAtres = aortic atresia; Interr Ao = interrupted aortic arch; HLV = hypoplastic left ventricle.

Reference: Greenwood, R.D., Rosenthal, A., Parisi, L., et al.: Pediatrics, *55*:485, 1975.

# COUNSELING YOUNG PATIENTS WITH HEART DISEASE ABOUT RECREATIONAL ACTIVITIES

It is frequently necessary to advise children and adolescents with heart disease about the recreational activities they may pursue. Recommendations are difficult to make because of the paucity of data. Guidelines have been proposed by the American Heart Association which are based on the combined experience of many physicians. These guidelines are based on the average functional state of patients with a certain defect and should be considered only as a part of the total evaluation. The accuracy of counseling will be improved by exercise testing that takes into account individual variations. Until such time as precise information is available, the guidelines of the American Heart Association can serve as a very useful source of advice.

Before using the table, the following categories should be appreciated:

### Mild Restriction

Advise against activities that would require maximal or near-maximal effort for a duration of more than one-half minute. Prohibited activities would include track (running events) and competitive basketball, swimming, soccer, hockey, skiing, and football.

### Moderate Restriction

Advise against competitive pressures generated by most team sports, except baseball and perhaps volleyball. These patients should not take part in a complete physical education program but may participate in noncompetitive activities and should be encouraged to stop when fatigued.

### Severe Restriction

Patients should be encouraged to take up activities that are enjoyable at low levels of energy expenditure and that allow the patient to set his own pace. Examples of such activities include golf with a cart, bowling, walking, and swimming.

*Guidelines for Recreational Activities*

| DEFECT | RECREATIONAL RESTRICTIONS | EXAMPLES OF ALLOWABLE RECREATION |
| --- | --- | --- |
| *Aortic Insufficiency* | | |
| Mild, with normal ECG and heart size | None | All recreational activity is allowed |
| Moderate, with cardiac enlargement | Mild | All but those requiring violent, prolonged exertion |
| Severe, without signs of QRS-T angle abnormality on ECG | Moderate | Baseball, volleyball, and noncompetitive activities |
| Severe, with signs of QRS-T angle abnormality on ECG | Severe | Golf with cart, bowling, walking, swimming at own pace |
| *Aortic Stenosis* | | |
| Mild, with or without surgery | None | All recreational activity is allowed |
| Moderate, with or without surgery | Mild | All but those requiring violent, prolonged exertion |
| Severe, with or without surgery | Moderate | Baseball, volleyball, and noncompetitive activities |
| *Atrial Septal Defect* | | |
| Unoperated or successfully operated, with normal pulmonary artery pressure | None | All recreational activity is allowed |
| Unoperated or successfully operated, with pulmonary hypertension but pulmonary artery pressure <0.50 systemic | None | All recreational activity is allowed |
| With severe pulmonary vascular disease | Moderate | Baseball, volleyball, and noncompetitive activities |
| *Chronic Congestive Heart Failure* | Severe | Golf with cart, bowling, walking, swimming at own pace |
| *Coarctation of the Aorta* | | |
| Unoperated, with severe systemic hypertension and no significant aortic valve disease | None | All recreational activity is allowed |
| Postoperative, with normal blood pressure and no significant aortic valve disease | None | All recreational activity is allowed |
| *Mitral Insufficiency* | | |
| With little or no cardiac enlargement | None | All recreational activity is allowed |
| With moderate to marked cardiac enlargement | Moderate | Baseball, volleyball, and noncompetitive activities |

*Table continued on the following page*

9

| DEFECT | RECREATIONAL RESTRICTIONS | EXAMPLES OF ALLOWABLE RECREATION |
|---|---|---|
| *Myocarditis, Active* | Severe | Golf with cart, bowling, walking, swimming at own pace |
| *Patent Ductus Arteriosus* | | |
| Unoperated or operated, with normal pulmonary artery pressure | None | All recreational activity is allowed |
| Unoperated or operated, with pulmonary hypertension (pulmonary artery pressure <0.50 systemic) | None | All recreational activity is allowed |
| Unoperated or operated, with severe pulmonary vascular disease | Moderate | Baseball, volleyball, and noncompetitive activities |
| *Prosthetic Valve Replacement* | Moderate | Baseball, volleyball, and noncompetitive activities |
| *Pulmonary Stenosis* | | |
| Mild to moderate (peak systolic gradient <50 mm Hg) with or without surgery | None | All recreational activity is allowed |
| Severe (peak systolic gradient >80 mm Hg) | Moderate | Baseball, volleyball, and noncompetitive activities |
| *Tetralogy of Fallot* | | |
| Postoperative, right ventricle–pulmonary artery gradient <50 mm Hg without outflow patch | None | All recreational activity is allowed |
| Postoperative, right ventricle–pulmonary artery gradient <50 mm Hg with outflow patch and pulmonary insufficiency | Mild | All but those requiring violent, prolonged exertion |
| *Ventricular Septal Defect* | | |
| Unoperated or operated, with normal pulmonary artery pressure | None | All recreational activity is allowed |

| | | |
|---|---|---|
| Unoperated or operated, with pulmonary hypertension (pulmonary artery pressure <50 mm Hg systolic) | None | All recreational activity is allowed |
| Unoperated or operated, with severe pulmonary vascular disease | Moderate | Baseball, volleyball, and noncompetitive activities |
| *Other Mild Forms of Heart Disease* not requiring surgery and without natural history of progressive disability | None | All recreational activity is allowed |
| *Other Severe Defects* not operated or amenable to surgery | Severe | Golf with cart, bowling, walking, swimming at own pace |

Reference: Recreational and occupational recommendations for use by physicians counseling young patients with heart disease. American Heart Association Bulletin, 1971.

9

## PROTECTION FROM BACTERIAL ENDOCARDITIS

What is the preferred method for the prevention of bacterial endocarditis in patients with congenital heart disease or rheumatic heart disease who must undergo surgical or dental procedures? The guidelines below have been proposed by the American Heart Association.

*For Dental Procedures and also for Tonsillectomy, Adenoidectomy, and Bronchoscopy*

I. For most patients:

*Penicillin*
  a. *Intramuscular*
600,000 units of procaine penicillin G mixed with 200,000 units of crystalline penicillin G one hour prior to procedure and once daily for two days* following the procedure.

OR  b. *Oral*
1. 500 mg of penicillin V or phenethicillin one hour prior to procedure and then 250 mg every six hours for the remainder of that day and for the two days* following the procedure.

OR

2. 1,200,000 units of penicillin G one hour prior to procedure and then 600,000 units every six hours for the remainder of that day and for the two days* following the procedure.

II. For patients suspected to be allergic to penicillin or for those on continual oral penicillin for rheumatic fever prophylaxis, who may harbor penicillin-resistant viridans streptococci:

*Erythromycin*
  *Oral*

*Adults:* 500 mg one and one-half to two hours prior to procedure and then 250 mg every six hours for the remainder of that day and for the two days* following the procedure.

*Children:* The dose for small children is 20 mg/kg orally one and one-half to two hours prior to the procedure and then 10 mg/kg every six hours for the remainder of that day and for the two days* following the procedure.

---

*Or longer in the case of delayed healing.

*For Gastrointestinal and Genitourinary Tract Surgery and Instrumentation and also for Any Surgery of Infected Tissues*

I. For most patients:

*Penicillin*

600,000 units of procaine penicillin G mixed with 200,000 units of crystalline penicillin G intramuscularly one hour prior to procedure and once daily for the two days following the procedure.

PLUS
*Streptomycin*

1 to 2 gm intramuscularly one hour prior to procedure and once daily for the two days following the procedure.

*For children:* 40 mg/kg intramuscularly one hour prior to the procedure and once daily for the two days following the procedure. (Not to exceed 1 gm/24 hours.)

OR
*Ampicillin*

25 to 50 mg/kg given orally or intravenously one hour prior to procedure and then 25 mg/kg every six hours for the remainder of that day and for the two days following the procedure.

PLUS
*Streptomycin*

(As above.)

II. For patients suspected to be allergic to the penicillins, *erythromycin* can be given (instead of penicillin or ampicillin)

(For dosage and duration for erythromycin, see suggested prophylaxis schedule for dental procedures.)

PLUS
*Streptomycin*

(As above.)

*Vancomycin* can be given as an alternative to erythromycin

0.5 to 1.0 gm intravenously one hour prior to procedure and then 0.5 gm intravenously every six hours for the remainder of that day and for the two days* following the procedure.

PLUS
*Streptomycin*

For children: 20 mg/kg one hour prior to procedure and then 10 mg/kg every six hours for the remainder of that day and for the two days following the procedure. (As above.)

---

*Or longer in the case of delayed healing.

Reference: American Heart Association Communications Division, American Heart Association.

# POTASSIUM DISORDERS AND THE ELECTROCARDIOGRAM

Electrocardiographic changes may be roughly correlated to degrees of hypo- or hyperkalemia as illustrated in Figure 9–1.

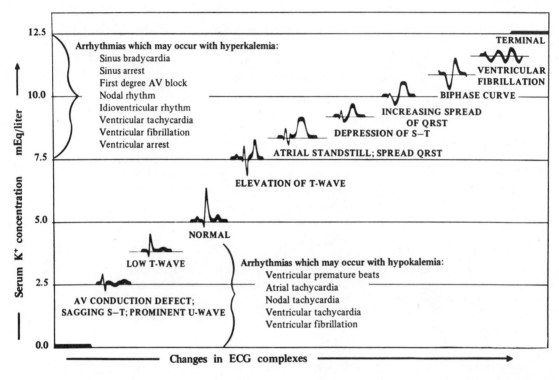

*FIG. 9–1*

The cardiac toxicity of hyperkalemia may be accentuated by low sodium levels. Severe hyponatremia may lead to advanced cardiac toxicity at a potassium level of 7.5 mg/liter.

Potassium depletion may accompany hypochloremic metabolic alkalosis. Until the chloride deficiency is corrected, the potassium that is administered will continue to be wasted by the kidneys. Administration of KCl corrects both disorders.

Reference: O'Brien, D.: *In* Kempe, C.H., Silver, H.K., and O'Brien, D. (Eds.): Current Pediatric Diagnosis and Treatment. Los Altos, California, Lange Medical Publications, 1976, p. 956.

# ASTHMA IN CHILDHOOD— CHARACTERISTICS AND PROGNOSIS

What is the natural history and the clinical and physiologic manifestations of asthma in children? A review of 315 children who were all evaluated at age 14 years provides many insights. The children were classified by history as follows:

| CLASS | DEFINITION |
|-------|------------|
| A | No more than five episodes of wheezing up to 14 years of age. |
| B | More than five episodes of wheezing but none within 12 months of their 14th birthday. |
| C | Continuing history of episodic asthma with attacks within 12 months of the 14th birthday. |
| D | History of very frequent or chronic unremitting asthma having either periods of severe or prolonged asthma during the 13th year of life with remissions of less than one month or more than 10 attacks within three months of 14th birthday. |

The following table describes the characteristics of these four groups of patients. From this table it can be seen that the characteristics of severe persistent asthma include onset usually in the first three years of life, a high frequency of attacks within the initial year, clinical and physiologic evidence of persisting airway obstruction and pulmonary hyperinflation, chest deformity, and impairment of growth. In contrast, mild asthma usually begins later in childhood, is episodic, and is not associated with evidence of airway obstruction between attacks. Most of the patients with mild asthma will have no further difficulty after age 10 years.

*Asthma — Prognosis and Characteristics*

| CLASS | FREQUENCY (%) | USUAL AGE OF ONSET | AGE AT REMISSION | SEX PREVALENCE | PHYSICAL CHARACTERISTICS AT AGE 14 | ASSOCIATED ALLERGIES (ANYTIME BEFORE AGE 14) | | |
|---|---|---|---|---|---|---|---|---|
| | | | | | | Hay Fever (%) | Eczema (%) | Urticaria (%) |
| A | 20 | After 3 | 8 | None | Normal | 44 | 14 | 55 |
| B | 28 | 2 to 3 | 5 to 14 | 60% males 40% females | Normal | 55 | 22 | 54 |
| C | 34 | 2 to 3 | After 10 | 68% males 32% females | 7% Pigeon chest 15% Barrel chest Decreased weight 10% pulmonary hyperinflation by x-ray | 72 | 56 | 57 |
| D | 18 | Before 2 (28% before 6 months) | After 10 | 79% males 21% females | 25% Pigeon chest 48% Barrel chest Decreased weight and height 27% pulmonary hyperinflation by x-ray | 80 | 67 | 57 |
| | | | | | *Controls* | 18 | 11 | 30 |

Reference: McNicol, K.N., and Williams, H.B.: Br. Med. J., 4:7, 1973.

| CLASS | POSITIVE SKIN TESTS AT AGE 14 YEARS (%) | BLOOD EOSINOPHIL COUNT (PER mm³) | PROPORTION OF EOSINOPHILS IN NASAL SMEAR (% eosinophils – % patients) | MEAN SERUM IgE AT AGE 14 (ng/ml) |
|---|---|---|---|---|
| A | 43 | $293 \pm 271$ ($2\% > 1000/mm^3$) | $>5 - 9$ $>20 - 3$ | $607 \pm 448$ |
| B | 45 | $300 \pm 290$ ($8\% > 1000/mm^3$) | $>5 - 11$ $>20 - 1$ | $607 \pm 448$ |
| C | 80 | $554 \pm 369$ ($18\% > 1000/mm^3$) | $>5 - 23$ $>20 - 3$ | $1005 \pm 508$ |
| D | 81 | $657 \pm 297$ ($27\% > 1000/mm^3$) | $>5 - 24$ $>20 - 7$ | $2163 \pm 1800$ |
| Control: 10 | | Control: $213 \pm 250$ ($0\% > 1000/mm^3$) | Control: $>5 - 7$ $>20 - 1$ | Control: $79 \pm 156$ |

9

## PULSUS PARADOXUS—A SIGN OF A SEVERE ASTHMA ATTACK

When the arterial pulse decreases in amplitude or actually disappears during inspiration, it is termed pulsus paradoxus. Pulsus paradoxus can be suspected by palpation of the radial pulse. Its presence can be confirmed by measuring changes in blood pressure at the brachial artery. The systolic pressure on expiration can be defined as the highest level at which the systolic pulse sounds can be heard during expiration. The systolic pressure on inspiration can be defined as the highest level at which these sounds could be heard with every pulse beat throughout the whole of inspiration. When the systolic pressure is 10 mm Hg lower during inspiration, this is pulsus paradoxus.

This sign is easily elicited and provides a valuable clue to the severity of the asthmatic attack. Its presence has been found to correlate quite well with the decrease in $FEV_1$, the peak expiratory flow rate, and the magnitude of the increase in the $P_aCO_2$. It is frequently difficult to determine the severity of an asthmatic attack adequately from physical examination alone. We often tend to underestimate the degree of pulmonary embarrassment. This simple test can provide you with quick information. When pulsus paradoxus is present, immediate, intensive treatment of the asthmatic attack is indicated.

Reference: Knowles, G.K., and Clark, T.J.H.: Lancet, 2:1356, 1973.

## THE TWENTY-NINE FACES OF CYSTIC FIBROSIS

Most pediatricians now appreciate the fact that juvenile rheumatoid arthritis may present in a variety of ways; this fact has been captured by the phrase, "the three faces of juvenile rheumatoid arthritis." Cystic fibrosis is a far more prodigious imitator. Are you aware of "the 29 faces of cystic fibrosis"?

Listed below are the 29 ways in which cystic fibrosis may initially manifest itself. Be suspicious and perform a sweat test when these problems are encountered without a suitable alternative explanation.

Meconium ileus and meconium peritonitis
Pancreatic insufficiency and growth failure
Recurrent pulmonary infections
Intestinal impaction and obstruction (may produce intussusception)
Rectal prolapse
Prolonged neonatal hyperbilirubinemia
Cirrhosis of the liver
Portal hypertension

Glucose intolerance
Diabetes
Acute and recurrent pancreatitis
Vitamin K deficiency with bleeding
Vitamin A deficiency
Vitamin E deficiency, muscle weakness, and creatinuria
Night cramps
Hypoproteinemia in infancy with edema and anemia (seen usually in
    infants fed soybean formulas or human milk)
Lactase deficiency
Duodenal ulcer
Cholelithiasis and cholecystitis
Chronic obstructive airway disease
Cor pulmonale
Recurrent episodes of asthma
Hypertrophic pulmonary osteoarthropathy
Nasal polyps
Optic neuritis
Salty taste of infant noted by mother
Hyponatremic dehydration in warm weather
Heat stroke
Infertility in males

## SARCOIDOSIS

Sarcoidosis is rare in children, but it should not be a difficult diagnosis to make. In the United States, 75 per cent of the children with sarcoidosis are black. Presenting symptoms and signs and appropriate laboratory findings are listed below in order of decreasing frequency.

| SYMPTOMS | SIGNS | LABORATORY FINDINGS |
|---|---|---|
| Fatigability, lethargy, malaise | Bilateral hilar adenopathy | Increased serum globulin |
| Cough | Parenchymal lung involvement | Eosinophilia |
| Fever | Peripheral adenopathy | Elevated alkaline phosphatase |
| Dyspnea | Liver enlargement | Leukopenia |
| Weight loss | Splenic enlargement | Hypercalcemia |
| Loss of visual acuity | Cutaneous lesions | |
| Anorexia | Uveitis | |
| | Parotid gland enlargement | |
| | Roentgenographic evidence of bone disease | |
| | Joint swelling | |

Some patients are asymptomatic at presentation and are diagnosed as a result of a chest roentgenogram taken for an unrelated cause.

The diagnosis is best verified by biopsy of a lymph node, although biopsy of any tissue or organ involved will provide the characteristic noncaseating granuloma.

Sarcoidosis should be considered strongly in any child presenting with bilateral hilar adenopathy. This finding is present in 97 per cent of children in whom sarcoidosis is diagnosed.

Reference: Kendig, E.L.: Pediatrics, *54*:289, 1974.

## A SIMPLE MEANS OF SELECTING THE APPROPRIATE ENDOTRACHEAL TUBE

The intubation of an infant or child should not be accomplished by trial and error. Age is not an appropriate criterion for the selection of the correct size endotracheal tube; the width of the patient's fifth finger appears to be a much better guide.

Figure 9–2 depicts the landmarks to be used in measurement of the little finger and provides a simple formula for converting this measurement into the selection of the endotracheal tube. This technique is most useful for the patient under 6 years of age.

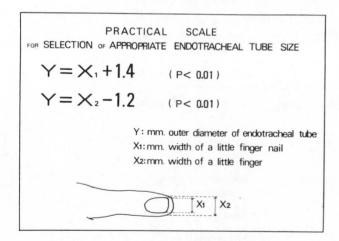

PRACTICAL SCALE
FOR SELECTION OF APPROPRIATE ENDOTRACHEAL TUBE SIZE

$$Y = X_1 + 1.4 \qquad (P < 0.01)$$

$$Y = X_2 - 1.2 \qquad (P < 0.01)$$

Y : mm. outer diameter of endotracheal tube
$X_1$: mm. width of a little finger nail
$X_2$: mm. width of a little finger

*FIG. 9–2*

Reference: Iwai, S., and Mukubo, Y.: Pediatr. News, October 1974, p. 14.

## TEXIDOR'S TWINGE OR THE PERICARDIAL CATCH SYNDROME

This type of pain is a common complaint of teenagers and normal individuals in their 20s and 30s. It is a very brief, very sharp needle-like pain near the apex of the heart. It is acutely localized to one point, seemingly inside the chest wall. Breathing sharpens it and results in a disinclination to take a deep breath while the pain persists.

It most commonly occurs while the subject is either seated or lying down.

Although it may frighten the individual, it is of no pathologic significance. The patient should be reassured. If the symptoms are classic, no diagnostic studies are indicated.

---

Reference: Miller, A.J., and Texidor, T.A.: J.A.M.A., *159*:1365, 1955.

# EVALUATION OF HYPERTENSION

The conventional wisdom is that most hypertension detected in infants, children, and adolescents is secondary to a definable disease. Recently, it has been suggested that essential hypertension also manifests itself in late childhood and early adolescence and may be responsible for as much as 30 per cent of all observed elevations in blood pressure.

When confronted with a patient with hypertension, one must determine the following:

1.  Is it transient or persistent?
2.  Is it secondary to another process?

It is unfortunate that most pediatric patients do not have their blood pressure recorded. A survey revealed that in only 5 per cent of all pediatric out-patient visits was the blood pressure recorded, and in only 62 per cent of hospital admissions was the blood pressure measured. In patients less than 1 year of age, blood pressure was recorded in 0.4 per cent of out-patients and 56 per cent of in-patients.

A complete physical examination must include a blood pressure measurement. The blood pressure should be measured in all acutely ill patients, particularly those with complaints referable to the heart, kidneys, or central nervous system.

### The Normal Blood Pressure

The following guidelines should be employed when obtaining a conventional office blood pressure.

1. The patient should be supine.
2. The cuff should be at least 20 per cent wider than the diameter of the arm and cover approximately two-thirds to three-quarters of the arm as measured from elbow to axilla.
3. The examiner should be at eye level with the manometer.

4. The meniscus of the manometer should be checked weekly for zero calibration.

5. While measuring, the rate of fall should be approximately 2 to 3 mm Hg per heart beat.

6. Readings should be made to the nearest 2 mm Hg.

Guidelines for the 95th percentile of acceptable blood pressure are:

| AGE (years) | SYSTOLIC (mm Hg) | DIASTOLIC (mm Hg) |
|:-----------:|:----------------:|:-----------------:|
| 0–3 | 110 | 65 |
| 3–6 | 120 | 70 |
| 6–11 | 125 | 78 |
| 11–15 | 140 | 80 |

## Conditions Associated with Acute Transient Hypertension or Intermittent Hypertension

### RENAL

Acute poststreptococcal glomerulonephritis
Hemolytic-uremic syndrome
Henoch-Schönlein purpura with nephritis
Genitourinary tract surgery
Post–renal transplantation
Following blood transfusion in patients with azotemia
Anephric patients

### OTHER

Burns
Leukemia
Bacterial endocarditis
Poliomyelitis
Mercury poisoning
Hypercalcemia
Guillain-Barré syndrome

Stevens-Johnson syndrome
Hypernatremia
Familial dysautonomia
Increased intracranial pressure
Corticosteroid therapy
Amphetamines

## Potentially Curable Forms of Hypertension

### RENAL

Unilateral hydronephrosis
Unilateral pyelonephritis
Unilateral dysplastic kidney
Traumatic damage
Tumors
Unilateral multicystic kidney
Unilateral ureteral occlusion
Ask-Upmark kidney (segmental dysplasia of small renal arteries)

**VASCULAR**

Coarctation of the aorta
Renal artery abnormalities
  Stenosis
  Arteritis
  Fibromuscular dysplasia
  Neurofibromatosis
  Fistula
  Aneurysm
Renal artery thrombosis

**ADRENAL**

Neuroblastoma
Pheochromocytoma
Adrenogenital syndrome
Cushing's disease
Primary aldosteronism
  Adenoma
  Hyperplasia

**OTHER**

Vascular or renal parenchymal abnormalities after irradiation
Ingestion of excessive amounts of licorice
Administration of glucocorticoids

*Incurable, but Therapeutically Controllable, Forms of Chronic Hypertension*

**RENAL**

Chronic glomerulonephritis
Chronic bilateral pyelonephritis
Congenital dysplastic kidneys (bilateral)
Polycystic kidneys
Medullary cystic disease
Post–renal transplantation

**VASCULAR**

Surgically irremediable main renal artery abnormalities
Surgically irremediable coarctation of the aorta
Generalized hypoplasia of the aorta

**MISCELLANEOUS**

Essential hypertension
Lead nephropathy (late)
Radiation nephritis

*The Diagnostic Evaluation*

### ACUTE OR CHRONIC? FAMILIAL OR ISOLATED?

Careful physical examination (lupus? Cushing's syndrome? neurofibromatosis? adrenogenital syndrome? abdominal mass?)
Blood pressure in all four extremities
Blood pressure measurements in parents and siblings
Examination of the ocular fundus
Examination of the heart
Chest roentgenogram for cardiac size
Electrocardiogram

### RENAL PARENCHYMAL?

Urinalysis
Blood urea nitrogen
Creatinine

If renal parenchymal disease is suspected, then a judgment must be made as to whether it is acute or chronic. Urine culture, measurements of serum complement components, and intravenous pyelogram are useful in reaching this decision. Renal biopsy may be required to establish a diagnosis.

### NONRENAL PARENCHYMAL?

Vascular abnormality
  Renal flow study: renal scan and arteriography
Endocrine abnormality
  Aldosteronism (serum electrolytes–hypokalemia, plasma renins)
  Neuroblastoma (catecholamines)
  Cushing's syndrome (plasma cortisol)
  High renin essential hypertension (plasma renin)

The physician should proceed with the premise that almost all hypertension in children under 6 years of age has an identifiable cause, and that 60 to 80 per cent of hypertension in children 6 to 12 years of age is secondary to a diagnosable disease.

---

References: Loggie, J.M.H., and McEnery, P.T.: *In* Rubin, M.I. (Ed.): Pediatric Nephrology. Baltimore, Williams & Wilkins Company, 1976, p. 417. Pazdrai, P.T., Lieberman, H.M., Pazdrai, W.E., et al.: J.A.M.A., *235*:2320, 1976. Lieberman, E., and Holliday, M.A.: Pediatric Portfolio, Vol. II, Number 2, 1972.

# ANTIHYPERTENSIVE DRUGS

The table below provides a concise summary of the agents available for the treatment of hypertension.

*Antihypertensive Drugs*

| DRUG | SUPPLIED | | DOSE | REMARKS |
|---|---|---|---|---|
| *Volume-Depleting Drugs* | | | | |
| Chlorthiazide (Diuril) | Tablets: | 250, 500 mg | 20 mg/kg/day orally divided every 12 hours | May cause hypokalemia, alkalosis. |
| Hydrochlorthiazide (HydroDiuril) | Tablets: | 25, 50 mg | 2 mg/kg/day orally divided every 12 hours | As above. |
| Spironolactone (Aldactone) | Tablets: | 25 mg | 2–3 mg/kg/day orally divided every 6–8 hours | Contraindicated in acute renal failure. May cause hyperkalemia. |
| Triamterene (Dyrenium) | Tablets: | 50 mg | *Adults:* 50 mg every 12 hours | May cause hyperkalemia and azotemia. |
| | Capsules: | 100 mg | *Children:* 2–4 mg/kg/day divided in 1–2 doses; max. 300 mg/day | |
| Ethacrynic Acid (Edecrin) | Tablets: | 40 mg | 2–3 mg/kg/day orally | Ototoxicity; may cause marked extracellular fluid depletion. |
| | Vials: | 50 mg | 1 mg/kg intravenously | |
| Furosemide (Lasix) | Tablets: | 40 mg | 2–3 mg/kg/day orally | As above. |
| | Ampules: | 10 mg/ml | 1–2 mg/kg intravenously | |
| *Renin-Lowering Drugs* | | | | |
| Propranolol (Inderal) | Tablets: | 10, 40 mg | 0.5–1.0 mg/kg/day orally divided every 6–8 hours; max. daily dose 60 mg (intravenous not established for hypertension) | Contraindicated in asthma and heart block. May cause heart failure. Discontinue before general anesthetic. |
| | Ampules: | 1 mg/ml | | |
| Methyldopa (Aldomet) | Tablets: | 125, 250, 500 mg | *Oral:* 10 mg/kg/day orally divided every 8–12 hours; increase as necessary every 2 days | May cause postural hypotension and sleepiness in large dose. Contraindicated for pheochromocytoma. May cause a positive Coombs' test. |
| | Ampules: | 50 mg/ml | *Intravenous:* (crises) 20–40 mg/kg/day intravenously divided every 6 hours; max. 65 mg/kg/day | |

*Table continued on the following page*

**9**

| DRUG | SUPPLIED | DOSE | REMARKS |
|---|---|---|---|
| Reserpine (Serpasil) | Tablets: 0.1, 0.25 mg<br>Ampules: 2.5 mg/ml | 0.02 mg/kg/day orally<br>*Crisis:* 0.07 mg/kg intramuscularly; repeat every 8–24 hours as necessary; max. 2.5 mg | May cause CNS depression, nasal congestion. |
| *Renin-Independent Direct Vasodilators* | | | |
| Hydralazine (Apresoline) | Tablets: 10, 25, 50, 100 mg<br>Ampules: 20 mg/ml | *Oral:* 0.75 mg/kg/day divided every 6 hours; max. dose 3.5 mg/kg/day<br>*Parenteral alone:* 0.15 mg/kg single dose intramuscularly, intravenously<br>*or*<br>1.7–3.5 mg/kg/day divided every 4–6 hours<br>*Parenteral with reserpine:* 0.15 mg/kg/dose intramuscularly, intravenously every 4–6 hours | May cause lupus-like syndrome. |
| Diazoxide (Hyperstat) | Ampules: 15 mg/ml | 5 mg/kg intravenously in 30 seconds or less. May repeat in 30 minutes | Use with caution with diabetes mellitus. Can cause hyperglycemia and hypertrichosis. |
| Sodium nitroprusside | | *Crisis:* 60 mg in 500 ml 5 per cent dextrose/water; titrate infusion rate with blood pressure. | Not available in a sterile solution. |
| Minoxidil | Tablets: 5, 10 mg | 2.5 mg every 6 hours; increase every 2–3 days; max. 40 mg/day | May cause tachyarrhythmias and thus require propranolol. |

*Renin-Independent Adrenergic Blockers*

| | | | |
|---|---|---|---|
| Guanethidine (Ismelin) | Tablets: 10, 25 mg | 0.2 mg/kg/day single dose orally; increase every 7–10 days by 0.2 mg/kg/day; effective dose may be 5–8 times initial dose | Causes postural hypotension. Contraindicated with pheochromocytoma and monoamine oxidase inhibitors. |
| Bethanidine (Esbaloid) | Tablets: 10, 25 mg | *Adult:* 5–10 mg every 8 hours; gradually increase by 5–10 mg every 8 hours; maintenance 20–150 mg/day. Dose for children not established. | Causes postural hypotension. |
| Pargyline (Eutonyl) | Tablets: 10, 25 mg | *Adult:* 25 mg once daily; increase weekly by 10 mg. Usual range 25–50 mg/day. | Causes orthostatic hypotension. A nonhydrazine monoamine oxidase inhibitor. Antidepressant. |

Reference:  Rance, C.P., Arbus, G.S., Balfe, J.W., et al.: Pediatr. Clin. North Am., *21*:801, 1974.

9

# PAROXYSMAL ATRIAL TACHYCARDIA

Paroxysmal atrial tachycardia (PAT) is rare in infancy and childhood, affecting not more than one in every 25,000 children. Studies have revealed patients fall into three groups: (1) patients with the Wolff-Parkinson-White syndrome (WPW); (2) patients whose attacks of PAT begin before 1 year of age; and (3) patients with onset of attacks later in childhood.

In patients with otherwise normal hearts, brief periods of PAT (6 to 24 hours) do not precipitate acute congestive heart failure. The patient who presents in heart failure, therefore, has suffered a prolonged attack of PAT or has an abnormal heart.

Characteristics of these three groups are delineated in the following table.

| | PAT PATIENTS WITH ONSET IN INFANCY | PAT PATIENTS WITH ONSET IN CHILDHOOD | PAT PATIENTS WITH WPW (ONSET AT ANY AGE) |
|---|---|---|---|
| Sex predominance | Male | None | None |
| Likelihood of recurrence | Low | High | High |
| Presentation at initial attack | Diagnosis frequently made only after patient presents in cardiac failure. Fever may be the presenting feature. | Usually rapid heart rate or palpitations noted by patient or parent. May present with loss of consciousness, vomiting with abdominal pain, or fever. | Characteristics of onset depend upon age of patient and are the same as for patients with PAT without WPW. |
| Response to treatment | The majority of patients suffer single attacks without recurrences. When attacks recur, they may frequently be treated successfully with digitalis alone or with digitalis and quinidine in combination. Rarely, attacks continue into the second year of life. | Recurrent attacks in this group are short and benign; however, control with digitalis, quinidine, and propranolol is often difficult. Physical means of aborting attacks (eyeball pressure or Valsalva maneuver) may have some success in older children. | Control with digitalis, quinidine, and propranolol is often not completely effective. |

Reference: Simcha, A., and Bonham-Carter, R.E.: Lancet, 1:832, 1971.

# 10

# GASTRO-INTESTINAL

# RECURRENT ABDOMINAL PAIN

It is all too common for the pediatrician to be presented with a child with recurrent abdominal pain. John Apley has studied this problem in detail and has accumulated facts that can be of use when evaluating such children.

## Definition

Children who complained of at least three episodes of pain, severe enough to affect their activities, over a period longer than three months.

## Incidence

In school-aged children:

| | |
|---|---|
| Overall incidence | 10.8% |
| Girls | 12.3% |
| Boys | 9.5% |

## Age at Onset

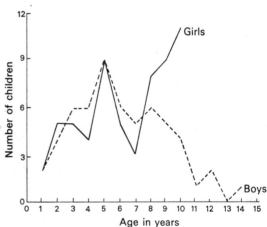

FIG. 10-1

Age at onset of pains.

## Characteristics of Pain

1. In two-thirds of patients it was referred to the region of the umbilicus.
2. In one-third of patients it was described as a dull ache; in about another one-third it was described as colicky. In the remainder it was described as sharp and stabbing.
3. Time of occurrence variable and duration ranged from minutes to days.
4. Abdominal pain associated with vomiting (66 per cent), headache (20 per cent), sleepiness after attack (25 per cent), pallor with the pain (50 per cent).

## Organic Causes

Only 8 of 100 children with recurrent abdominal pain were found to have an associated organic disorder. These were single cases of vulvovaginitis, urethral cyst, hydronephrosis, recurrent pyelonephritis, duodenal ulcer, Meckel's diverticulum, displaced colon, and calcification of the pancreas.

*Family History*

In 46 per cent of the families of children with recurrent abdominal pain, another member had similar complaints (sibling, 18 per cent; mother, 17 per cent; father, 11 per cent). In families of the control patients, only 8 per cent had a history of recurrent abdominal pain. Peptic ulcer, migraine, "nervous breakdowns," and seizure disorders also occurred with greater frequency in the families of affected children.

*Conclusions*

**Apley's Rule:**

*"The farther the localization of the pain from the umbilicus, the more likely is there to be an underlying organic disorder."*

Always try to make a positive diagnosis of an emotional basis for the disorder with a careful history. Do not rely on extensive laboratory tests to make the diagnosis by exclusion.

Reference: Apley, J.: The Child with Abdominal Pains. 2nd Ed. Oxford, Blackwell Scientific Publications Ltd., 1964.

# DIARRHEA—CLUES TO THE DIAGNOSIS

Certain features of the patient's history in conjunction with physical findings and the appearance of the stool will allow you to make the correct etiologic diagnosis in approximately 75 per cent of all patients you see with diarrhea. The important clinical features of acute diarrheal disease that are useful in differential diagnosis are describe' on page 279.

Reference: Nelson, J., and Haltalin, K.: J. Pediatr., *78*:519, 1971.

*Diaper*—From the old French. *Diaspre* means ornamental cloth. The word originally came from the Greek *dia*, meaning through, and the Byzantine *aspros*, meaning white. The word aspros appears in the Greek aspropatos, which means "bottoms up" and suggests the transparent bottom of the bottle as the last of the wine is drunk. Bottoms up is, of course, applicable to the baby as the diaper is being applied.

*Clinical Features of Acute Diarrheal Disease Useful in Differential Diagnosis*

| CLINICAL FEATURES | SHIGELLA | ENTEROPATHOGENIC E. COLI | SALMONELLA (EXCLUDING TYPHOID FEVER) | NONBACTERIAL |
|---|---|---|---|---|
| Age | 6 months to 5 years (rare in neonate) | Less than 2 years | Any age | Any age |
| Diarrhea in household | Common (>50%) | No | Variable | Variable |
| Onset | Abrupt | Gradual | Variable | Abrupt |
| Vomiting as a prominent symptom | Absent | Uncommon | Common | Common |
| Fever (over 102° F) | Common | Absent | Variable | Uncommon |
| Respiratory symptoms | Common (bronchitis) | Absent | Uncommon (except in septicemia form) | Common (upper respiratory) |
| Convulsion | Common | Rare | Rare | Rare |
| Anal sphincter | Lax tone (rarely, rectal prolapse) | Normal | Normal | Normal |
| Stools: | | | | |
| Consistency | Watery | Loose, slimy | Loose, slimy | Loose |
| Odor | Relatively odorless | Foul | Foul (rotten egg) | Unpleasant |
| Blood | Common | Rare | Rare | Rare |
| Color | Yellow-green (almost colorless in severe cases) | Green | Green | Variable |
| Mucus | Present | Variable | Variable | Absent |
| Time after onset when seen by physician | Early | Several days | Several days | Early |
| Early course, untreated | Slight or no improvement | Persistent or relapsing | Persistent | Daily improvement |

10

# THE PATIENT WITH CHRONIC DIARRHEA

The infant or child with chronic diarrhea always poses a diagnostic and therapeutic challenge. In such patients in whom a number of diagnostic possibilities exist, an orderly and relatively simple and inexpensive approach to investigation should be pursued. One such approach, employing three stages of diagnostic procedures, is outlined below.

**STAGE 1**

| DIAGNOSTIC TEST | DIAGNOSTIC INFORMATION |
|---|---|
| Examination of the stool | A mucoid stool with blood suggests infection. |
| | A mucoid stool without blood suggests an irritable colon. |
| | White flecks and beanlike curds are seen in protein allergies. |
| | Soufflelike stools, with the smell of vinegar, suggest disaccharide intolerance. |
| | Oil droplets in the stool suggest steatorrhea. |
| Test for reducing substances | Positive test suggests disaccharide intolerance. |
| pH | Stool pH below 6.0 suggests disaccharide intolerance. |
| Stool trypsin | If no digestion of gelatin in dilution of 1:100, it suggests pancreatic insufficiency. |
| Stool supernatant tested for precipitins to milk, soy, and gluten | Protein intolerance. |
| Stool for ova and parasites | Parasitic infection. |
| Smear of stool for leukocytes | If leukocytes present, it suggests presence of bacterial infection or ulcerative colitis. |
| Stool culture | |
| Sweat test | Cystic fibrosis. |
| Complete blood count | Neutropenia suggests pancreatic insufficiency. |
| | Macrocytic anemia suggests small bowel disease with folic acid deficiency. |
| | Hypochromic anemia suggests iron deficiency with gastrointestinal bleeding as a result of protein allergy or ulcerative colitis. |
| Serum carotene | If low, suggests presence of fat malabsorption. |
| Serum folate | If low, suggests presence of small bowel disease. |

*If No Diagnosis Is Established or Tests Suggest Presence of Malabsorption, then Proceed to Stage 2 Tests*

| STAGE 2 | DIAGNOSTIC TEST | DIAGNOSTIC INFORMATION |
|---------|-----------------|------------------------|
| | 72-hour stool collection for quantitative fat determination | Steatorrhea documents the presence of malabsorption. Common causes include cystic fibrosis, celiac syndrome, and inflammatory disease of the small bowel. |
| | Disaccharide tolerance test. Perform in patients with acid stools or patients with reducing substance in stool | Administer 2 gm/kg of disaccharide — start with lactose. Should produce a rise in blood glucose of at least 20 mg/dl in 20 to 60 minutes. Lack of appropriate response indicates disaccharidase deficiency. |
| | Xylose tolerance test. Administer 0.5 gm/kg after a 4-hour fast. Collect all urine for 5 hours | Infants 0 to 6 months of age should excrete 8 to 16 per cent of dose; infants and children over 6 months of age should excrete 20 to 25 per cent of dose. Impaired absorption indicates impaired small bowel function. Falsely low values seen with gastric retention, impaired renal function, or inadequate hydration. |
| | Radiologic examination of small and large bowel. Begin with barium enema | Look for malrotation, Hirschsprung's disease, colitis, chronic granulomatous disease, small bowel pattern of malabsorption. |
| | Sigmoidoscopy. Consider in patients with diarrhea accompanied by occult or gross gastrointestinal bleeding | Ulcerative colitis. Chronic granulomatous disease. |

10

*If No Diagnosis Has Been Established or Definitive Proof Is Required, then Proceed to Stage 3 Tests*

These include:

Small bowel biopsy
Duodenal intubation for collection of pancreatic enzymes and bile acids, and for culture of small bowel flora
Urine collection for catecholamines, amino acids, and keto acids

---

Reference: Gryboski, J.: Gastrointestinal Problems in the Infant. Philadelphia, W.B. Saunders Company, 1975, p. 676.

## CHRONIC DIARRHEA IN INFANCY

The list below may be consulted when you are confronted with a patient with chronic diarrhea. Both the common and uncommon causes are included. It may help to remind you of a diagnosis you have overlooked.

*Infectious*

Bacterial
Parasitic
Fungal
Tuberculosis

*Immunologic*

Dysgammaglobulinemia (e.g., IgA deficiency)
Agammaglobulinemia
Secondary hypogammaglobulinemia

*Anatomic*

Hirschsprung's disease
Malrotation
Intermittent volvulus
Small bowel stenosis
Polyps or tumor of the small bowel
Enteric fistulas
Short gut syndrome
Blind loop syndrome

*Autoimmune (?)*

Regional enteritis
Ulcerative colitis

*Vascular*

> Mesenteric artery insufficiency
> Intestinal ischemia, necrotizing entercolitis
> Portal hypertension (early)

*Lymphatic*

> Intestinal lymphangiectasia

*Hepatic*

> Chronic hepatitis, biliary atresia
> Deficiency of bile acids

*Allergic*

> Milk and wheat protein allergies

*Metabolic and Malabsorptive Diseases*

> Disaccharide intolerance
> Monosaccharide intolerance
> Familial chloride diarrhea
> Celiac disease
> Cystic fibrosis
> Enterokinase deficiency
> Pancreatic insufficiency
> Methionine malabsorption
> Abetalipoproteinemia
> Selective malabsorption of vitamin $B_{12}$
> Folic acid malabsorption
> Primary hypomagnesemia
> Amino acid malabsorption

**10**

*Nonspecific*

> Starvation
> Antibiotic-induced diarrhea
> High mineral content of water
> Dietetic candies

*Extraintestinal*

> Ganglioneuroma

---

Reference: Gryboski, J.: Gastrointestinal Problems in the Infant. Philadelphia, W.B. Saunders Company, 1975, p. 566.

# IRRITABLE COLON SYNDROME OF CHILDHOOD

The infant or young child with persistent or recurrent diarrhea who has adequate weight gain may have the irritable colon syndrome. The irritable colon syndrome is characterized by the following facts:

Onset is usually between 6 and 20 months of age, but diarrhea may begin at an earlier age.

Bowel movements occur usually in the early hours of the day. There are usually no more than three or four bowel movements per day.

The first stool of the day may be large and sometimes totally or partially formed, but subsequent stools are smaller, looser, and contain more vegetable fibers and mucus. A small amount of blood may be present.

Malabsorption is not an etiologic factor. Starch granules may be present in the stool, but these are a result of premature evacuation of the colon.

The condition is not influenced by diet.

The diarrhea is not caused by infection, but exacerbations do seem to be associated with respiratory infections and teething.

Affected children often have a history of constipation prior to the onset of diarrhea, and many suffered from infantile colic. Following clearance of diarrhea, many affected children develop constipation.

There is frequently a family history of functional bowel complaints.

Clearance of diarrhea is gradual and occurs in 90 per cent of cases by 36 to 39 months of age.

Etiology is unknown, but hypotheses include a psychosomatic origin and hereditary predisposition.

Treatment consists of maintaining a normal diet with elimination of chilled liquids (these seem to promote colonic motility). Diodoquin may be helpful for some patients but should be used for very limited periods of time because it may produce optic atrophy.

Infection may be ruled out by examination of the stool for leukocytes. Malabsorption must be considered in the child who fails to gain weight.

---

Reference: Davidson, M., and Wasserman, R.: J. Pediatr., *69*:1027, 1966.

# ENCOPRESIS

The vast majority of children who experience fecal incontinence will be found on physical examination to have impacted stool in the rectum. A few of these children will be found to have an organic or neurogenic cause for their chronic constipation, but the mechanism in most cases is one or more of the following:

1. A constitutional predisposition to constipation which may be first demonstrated in the newborn period when the infant becomes constipated on a formula that allows normal bowel movements in most infants.

2. Dietary factors — large quantities of milk may produce constipation because of the low residue and high calcium content of milk. The mother may feel

that an increased fruit intake is indicated in the constipated child, but she may feed the child bananas, apples, or pears, which tend to have a constipating effect.

3. The young child may have difficulty in passing a large stool because he lacks a firm surface on which to place the feet, creating inadequate leverage during attempted bowel movements.

4. Pain and voluntary resistance to bowel movements may cause stool retention. This may be initiated by an anal fissure.

The chronic constipation caused by these mechanisms may lead to incontinence of relatively liquid stool that leaks around an impacted mass in the rectum. This incontinence may be referred to as paradoxical diarrhea. The child may even be treated with antidiarrheal drugs for a time.

The characteristic history of the child with chronic constipation and fecal incontinence often includes the following:

Fecal incontinence occurs predominantly in the late afternoon or evening.

Children often state that they do not feel the stools coming.

Accompanying symptoms may be chronic abdominal pain (often peri-umbilical), poor appetite, and lethargy.

A few of these children may report daytime enuresis.

The history may include large caliber stools when the child does have a bowel movement on the toilet. Parents often report the mechanical breaking up of these stools was necessary in order to flush the toilet.

There may be a history of stool retention or constipation during infancy.

The child may have periods of normal bowel pattern alternating with constipation and incontinence.

### Diagnostic Procedures

Minimal diagnostic procedures should include the following:

1. A rectal examination.
2. A neurologic examination testing for anal reflex and deep tendon reflexes in lower extremities.
3. A barium enema (without preparation).
4. A urinalysis (if abnormal, an intravenous pyelogram should be obtained).

### Treatment

1. Removal of the impaction; this is done by the performance of pairs of phosphate enemas one hour apart in the morning and the evening of the first day of treatment. If the impaction is not successfully removed, this procedure may be repeated on the second day. The mother should be instructed to give no more enemas following this initial period.

2. Large doses of mineral oil should be given (2 ounces) twice a day between meals to avoid interference with vitamin absorption. The diet should be adjusted at this time to include fruits such as melons, berries, cherries, plums, dates, figs, and prunes instead of bananas, apples, and pears. Milk intake should be reduced to less than 1 pint of whole milk per day.

3. Results should be reviewed after two to three weeks. Poor results should provoke evaluation for organic or neurogenic cause for constipation.

4. If treatment with mineral oil has been met with some success, the institution of regular bowel habits should begin. The child over 4 years of age should be encouraged to take responsibility for his own treatment in this regard. A potty chair should be provided so that the feet may touch the ground for leverage. In the larger child, a stool may be placed under the feet in front of the toilet. There should be a toileting period of 15 to 20 minutes twice each day during which the child is allowed to read or play on the toilet. Performance is not necessary each time, but institution of the habit should begin. The physician may feel that this is the time to discourage undue pressure by the mother and to discuss appropriate attitudes toward bowel function.

5. Following two full months of success with this regimen, the mineral oil may be tapered very gradually. Treatment with a stool softener may be instituted.

6. Both mother and child should understand that "regularity" need not mean one bowel movement each day. The continuation of regular habits should be encouraged. The mother may resort to mineral oil on occasion if the child reports that there has been no bowel movement for several days.

Failure of the above treatment in the child with no organic or neurogenic disease may result from one of two causes:

1. Mineral oil may have been discontinued too rapidly or too early.

2. The child may be hostile to the entire procedure. In this case, psychiatric evaluation and treatment should be instituted.

Urinary tract disease has been associated with chronic constipation. The urinary tract should be evaluated if constipation has been present for some time.

---

References: Fitzgerald, J.F.: Pediatrics, *46*:349, 1975. Levine, M.D.: Pediatrics, *56*:412, 1975. Davidson, M.: Pediatr. Clin. North Am., *5*:749, 1958.

# THE DIAGNOSIS OF REGIONAL ENTERITIS (CROHN'S DISEASE)

The diagnosis of regional enteritis is often unnecessarily delayed. The physician is frequently misled by the nongastrointestinal manifestations of the disease. In over one-third of patients, an initial diagnosis of an infection or collagen vascular disease is incorrectly made. In another one-third of patients, the initial diagnosis is appendicitis or other gastrointestinal disease. The average delay in correct diagnosis may be one full year.

The table below illustrates the more common clinical manifestations of regional enteritis in children and young adolescents.

| CLINICAL MANIFESTATIONS | PER CENT OF PATIENTS |
|---|---|
| Abdominal pain | 86 |
| Fever | 83 |
| Weight loss | 80 |
| Diarrhea | 72 |
| Growth retardation | 30 |
| Joint symptoms (polyarthritis and arthralgia) | 25 |
| Anorectal disease | 24 |
| Gastrointestinal bleeding | 14 |
| Nonspecific rash or erythema nodosum | 10 |
| **NONSPECIFIC LABORATORY ABNORMALITIES** | |
| Increased erythrocyte sedimentation rate | 84 |
| White cell count over 10,000/mm$^3$ | 70 |
| Decreased serum albumin | 64 |
| Hypochromic, microcytic anemia | 50 |
| Stools positive for occult blood | 36 |

Regional enteritis should be considered in the differential diagnosis of all children with prolonged fever and arthralgia even in the absence of gastrointestinal symptoms. On some occasions, the nongastro-intestinal manifestations of the disease may precede the radiographic evidence of disease in the bowel by as much as 2 years.

Reference: Burbige, E.J., Huang, S.S., and Bayless, T.M.: Pediatrics, *55*:866, 1975.

## PROTEIN-LOSING ENTEROPATHY

The hypoalbuminemic, edematous infant or child may be losing his protein from the gastrointestinal tract. Over 40 different clinical entities have now been identified in which protein losses exceed the synthetic capacity of the liver and the patient becomes hypo-albuminemic. Those that have been observed in pediatric patients are listed below.

Giant hypertrophy of gastric mucosa
Gluten enteropathy
Regional enteritis
Lymphosarcoma of the bowel
Gastrointestinal tuberculosis
Acute infection
Lymphangiectasia
Angiomas of the bowel
Pancreatitis, chronic

Ulcerative colitis
Megacolon
Hypogammaglobulinemia
Nephrosis
Congestive heart failure
Constrictive pericarditis
Allergic gastroenteropathy
Iron deficiency

The most common cause of this disorder in infants and children appears to be cow's milk sensitivity. Dramatic improvement may be anticipated within 48 to 72 hours after the removal of all milk and milk products from the diet. In some instances, all proteins of cow origin, such as beef, must also be eliminated as well. In the cow milk–allergic child, gastrointestinal intolerance to soy protein and wheat and gluten may also occur. In the therapeutic trial, it is best to eliminate all potential allergens. When a response is produced, these other protein sources may be reintroduced, one at a time, with careful clinical observations.

## CELIAC DISEASE, CYSTIC FIBROSIS, OR GASTROINTESTINAL ALLERGY

|  | CELIAC DISEASE | CYSTIC FIBROSIS | GASTROINTESTINAL ALLERGY |
|---|---|---|---|
| Family history | Occasionally + | Often + | Often + |
| Onset | Usually 8 months to 2 years | <6 months | 1 to 6 months |
| Respiratory symptoms | — | 95% by 1 year | Asthma, bronchitis 4 years or so |
| Appetite | Poor | Excessive | Normal |
| Stools | Bulky, foul, liquid | Greasy, bulky | Soft to watery, mucoid |
| Blood in stools | — | — | + |
| Growth | Normal to 8 to 10 months | Retarded | Variable |
| Sweating | — | + | — |
| Vitamin deficiencies | Unusual | Sometimes | Sometimes |
| Calcium deficiency | + | Rare | Sometimes |

*Celiac*—From the Greek word *koilia*, which means belly. The name celiac disease is derived from the enlarged belly these children normally demonstrate.

| | CELIAC DISEASE | CYSTIC FIBROSIS | GASTROINTESTINAL ALLERGY |
|---|---|---|---|
| Glucose tolerance | Flat | Normal to ↑ | Normal |
| Vitamin A | Low normal | Below normal 80% | Variable |
| Proteins | May be low | Often low | Often low |
| Carotene | Very low | Very low | Usually normal |
| Finger clubbing | + | + | — |

Reference: Gryboski, J.: Gastrointestinal Problems in the Infant. Philadelphia, W.B. Saunders Company, 1975, p. 653.

# THE BLACK STOOL

When you test a black stool for occult blood and it proves to be negative, do not be frustrated — get more history. Other causes of a black stool include:

Ingestion of iron preparations
Ingestion of bismuth (Pepto-Bismol)
Ingestion of lead
Eating licorice
Eating charcoal, coal, or dirt

If the patient is taking large quantities of ascorbic acid, you may get a false-negative test for occult blood even with significant bleeding. The vitamin C interferes with the color change normally produced by the peroxidase activity of the heme.

Reference: Jaffe, R.M.: Ann. Intern. Med., *83*:824, 1975.

*"A baby is God's opinion that the world should go on."*

Carl Sandburg

# GASTROINTESTINAL HEMORRHAGE

Gastrointestinal hemorrhage in infants and children has many causes. Some forms of bleeding can present an immediate threat to life. Management includes prompt diagnosis. It is important to be aware of the more common causes of gastrointestinal bleeding and the fact that the relative frequency of different lesions changes with the age of the patient.

*Lesions Producing Gastrointestinal Hemorrhage*

| | RELATIVE FREQUENCY (%) | |
| --- | --- | --- |
| | *Under 1 Year of Age* | *Over 1 Year of Age* |
| Anal fissure | 43.0 | 12.5 |
| Duodenal ulcers | 6.0 | 6.0 |
| Duplication of colon | 0.7 | 0.0 |
| Esophageal varices | 0.0 | 10.5 |
| Gastric ulcers | 5.6 | 8.0 |
| Gangrenous bowel | 9.0 | 0.0 |
| Hemorrhoids | 0.0 | 0.8 |
| Intussusception | 31.9 | 9.0 |
| Meckel's diverticulum | 3.8 | 1.2 |
| Polyps | 0.0 | 50.0 |
| Ulcerative colitis | 0.0 | 2.0 |

Reference: Spencer, R.: Surgery, *55*:718, 1964.

# NONSURGICAL CAUSES OF GASTROINTESTINAL BLEEDING

Gastrointestinal bleeding is not always produced by lesions requiring surgery. Nonsurgical causes of both melena and occult gastrointestinal bleeding include:

Hematologic Disorders
   Vitamin K deficiency
   Thrombocytopenia
   Hemophilia
   Iron deficiency

Systemic Disorders
   Henoch-Schönlein purpura
   Milk allergy
   Shigellosis
   Idiopathic pulmonary hemosiderosis
   Pseudoxanthoma elasticum
   Turner's syndrome
   Uremia
   Scurvy

Drugs or Toxins
  Aspirin
  Steroids
  Potassium chloride tablets
  Iron poisoning

It is also important to remember:

1. In a newborn with blood in the stool, always eliminate the possibility that the blood was of maternal origin and swallowed during the delivery process before seeking other causes for the bleeding.

Vomitus, gastric aspirate, or stool containing red blood may be used for this purpose, employing the alkali denaturation test.

**Technique.** To lyse the erythrocytes and to prepare the hemoglobin solution, a small amount of stool or vomitus is mixed with water. Generally, one part of stool or vomitus is mixed with five to ten parts of water. The test tube is centrifuged for several minutes at approximately 2000 rpm to separate the debris. The supernatant solution, which must be pink, is then decanted or filtered. About 1 ml of 0.25 N (1 per cent) sodium hydroxide is then mixed with 5 ml of the hemoglobin solution.

The color change is read in two minutes. Blood containing adult hemoglobin (HbA) changes from pink to brown-yellow, while blood containing predominantly HbF remains pink. It is helpful to run a control tube containing the peripheral blood of the infant being studied.

2. Always eliminate recent aspirin ingestion as a cause of upper gastrointestinal bleeding before seeking other explanations.

3. Remember that nutritional iron deficiency may produce occult blood in the stools. Correct the iron deficiency anemia and recheck the stools before further gastrointestinal studies.

4. In children with portal hypertension and esophageal varices, hemorrhage may produce a disappearance of the previously existing splenomegaly. Do not discard the diagnosis until the blood volume has been restored.

5. Always consider the possibility that blood swallowed from a nosebleed or coughed up from the lungs may produce a positive test for occult blood in the stool.

6. Bleeding secondary to an intussusception may be the initial manifestation of anaphylactoid purpura.

References: Oski, F.A.: Pediatric Portfolio, *1*:21, 1971. Oski, F.A., and Naiman, J.L.: Hematologic Problems in the Newborn. Philadelphia, W.B. Saunders Company, 1972, p. 240.

# THE USE OF ALGORITHMS FOR THE DIAGNOSIS OF JAUNDICE IN CHILDHOOD

Jaundice in the neonatal period has multiple causes that are unique to that period of life (see pages 123 and 126). The algorithms on the following pages are designed to provide a diagnostic guide to the evaluation of jaundice when it presents in late infancy and childhood.

Some points that should prove useful in employing these algorithms include the following:

1. Begin the differential diagnosis of jaundice with an examination of the urine. A positive urine test for bilirubin indicates the retention of conjugated bilirubin in the serum. The urine tests are positive in approximately 70 per cent of patients with conjugated bilirubin levels in the range of 1 to 2 mg/100 ml and in virtually all patients with serum conjugated bilirubin levels in excess of 2 mg/100 ml. The Ictotest (Ames Laboratories) is negative in patients with unconjugated hyperbilirubinemia.

2. Confirm the urinary findings with a measurement of the serum fractions of both conjugated and unconjugated bilirubin. The upper limit of normal for total bilirubin is 1.0 mg/100 ml with a conjugated (direct reacting fraction) of less than 0.2 mg/100 ml.

3. In pure unconjugated hyperbilirubinemia, at least 85 per cent of the total bilirubin should be of the unconjugated form. In conjugated hyperbilirubinemia, there is at least 30 per cent, and usually close to 50 per cent, of the total bilirubin in the direct or conjugated form.

4. Obstructive jaundice and acute hepatocellular disease tend to give values greater than 50 per cent direct reacting bilirubin, while in chronic liver disease the conjugated fraction is usually in the 30 to 50 per cent range.

5. Patients with 15 to 30 per cent conjugated bilirubin generally have hepatocellular or cholestatic jaundice complicated by hemolysis.

6. Unconjugated hyperbilirubinemia can be arbitrarily separated into patients with indirect bilirubin levels of above and below 6.0 mg/100 ml. This is not a precise distinction. Some patients with Gilbert's syndrome may have unconjugated bilirubin levels as high as 8.0 mg/100 ml, while patients with Arias Type II syndrome may have values as low as 3.0 mg/100 ml.

7. Gilbert's syndrome has multiple causes. The unconjugated hyperbilirubinemia is always in excess of that which would be expected for the red cell life span.

8. In both Gilbert's syndrome and Arias Type II conjugation defect, there is impaired conjugation of bilirubin with glucuronic acid. The Type I defect (Crigler-Najjar syndrome) presents no diagnostic difficulty because in this syndrome the unconjugated hyperbilirubinemia first develops in the neonatal period and the conjugation defect is complete.

9. Cholestatic jaundice can usually be distinguished from hepatocellular jaundice by the measurement of alkaline phosphatase. Approximately 90 per cent of patients with cholestasis will have alkaline phosphatase values that are more than three times normal, while 90 per cent of patients with hepatocellular jaundice will have elevations of alkaline phosphatase that do not exceed three times normal. Patients with drug-induced cholestasis tend to have values one to three times normal.

10. Although the diagnosis of Dubin-Johnson syndrome can be confirmed by liver biopsy that demonstrates the characteristic finding of brown to black centrilobular granular pigment, this is seldom necessary. Sulfobromophthalein (BSP) kinetic studies will identify the minuscule transfer maximum for BSP into bile. In addition, analysis of the isomers of coproporphyrin in the urine will show the characteristic increases in the total quantity of the isomer 1 and in the ratio of isomer 1 to isomer 3.

---

Reference: Ostrow, J.D.: J.A.M.A., *234*:522, 1975.

*Diagnosis of Unconjugated Hyperbilirubinemia*

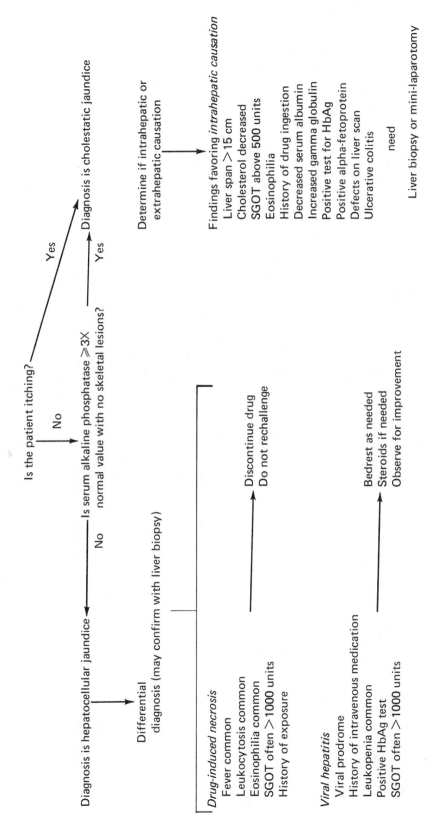

Is the patient itching?

No — Yes

Diagnosis is cholestatic jaundice

Is serum alkaline phosphatase ≥3X
normal value with no skeletal lesions?

No — Yes

Diagnosis is hepatocellular jaundice

Determine if intrahepatic or
extrahepatic causation

Differential
diagnosis (may confirm with liver biopsy)

Findings favoring *intrahepatic causation*
  Liver span >15 cm
  Cholesterol decreased
  SGOT above 500 units
  Eosinophilia
  History of drug ingestion
  Decreased serum albumin
  Increased gamma globulin
  Positive test for HbAg
  Positive alpha-fetoprotein
  Defects on liver scan
  Ulcerative colitis

  need

  Liver biopsy or mini-laparotomy

*Drug-induced necrosis*
  Fever common
  Leukocytosis common
  Eosinophilia common
  SGOT often >1000 units
  History of exposure

Discontinue drug
Do not rechallenge

*Viral hepatitis*
  Viral prodrome
  History of intravenous medication
  Leukopenia common
  Positive HbAg test
  SGOT often >1000 units

Bedrest as needed
Steroids if needed
Observe for improvement

**10**

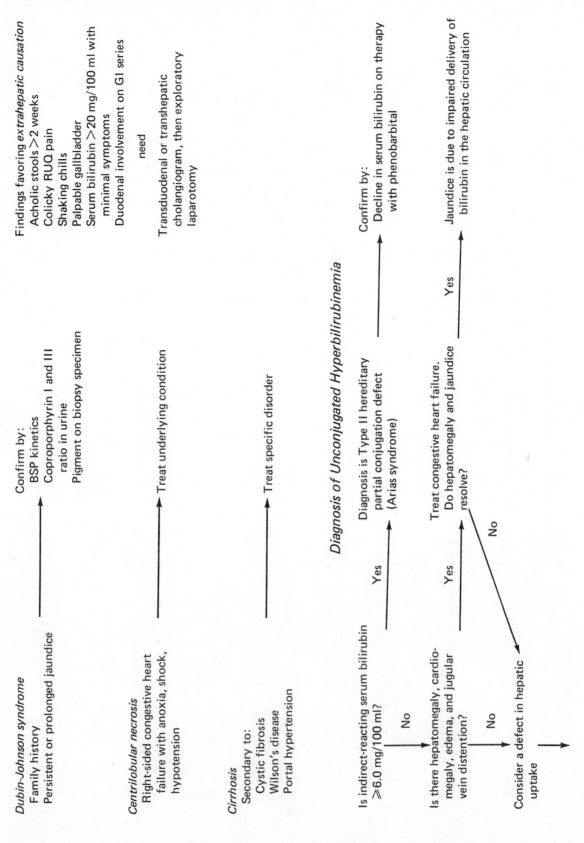

*Dubin-Johnson syndrome*
Family history
Persistent or prolonged jaundice
→ Confirm by:
BSP kinetics
Coproporphyrin I and III ratio in urine
Pigment on biopsy specimen

*Centrilobular necrosis*
Right-sided congestive heart failure with anoxia, shock, hypotension
→ Treat underlying condition

*Cirrhosis*
Secondary to:
Cystic fibrosis
Wilson's disease
Portal hypertension
→ Treat specific disorder

Findings favoring *extrahepatic causation*
Acholic stools >2 weeks
Colicky RUQ pain
Shaking chills
Palpable gallbladder
Serum bilirubin >20 mg/100 ml with minimal symptoms
Duodenal involvement on GI series

need

→ Transduodenal or transhepatic cholangiogram, then exploratory laparotomy

## Diagnosis of Unconjugated Hyperbilirubinemia

Is indirect-reacting serum bilirubin ≥6.0 mg/100 ml?
Yes → Diagnosis is Type II hereditary partial conjugation defect (Arias syndrome)
Confirm by: Decline in serum bilirubin on therapy with phenobarbital
No ↓

Is there hepatomegaly, cardiomegaly, edema, and jugular vein distention?
Yes → Treat congestive heart failure. Do hepatomegaly and jaundice resolve?
Yes → Jaundice is due to impaired delivery of bilirubin in the hepatic circulation
No
No ↓

Consider a defect in hepatic uptake →

10

Did the patient recently receive any of these drugs: biliary contrast agents, rifamycin, progestational steroids, or flavaspidic acid?

Yes → Discontinue use of the drug. Does the jaundice resolve?

Yes → Jaundice was due to inhibition of hepatic uptake of bilirubin by the drug.

No

No ↓

Does patient have hyperthyroidism?

Yes → Treat hyperthyroidism. Does the jaundice resolve?

Yes → Jaundice was due to impairment of hepatic uptake of bilirubin by hyperthyroidism.

No

No ↓

Perform red cell survival. Is serum bilirubin disproportionately high for red cell life span?

Yes → Diagnosis is Gilbert's syndrome (familial hepatic uptake defect)

Confirm by:
Increase in serum bilirubin >3.0 mg/100 ml after 24 hour fast

No →

Is there: Anemia, reticulocytosis, abnormal red cell morphology, hemoglobin electrophoresis, decreased serum haptoglobin level, increased fecal urobilinogen level, or disproportionately elevated LDH?

No → Probably no bilirubin overproduction

Yes ↓

Overproduction of bilirubin is contributing to the hyperbilirubinemia (hemolysis or ineffective erythropoiesis)

# 11
# GENITO-URINARY

# DEVELOPMENT OF RENAL FUNCTION

In the evaluation of the newborn or young infant for possible renal disease, one must be aware of the normal kidney function during this early period of life in order to appropriately interpret the laboratory values. The following table should prove useful.

*Functional Development of the Kidney*

| | PREMATURE INFANT | FULL-TERM NEONATE | ADULT | AGE OF MATURATION (IN MONTHS) |
|---|---|---|---|---|
| Glomerular filtration rate (ml/min/1.73 m$^2$) | 30–50 | 40–60 | 120 | 12–24 |
| Renal plasma flow (ml/min/1.73 m$^2$) | | 120–150 | 630 | 3–6 |
| Filtration fraction (per cent) | | 30–40 | 20 | 6–36 |
| Tm PAH (mg/min/1.73 m$^2$) | | 12–30 | 75 | 12–24 |
| Tm glucose (mg/min/1.73 m$^2$) | | 35–100 | 300 | 12–24 |
| Urea clearance (ml/min/1.73 m$^2$) | 15–30 | 20–50 | 75 | 12–24 |
| Extreme dilution of urine (mOsm/liter) | 50 | 50 | 50 | |
| Maximal concentration of urine (mOsm/liter) | 400–600 | 400–600 | 1400 | 3 |
| Maximal U/P osmolar ratio | 2.5 | | 4 | 3 |
| Ammoniogenesis | Lowered | Normal | | |
| Lowering of urinary pH | Normal | Normal | | |
| Hydrogen ion excretion | Lowered | Normal or lowered | | |

Tm, Maximal tubular reabsorption; PAH, para-aminohippurate; U/P, urine/plasma.

---

Reference: Royer, P., Habib, R., Mathieu, H., and Broyer, M.: *In* Pediatric Nephrology. Philadelphia, W.B. Saunders Company, 1974, p. 118.

# NOCTURNAL ENURESIS—NATURAL HISTORY

At what age do children normally stop wetting their bed? Most parents, as well as physicians, have unrealistic expectations and assume that most bed-wetting after age 4 years suggests the presence of underlying renal disease. Not true!

Age by which bed-wetting stopped:

| AGE | BOYS | | GIRLS | |
|:---:|:---:|:---:|:---:|:---:|
| | White (%) | Black (%) | White (%) | Black (%) |
| <2 | 28 | 37 | 37 | 35 |
| 2–3 | 70 | 73 | 80 | 77 |
| 4–5 | 85 | 83 | 89 | 90 |
| 6–7 | 91 | 89 | 92 | 92 |

Bed-wetting after age 4 years is more common in boys, in children from large families, and in children from lower socioeconomic groups and occurs more commonly in families where one of the parents may have been a bed-wetter.

When bed-wetting recurs after a period of dryness, then an explanation should be sought. The polyuria of diabetes mellitus may frequently present in this way. Also rule out urinary tract disease and diabetes insipidus.

Reference: Dodge, W.F., West, E.F., Bridgforth, E.B., et al.: Am. J. Dis. Child., *120*:32, 1970.

## A TREATMENT FOR PRIMARY ENURESIS

By the time they are 4½ years of age, most children are able to sense the need to urinate, to "hold" their urine until urination is convenient, both day and night, and to stop the urinary stream at will. This control is accomplished when the child learns to coordinate the contraction of the diaphragm, the abdominal muscles, and the detrusor muscle, with the relaxation of the levator ani at will. If the child does not accomplish this control, the bladder may not develop the capacity to hold the entire nighttime urine.

Primary enuresis is a problem for approximately 12 per cent of children. Many children develop control with age, and by 7¾ years of age, only 7 per cent of children remain enuretic. Parents, children, and physicians develop elaborate schemes to conquer the problem. A training program that allows the child to measure achievement daily is outlined below.

1. The child and the parents maintain a "voiding chart" on which the child's fluid intake and output are recorded. The child voids into a glass measuring cup and records the volume of each voiding. A voiding volume of 8 to 10 ounces is usually sufficient to eliminate enuresis, but a goal of 14 ounces is more likely to ensure permanent cure. It should be emphasized that an occasional large voiding does not signify real increases in bladder capacity.

2. The child is instructed to force fluids during the day and to attempt to hold the urine as long as possible. Bed-wetting should be strictly ignored during this period.

3. Anticholinergic drugs (e.g., Pro-Banthine or Daricon) may be used during the day and at bedtime for relaxing the detrusor and allowing the bladder to distend and hold large amounts of urine.

4. The process may take three to six months, depending on the initial capacity of the bladder and the cooperation and presistence of the patient and the parents.

Failure of this program after a reasonable trial suggests the need for urine culture, voiding cystourethrogram, and intravenous pyelogram.

Reference: Meullner, S.R.: J.A.M.A., *172*:1256, 1960.

# THE CHILD WITH EXCESSIVE URINATION

The concern of parents about urinary frequency or excessive urine volume in their child should be approached in a systematic manner. After a thorough history and physical examination, the next step should be a comparison of the number of the child's voids per 24 hours with the normal values.

| AGE | NORMAL NUMBER OF VOIDS PER 24 HOURS |
|---|---|
| 3–6 months | 20 |
| 6–12 months | 16 |
| 1–2 years | 12 |
| 2–3 years | 10 |
| 3–4 years | 9 |
| 12 years–adulthood | 4–6 |

This step alone may be sufficient to allay parental and physician concern.

If, however, the number of voids is above normal or if the initial concern was excessive urine volume, then a urinalysis and 24-hour urine volume will further clarify the situation, as illustrated in the accompanying algorithm.

References: Hollerman, C.E., Jose, P., and Calcagno, P.L.: *In* Neonatology, Pathophysiology and Management of the Newborn. Philadelphia, J.B. Lippincott Company, 1975, p. 487. Illingworth, R.S.: *In* Common Symptoms of Disease in Childhood. 5th Ed. Oxford, Blackwell Scientific Publications, 1975, p. 299.

*An Approach to Polyuria and/or Frequency*

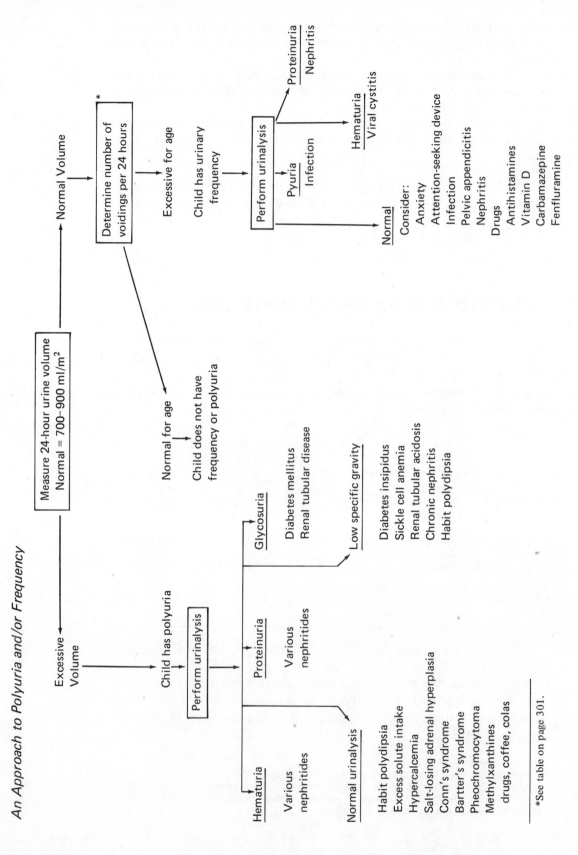

Measure 24-hour urine volume
Normal = 700–900 ml/m$^2$

Normal Volume

*
Determine number of voidings per 24 hours

Excessive for age
Child has urinary frequency

Perform urinalysis

Proteinuria
Nephritis

Pyuria
Infection

Hematuria
Viral cystitis

Normal
Consider:
Anxiety
Attention-seeking device
Infection
Pelvic appendicitis
Nephritis
Drugs
Antihistamines
Vitamin D
Carbamazepine
Fenfluramine

Normal for age
Child does not have frequency or polyuria

Excessive Volume

Child has polyuria

Perform urinalysis

Glycosuria
Diabetes mellitus
Renal tubular disease

Low specific gravity
Diabetes insipidus
Sickle cell anemia
Renal tubular acidosis
Chronic nephritis
Habit polydipsia

Proteinuria
Various nephritides

Hematuria
Various nephritides

Normal urinalysis
Habit polydipsia
Excess solute intake
Hypercalcemia
Salt-losing adrenal hyperplasia
Conn's syndrome
Bartter's syndrome
Pheochromocytoma
Methylxanthines
drugs, coffee, colas

*See table on page 301.

# THE CHEST ROENTGENOGRAM IN ACUTE GLOMERULONEPHRITIS

It is not generally appreciated that patients with acute glomerulonephritis will have abnormalities on their chest films. In fact, approximately 85 per cent of patients will have one or more abnormal findings. These include:

| FINDING | PER CENT OF PATIENTS |
|---|---|
| Increased pulmonary vascularity | 74 |
| Cardiomegaly | 62 |
| Edema of the skin of chest wall | 60 |
| Pleural fluid, often infrapulmonary | 55 |
| Pulmonary edema | 25 |
| Pulmonary consolidation | 25 |

These findings are not related to the degree of hypertension or azotemia and more probably reflect increased vascular permeability, excessive renal reabsorption of water and salt, or pulmonary hypertension.

Reference: Kirkpatrick, J.A., and Fleisher, D.S.: J. Pediatr., *64*:492, 1964.

# THE NEPHROTIC SYNDROME—PROGNOSIS

What is the expected course for a child with nephrosis? The following data can provide you with some reasonable expectations.

*Adjusted Survival Rates*

| TIME FROM DIAGNOSIS | SURVIVAL RATE |
|---|---|
| 1 year | 94% |
| 2 years | 90% |
| 5 years | 85% |
| 10 years | 79% |
| 15 years | 77% |

The nephrotic syndrome represents a diverse clinical spectrum. The clinical course can be characterized in the following manner.

| 20% | 45% | 10% | 15% | 10% |
| :---: | :---: | :---: | :---: | :---: |
| ↓ | ↓ | ↓ | ↓ | ↓ |
| One episode with no further activity after first year | Relapsing disease with ultimate cure | Relapsing disease with continued activity for 10 years or more | Relapsing disease with death | Death within 2 years of onset |

Unfavorable prognostic factors at time of diagnosis include:

1. Azotemia (BUN >25 mg/100 ml)
2. Hematuria (>10 RBCs/HPF)
3. Hypertension (diastolic pressure >90 mm Hg)

---

Reference: Schwartz, M.W., Schwartz, G.J., and Cornfeld, D.: Pediatrics, *54*:547, 1974.

# THE NEPHROTIC SYNDROME IN YOUNG INFANTS

Approximately 5.5 per cent of children with nephrotic syndrome are below 6 months of age at the time of diagnosis. The following chart lists characteristics of the nephrotic syndrome in young infants and the condition that may cause the nephrotic syndrome.

| PRIMARY | CHARACTERISTICS |
| :--- | :--- |
| Congenital | Family history positive |
| | Usually begins at less than 3 months of age |
| | Large placenta |
| | Reduced complement, elevated IgM |
| | Fatal illness |
| | Histologic findings: from minimal change to chronic glomerulonephritis; tubular changes prominent |
| Idiopathic infantile | Family history negative |
| | Later onset |
| | Normal placenta |
| | Normal complement and IgM |
| | Histologic findings: variable — prognosis depends on severity of glomerular lesions |

SECONDARY TO:

Congenital syphilis

Nephrotoxin, e.g., mercury

Cytomegalic inclusion body disease

Renal vein thrombosis

Nephroblastoma

Reference: McDonald, R., Wiggelinkhuizen, F.C.P., and Kaschula, R.O.C.: Am. J. Dis. Child., *122*:507, 1971.

# RENAL SCANNING

There are a number of situations in which radionuclide imaging of the urinary tract can provide useful information which is either not available from excretory urography (IVP) or which supplements the information provided by IVP. Radiation exposure during a renal scan is significantly less than during IVP. A variety of radionuclides are available for use. Their selection is determined by the renal function to be evaluated, i.e., glomerular filtration rate, tubular secretion, or tubular reabsorption.

Indications for renal scanning include:

| INDICATION | COMMENT ON SCAN |
|---|---|
| Contrast media sensitivity | No adverse reactions to radionuclides used in renal scanning reported |
| Uremia | May be used even in severe uremia (BUN $\geq$ 100) |
| Trauma | Provides additional and supplementary information to IVP |
| In preparation for radiotherapy port placement or for renal biopsy | Significantly less radiation than fluoroscopy |
| Congenital anomalies | Complements IVP |
| Pyelonephritis | IVP often normal in acute situation; cortical scan may be useful in diagnosis and follow-up; especially useful in chronic pyelonephritis |
| Transplant evaluation | Baseline study crucial for follow-up; very sensitive in detecting early rejection |
| Quantitative or differential renal function studies | May replace ureteral catheterization, which is a difficult procedure |
| Obstructive disease | Superior to IVP in situations of poor renal concentrating ability. Can illustrate intact cortical tissue in patients with major hydronephrosis |

11

| INDICATION | COMMENT ON SCAN |
|---|---|
| Azotemia in the newborn | Because of decreased concentrating ability, the IVP may not be helpful in the neonate |
| Bladder abnormalities (including reflex and residual volume) | Equal to or superior to IVP; 100 to 1000 times less gonadal radiation exposure |

Reference: Handmaker, H., and Lowenstein, J.M.: Curr. Probl. Pediatr., 6:29, 1975.

## RENAL STONES

Kidney stones are responsible for both urinary tract infections and progressive renal failure in infants and children. Kidney stones are far more common than is generally appreciated and have been found in 1 per cent of autopsies in infants and children.

Approximately 30 per cent of all recognized cases occur in children before the age of 2 years, and over one-half occur before the age of 4. Stones may be found in neonates.

In young infants the stones tend to be bilateral, while they are unilateral in about 90 per cent of older children. Boys are affected in 80 to 85 per cent of cases under 2 years of age; 60 to 65 per cent of patients 4 to 10 years of age are male; and 55 per cent of adult patients with stones are male.

Stones may produce pyuria, hematuria, abdominal distention, vomiting, disturbances of micturition, urinary retention, and even anuria.

In approximately 50 per cent of patients, a cause for the stone can be determined. About 25 per cent of stones are associated with malformations of the urinary tract, and 25 per cent are a result of a metabolic disorder.

The evaluation of patients with renal stones should include the following:

1. Plain film of the abdomen.
2. Intravenous urography.
3. Measurement of both urine and plasma concentration of: calcium, magnesium, oxalic acid, and uric acid.
4. Chemical analysis of the stone.
5. Urinary amino acid chromatogram (if other chemical analyses have been nondiagnostic).

Some characteristics of the various disorders associated with stone formation are described in the accompanying table.

*Diagnostic Features of Renal Stone Diseases in Infants and Children*

| ETIOLOGY | X-RAY FILM APPEARANCE | DIAGNOSTIC FEATURES |
|---|---|---|
| Urinary tract malformations | Radiopaque | Obstruction at ureteropelvic junction most common abnormality. Frequently associated with infections. Stones usually composed of calcium phosphate and magnesium ammonium phosphate. |
| Metabolic Disorders Calcium stones | Radiopaque | Responsible for approximately one-half of stones of metabolic origin. Hypercalciuria present. Usually single stones. May be associated with nephrocalcinosis. |
| Cystine stones | Radiopaque | Account for 1 to 5 per cent of stones. Most common stone formed in renal tubular disorders (cystinuria and hypercystinuria). Calculi are generally large, multiple, and molded to the outline of the calyces and pelvis. Stones are soft, yellow, and waxy. Urinary cystine concentration increased. |
| Uric acid stones | Slightly radiopaque | Less common in children than adults. Most commonly associated with hyperuricemia due to a variety of causes. Hereditary form exists without either hyperuricemia or hyperuricosuria. |
| Oxalic stones | Radiopaque | Stones are large and regular in outline, and bristle with tiny spikes. Often produce hematuria. May be associated with primary hyperoxaluria or oxalosis. Oxaluria seen in glycinuria and hypercalciurias. Oxaluria may be caused by large consumption of vitamin C. |
| Xanthine stones | Radiolucent | Rare disorder. Stones are yellowish-brown and friable. Urine xanthine concentration increased. May be associated with xanthine oxidase deficiency. In this disorder, blood and urine uric acids are low. |
| Syndrome of lithiasis, psychomotor retardation, and hip malfunction | Radiopaque | Stones of calcium phosphate. Stones numerous and bilateral. Retardation of both growth and psychomotor development. Hip disorder simulates osteochondritis. No biochemical or histologic renal disease. Prognosis excellent for mental, renal, and hip function. Etiology unknown. |

11

| ETIOLOGY | X-RAY FILM APPEARANCE | DIAGNOSTIC FEATURES |
|---|---|---|
| Unknown origin | Radiopaque | Stones of calcium phosphate or magnesium ammonium phosphate. Prognosis good if no serious renal damage. Usually do not recur. |

Reference: Royer, P., Habib, R., Mathieu, H., and Broyer, M.: Pediatric Nephrology. Philadelphia, W.B. Saunders Company, 1974, p. 193.

# RENAL TRAUMA AND HEMATURIA

It is frequently forgotten that renal trauma, sometimes of a trivial nature, may produce hematuria. In almost 25 per cent of children with traumatic hematuria, an underlying abnormality of the kidney may be present. All children with traumatically induced hematuria deserve a radiologic evaluation of their kidneys.

The cause of the trauma to the kidneys can be broadly classified into the following categories:

| | |
|---|---|
| Falls | 34% |
| Automobile accidents | 29% |
| Direct blows (fists) | 15% |
| Athletic accidents | 11% |
| Sledding | 9% |

The nature of the injury and its clinical manifestations are:

| | |
|---|---|
| Contusion | Accounts for about 75 per cent of all injuries. Hematuria always present and often microscopic. Only rarely does it produce even minor changes in the urogram. Physical examination may reveal minor tenderness over the injured kidney. |
| Laceration | Observed in about 15 per cent of all injuries. Gross hematuria always present. Excretory urography may demonstrate severe distortion and even perirenal extravasation of dye. Physical examination may disclose a palpable mass. |
| Rupture | Seen in 10 per cent of patients. Gross hematuria frequently present. Patient may present in shock. |

Associated renal anomalies may include hydronephrosis, ectopia, tumor, megaloureter, and hypoplasia.

About two-thirds of patients can be successfully managed by conservative measures. Patients with rupture require nephrectomy after it has been established that another normal kidney is present. Operative procedures may be required because of the underlying renal abnormality rather than the trauma itself.

Reference: Persky, L., and Forsythe, W.E.: J.A.M.A., *182*:709, 1962.

# PROXIMAL OR DISTAL RENAL TUBULAR ACIDOSIS

Renal tubular acidosis is a syndrome consisting of metabolic acidosis that is out of proportion to the impairment of glomerular filtration and is associated with a paradoxically alkaline urine.

Patients with this disturbance can be separated into a proximal and a distal form, either of which may be primary or secondary.

The course, complications, and treatment of the two forms of the disorder are very different. It is important to distinguish between them. The table below provides some help.

*Renal Tubular Acidosis*

|  | PROXIMAL | DISTAL |
| --- | --- | --- |
| Primary | Idiopathic | Idiopathic |
| Usual age at diagnosis | 0 to 2 years | >2 years |
| Sex | Male predominance | Female predominance (?) |
| Presenting complaint | Growth failure | Growth failure, polydipsia, polyuria, vomiting, dehydration |
| Secondary to | Fanconi syndrome Cystinosis Lowe's syndrome Hereditary fructose intolerance Various states of renal insufficiency | Primary hyperparathyroidism Vitamin D intoxication Amphotericin B Hyperglobulinemia Medullary sponge kidney Renal tubular necrosis |
| Urine pH | 4.5 to 7.8, depending on plasma bicarbonate level | Always above 6.0 |
| Bicarbonate threshold | Decreased | Normal |
| Hydrogen excretion | Normal, below bicarbonate threshold | Impaired, below bicarbonate threshold |
| Therapy | Resistant to alkali therapy; diuretics effective | Sensitive to alkali therapy; no effect of diuretics |
| Spontaneous remission in primary form | Yes | No |
| Complications | Growth failure acidemia | Nephrocalcinosis Hypokalemia Bone lesions Ricketts |

11

Reference: Nash, M.A., Torrodo, A.D., Greifer, I., et al.: J. Pediatr., *80*:738, 1972.

# MYOGLOBINURIA, HEMOGLOBINURIA, OR PORPHYRIA?

The passage of large quantities of pigment in the urine often produces diagnostic confusion. Many substances may color the urine, but few mimic the appearance of hemoglobin. Hemoglobinuria must be most commonly distinguished from myoglobin or porphyrin compounds. Both myoglobin and hemoglobin will give positive results on the commonly employed dipstick (Labstix) for heme. The following table should provide a guide in the initial differential diagnosis of the three major causes of pigmenturia.

### Physical and Biochemical Features of the Pigmenturias

| PHYSICAL EXAMINATION | MYOGLOBINURIA | HEMOGLOBINURIA | PORPHYRIA |
|---|---|---|---|
| Muscles | | | |
|   Weakness | + | − | ± |
|   Pain | ± | − | ± |
|   Edema | + | − | − |
| Neuropathy (peripheral and autonomic) | − | − | + |
| CNS dysfunction | − | − | ± |
| Skin lesion | − | − | ± |
| Abdominal pain | Rare | − | + |
| **LABORATORY TESTS** | | | |
| Urine | | | |
|   Color | Brown | Red-brown | Burgundy |
|   Benzidine | + | + | − |
|   Hematest-orthotoluidine | + | + | − |
|   80% $(NH_4)_2SO_4$PPT | − | + | ? |
|   80% $(NH_4)_2SO_4$SUPER | + | − | ? |
|   Porphobilinogen | − | − | + |
|   Spectrophotometry ($\alpha$ band) | 582 (oxymyo) | 577 (oxyhemo) | 594 to 624* |
|   Taurine | Increased | Normal | ? |
|   Immunodiffusion | Specific | Specific | − |
| Serum | | | |
|   Appearance | Clear | Pink | Clear |
|   Haptoglobin | Normal | Low | Normal |
|   Creatine phosphokinases | Marked increase | Normal | Normal |
|   Carnitine | Increased | Normal | Normal |
|   Immunodiffusion | Specific | Specific | − |
|   Triglycerides | ↑In specific defects | − | − |

*Varies with type.

Reference: Robotham, J.L., and Haddow, J.D.: Pediatr. Clin. North Am., *23*:279, 1976.

# PSEUDOPROTEINURIA

When sulfosalicylic acid is employed for the determination of urine protein, false-positive reactions may be observed. False-positive reactions occur in:

1. Patients receiving large doses of nafcillin, penicillin G, and oxacillin. Urine antibiotic concentrations must be in the range of 100 mg/100 ml with nafcillin, and 250 to 500 mg/100 ml with penicillin G and oxacillin.
2. Patients taking tolbutamide.
3. Patients who have received organic iodine compounds for diagnostic x-ray procedures. In this circumstance, the "pseudoproteinuria" is usually observed on the day after the procedure but may occur as late as three days after the diagnostic study.

Urines tested with dipsticks will be negative under all of these circumstances.

---

References: Seedorf, E.E., Powell, W.N., Greenlee, R.G., et al.: J.A.M.A., *152*:1332, 1953. Line, D.E., Adler, S., Fraley, D.S., et al.: J.A.M.A., *235*:1259, 1976.

# HEMATURIA—AN ETIOLOGIC CLASSIFICATION

**11**

The causes of hematuria could easily fill a book. They can certainly fill a page, as a glance at the list below clearly indicates. A shopping list of this type has been provided to serve as a reminder of the things to consider the next time one observes red cells in the urine.

*Immunologic Injury*

Acute glomerulonephritis
Primary persistent glomerulonephritis
  Focal proliferative
  Membranous
  Membranoproliferative
  Diffuse proliferative
Henoch-Schönlein nephritis
Collagen vascular diseases
  Systemic lupus erythematosus
  Polyarteritis nodosa
Subacute bacterial endocarditis
Goodpasture's syndrome
Nephrotic syndrome

*Infectious Diseases of Urinary Tract*

Acute pyelonephritis
Renal tuberculosis

Hemorrhagic cystitis secondary to viral infection of the bladder
Varicella; rubeola, mumps
Schistosomiasis
Malaria

## Familial and Congenital Urinary Tract Disorders

Chronic hereditary nephritis (Alport's)
Benign familial hematuria
Polycystic disease of the kidney
Congenital urinary tract abnormalities

## Bleeding or Vascular Disorders

Coagulation disorders
  Coagulation factor deficiencies
  Platelet deficiencies
Hemoglobinopathies
Vascular abnormalities
  Hemangiomas
  Hereditary hemorrhagic telangiectasia
  Renal vein thrombosis
  Varices of the renal pelvis or ureter

## Neoplastic Disease

Renal neoplasms
Leukemia

## Renal Trauma

Direct trauma
Indirect trauma from shock, anoxia, and so on
Renal stones
Foreign bodies
Penile excoriations

## Drug or Chemically Induced

## Miscellaneous

Exercise
Hemolytic-uremic syndrome
Scurvy
Allergy
Menstruation
Congestive heart failure
Polyps

## Recurrent Monosymptomatic Hematuria (essential, idiopathic, or benign)

## Mimics of Hematuria

Urate crystals
Beet uria
Porphyrinuria
Hemoglobinuria
Myoglobin
Bile

---

Reference: Tunnessen, W.W., Jr.: Personal communication.

*"We of this self-conscious, incredulous generation sentimentalize our children, analyze our children, think we are endowed with a special capacity to sympathize and identify ourselves with children. And the result is that we are not more childlike, but our children are less childlike."*

Francis Thompson

**11**

## NEONATAL HEMATURIA

Gross hematuria is a rare presentation during the first month of life. The findings in one series of 35 patients are demonstrated below.

| CAUSE | NO. OF PATIENTS | AGE AT ONSET | | | | DURATION (DAYS) | REMARKS |
|---|---|---|---|---|---|---|---|
| | | 1st WEEK | 2nd WEEK | 3rd WEEK | 4th WEEK | | |
| Unknown | 11 | 8 | 2 | 1 | ... | 1-3 | 1 died of hyaline membrane disease and pneumothorax; normal BUN level in 9, elevated in 2 |
| Renal vein thrombosis | 7 | 3 | 1 | 3 | ... | 2-5 | 3 had diabetic mothers; Bun level >40 mg/100 ml in all; 4 had thrombocytopenia |
| Polycystic disease of kidney | 6 | 6 | ... | ... | ... | 2-4 | 5 died in neonatal period, one at 4 months; all had increased BUN, 40 to 80 mg/100 ml |
| Obstructive uropathy | | | | | | | |
| Hydronephrosis | 3 | 1 | ... | 2 | ... | 1-5 | BUN level 25 to 30 mg/100 ml; 2 with hydronephrosis underwent difficult delivery; 3 had pyuria and bacteriuria; palpable mass present in 2 |
| Ureteral valve | 3 | 2 | ... | ... | ... | 2-4 | |
| Bladder neck | 1 | 1 | ... | ... | 1 | 4 | |
| Sponge kidney | 3 | ... | ... | 2 | 1 | 1 | Death within 4 to 6 months of age |
| Wilms' tumor | 1 | ... | ... | ... | 1 | 2 | Survived, patient doing well 4 years later |

Abdominal masses were palpated in all patients later found to have renal vein thrombosis or polycystic kidneys. Intravenous pyelograms were normal in all patients in whom no cause was found for the hematuria, in the patients with posterior urethral valves, and in the one with bladder neck obstruction. IVP was abnormal in all other patients. Voiding cystourethrogram demonstrated the abnormality in the patients with obstruction.

**Conclusion:** Abdominal palpation, IVP, and blood urea nitrogen levels are warranted in all newborns presenting with gross hematuria. If the diagnosis is still unavailable, voiding cystourethrogram is in order. A significant number of these patients, however, will have no evident cause for their hematuria, and will recover spontaneously.

---

Reference: Emanuel, B., and Aronson, N.: Am. J. Dis. Child., 128: *204*, 1974.

# DECREASED SGOT ACTIVITY IN UREMIA

Be careful — do not rely on the serum glutamic oxaloacetic transaminase for the diagnosis of liver disease in patients with elevations in their blood urea nitrogen levels. It may be falsely low. This depression of SGOT values is most evident when the determinations are performed by the SMA technique on the AutoAnalyzer, but can also be observed when the assay is performed by the Karmen kinetic technique. Values of less than 10 units SGOT may be observed with blood urea nitrogen values exceeding 50 mg/100 ml. The mechanism of this inhibition is unknown, but it is not caused by the urea in the plasma. The inhibition if rapidly reversed when the patient is dialyzed.

---

Reference: Cohen, G.A., Goffinet, J.A., Donabedian, R.K., et al.: Ann. Intern. Med., *84*:275, 1975.

# THE DESCENT OF THE TESTIS

How frequent is an undescended testis? How long should it take for the testis to descend if it is not in the appropriate position at birth?

> *Masturbation*—From the Latin word *manustupratio*; from *manus*, or hand, and *stuprare*, which means to defile.

Here are some guidelines.

1. A testis 4 cm below the pubic crest in a term infant may be considered descended. In the infant weighing less than 2500 grams, a distance of 2.5 cm below the pubic crest may be used as a criterion for descent.

2. In approximately 97 per cent of term infants, the testes are in the correct position. In males who weigh less than 2500 grams at birth, the incidence of descended testes is 79 per cent.

3. In the term infant, the testis, if it is to descend, will have done so by 6 weeks of age. In the premature infant, this descent should be completed at the same gestational age — approximately 46 weeks.

4. The ultimate incidence of undescended testis in term infants is approximately 0.8 per cent or about 1 per 1000.

5. The testis that has not completely descended by 6 weeks of age in the term infant will always remain higher than its mate and will always remain smaller. There is no justification for deferring surgery beyond 4 years of age in the expectation that descent will eventually occur.

6. Ten per cent of patients with cryptorchidism have upper urinary tract abnormalities, such as duplication, hydroureter, hydronephrosis, horseshoe kidney, and hypoplastic kidney. The anomalies are more common when associated with unilateral cryptorchidism.

References: Grossman, H., and Ririe, D.G.: Am. J. Roentgenol., *103*:210, 1968. Scorer, C.G.: Arch. Dis. Child., *39*:605, 1974.

# THE $FE_{Na}$ TEST: USE IN THE DIFFERENTIAL DIAGNOSIS OF ACUTE RENAL FAILURE

The physician is frequently faced with the problem of distinguishing prerenal azotemia from acute tubular necrosis in patients with acute renal failure.

In the oliguric phase of these two conditions, the renal tubule handles sodium in distinctly different fashions. In prerenal azotemia, the renal tubule avidly reabsorbs the filtered sodium; in acute tubular necrosis, the reabsorption of sodium is restricted.

These observations provide the basis for a simple test for differentiating these two conditions — the "$FE_{Na}$ test" ($FE_{Na}$ is the excreted fraction of the filtered sodium).

The test is performed by measuring both sodium and creatinine in simultaneously collected samples of plasma and urine.

The $FE_{Na}$ is calculated as follows:

$$\frac{\dfrac{[Sodium]_U}{[Sodium]_P}}{\dfrac{[Creatinine]_U}{[Creatinine]_P}} \times 100$$

U and P represent concentrations in urine and plasma, respectively.

In general, an $FE_{Na}$ of less than 1 indicates prerenal azotemia, and an $FE_{Na}$ of more than 3 indicates acute tubular necrosis.

Reference: Espinel, C.H.: J.A.M.A., *236*:579, 1976.

# 12
# NEUROLOGY

# NEUROLOGIC SIGNS OF INFANCY

The appearance and disappearance of certain neurologic signs of infancy have been well delineated. Neurologic abnormality should be suspected when these responses are not present at the appropriate time. Equal significance may be attached to the failure of certain responses to disappear. The chart below gives the age of expected appearance and disappearance of some of the more important neurologic signs in infancy.

| RESPONSE | AGE AT TIME OF APPEARANCE | AGE AT TIME OF DISAPPEARANCE |
|---|---|---|
| **Reflexes of position and movement** | | |
| Moro reflex | Birth | 1–3 months |
| Tonic neck reflex (unsustained) | Birth | 5–6 months (partial up to 2–4 years) |
| Neck righting reflex | 4–6 months | 1–2 years |
| Landau response | 3 months | 1–2 years |
| Palmar grasp reflex | Birth | 4 months |
| Adductor spread of knee jerk | Birth | 7 months |
| Plantar grasp reflex | Birth | 8–15 months |
| Babinski response | Birth | Variable |
| Parachute reaction | 8–9 months | Variable |
| **Reflexes to sound** | | |
| Blinking response | Birth | |
| Turning response | Birth | |
| **Reflexes of vision** | | |
| Blinking to threat | 6–7 months | |
| Horizontal following | 4–6 weeks | |
| Vertical following | 2–3 months | |
| Optokinetic nystagmus | Birth | |
| Postrotational nystagmus | Birth | |
| Lid closure to light | Birth | |
| Macular light reflex | 4–8 months | |
| **Food reflexes** | | |
| Rooting response — awake | Birth | 3–4 months |
| Rooting response — asleep | Birth | 7–8 months |
| Sucking response | Birth | 12 months |
| **Handedness** | 2–3 years | |

12

| RESPONSE | AGE AT TIME OF APPEARANCE | AGE AT TIME OF DISAPPEARANCE |
|----------|--------------------------|------------------------------|
| *Spontaneous stepping* | Birth | |
| *Straight line walking* | 5–6 years | |

Reference: Children Are Different. Columbus, Ohio, Ross Laboratories, 1967, p. 67.

## EVALUATION OF "SOFT" NEUROLOGIC SIGNS IN THE SCHOOL-AGE CHILD

The traditional neurologic examination does not evaluate "soft" neurologic signs that may reflect abnormalities in the development or maturation of the central nervous system of the child. These differences in development may lead to learning and reading disabilities, but do not necessarily indicate pathologic changes or injury. Evaluation of these soft signs is difficult. The following examination has been used by the Child Study Unit of the Department of Pediatrics at the University of California at San Francisco. Poor results on this examination have been found to correlate with reading disability in the child of average intelligence.

### Evaluation of Fine-Motor Coordination

Observe the child during:

A. Undressing, unbuttoning.
B. Tying shoes.
C. Rapid alternating touch of fingertips by thumb.
D. Rattle of an imaginary doorknob.
E. Unscrewing of an imaginary light bulb.
F. Pencil grasp and use; penmanship.
G. Rapid tongue movements.
H. Hand grip.
I. Inversion of both feet. (Look for similar movements of the hands. See below.)
J. Repeating several times rapidly: kitty, kitty, kitty; pa, ta, ka. (Accurate reproduction of these sounds generally indicates adequate articulatory coordination.)

Note:

a. The child's general facility and coordination with these small muscle tasks.
b. On items C, D, E, H, and I, any marked movement of other parts of the body that mirror or duplicate movements of the test side. Such movements are called associated motor movements, mirror movements, adventitious overflow movements, or synkinesia. When marked they are felt to represent, particularly after 8 to 10 years, a lack of normal cortical inhibition.

c.  Excessive pressure on the pencil point or a pencil held too lightly. Fingers placed directly over the point, or fingers placed too far (greater than 1 inch) from the point may all indicate difficulty with the coordination of fine musculature within the hands.

d.  Presence of dysdiadochokinesia, noting speed, accuracy, and sequencing of maneuvers.

## Evaluation of Special Sensory Skills

**A.  Dual Simultaneous Sensory Tests (face-hand testing).**  With the patient's eyes closed (but first demonstrating items 1 and 2 below with patient's eyes open), simultaneously:

1.  Touch both cheeks.
2.  Touch both hands.
3.  Touch right cheek and contralateral hand.
4.  Touch right cheek and homolateral hand.
5.  Touch left cheek and contralateral hand.
6.  Touch left cheek and homolateral hand.

*Note:*

a.  Rostral dominance:  failure to perceive hand stimulus when the face is simultaneously touched. Approximately 80 per cent of normal children are able to perform this test without rostral dominance by age 8 years.

**B.  Finger Localization Test (finger agnosia test).**  Touch two fingers or two spots on one finger simultaneously with the patient's eyes closed, after demonstrating first with eyes open. Ask the patient: "How many fingers am I touching — one or two?"

*Note:*

a.  The number of correct responses in four trials for each hand; six correct answers out of eight are accepted as a "pass." Half of all children pass this test by age 6 years, 90 per cent by age 7½ years. This test reflects a child's orientation in space, concept of body image, praxic ability, and sensation to touch and position sense.

## Evaluation of Child's Laterality and Orientation in Space

**A.  Imitation of Gestures.**  Have the child imitate the following gestures performed by the examiner, emphasizing first that the child must use the same hand as the examiner:

1.  Extend index finger.
2.  Extend little and index finger.
3.  Extend index and middle finger.
4.  Touch two thumbs and two index fingers together simultaneously.
5.  Form two interlocking rings, thumb and index finger of one hand with thumb and index finger of other hand.

**12**

6. Point index finger of one hand down toward the cupped fingers of the opposite hand held below.

*Note:*

a. Difficulty with fine finger movements, manipulation, and/or reproduction of correct gesture.
b. After approximately age 8 years, marked right-left confusion with regard to examiner's right and left. This test reflects a child's ability with finger discrimination, postural praxis, awareness of self-image, and right-left, front-back, up-down orientation.

B. **Following Directions.** Ask the child to:

1. Show me your left hand.
2. Show me your right ear.
3. Show me your right eye.
4. Show me your left elbow.
5. Touch your left knee with your left hand.
6. Touch your right ear with your left hand.
7. Touch your left elbow with your right hand.
8. Touch your right cheek with your right hand.
9. Point to my left ear.
10. Point to my right eye.
11. Point to my right hand.
12. Point to my left knee.

*Note:*

a. Items 1 through 8 are mastered by approximately age 6 years; items 9 through 12 are mastered by approximately age 8 years.
b. Aside from correct versus incorrect responses, any difficulty with following the sequence of directions.

The above examination constitutes only a small part of the complete evaluation of a child with learning disabilities. The school and family should take part in the complete evaluation and treatment of the child along with the physician, psychologist, and counselor so that all resources may be mobilized, with the goal being the sustained and successful education of the child.

Reference: Gofman, H.P., and Allmond, B.W., Jr.: Curr. Probl. Pediatr., *1*:3, 1971.

# A RATIONAL DIAGNOSTIC EVALUATION OF THE CHILD WITH MENTAL DEFICIENCY

There are hundreds of recognized disorders accompanied by mental deficiency. Given a patient with mental deficiency, what is a rational diagnostic evaluation? All too frequently, inappropriate procedures are ordered in a seemingly random fashion. One suggested approach to the problem is as follows.

A. *Appropriate History*

1. *Family history*

   About 50 per cent of patients with mental deficiency will have a genetically determined disorder. Similarly affected individuals may be present in 9 to 10 per cent of families.

   a. Pedigree:  Search for a similar problem in both first and second degree relatives.
   b. Parental ages at birth of patient:  Older maternal age is a factor in trisomy syndromes, while paternal age is a factor in certain fresh mutant gene disorders.
   c. Parental levels of intelligence and head circumference:  Both mild mental deficiency and microcephaly may be familial.

2. *Cultural-Social History*

   Unfortunately, certain diseases occur more frequently among the poor.  These include prematurity, prenatal cytomegalovirus infections, maternal alcoholism, and emotional deprivation.

3. *Prenatal History*

   Fetal activity in utero, complications of pregnancy, maternal weight gain, duration of pregnancy, and drug ingestion should all be noted.

4. *Perinatal History*

   a. Birth presentation — problems of morphogenesis and neurologic function are more common among infants who fail to assume the vertex position.
   b. Amount and character of amniotic fluid. Polyhydramnios may suggest difficulty in swallowing. Meconium staining suggests perinatal distress.
   c. Head circumference and body weight and length at birth. Small size often associated with problems of morphogenesis and brain development.
   d. Apgar score at 5 minutes.
   e. Problems such as placenta previa, traumatic delivery, prolonged hypoxia, apneic episodes, seizures, hyperbilirubinemia, hypoglycemia, and sepsis should be recorded.

5. *Postnatal Events*

   a. Developmental progress
   b. Growth rate
   c. Postnatal events — central nervous system infections, head trauma.

B. *Physical Examination*

1. *Indirect assessment of brain and brain function*

   Head circumference, transillumination, scalp hair pattern (aberrant scalp hair pattern may be used as a clue to early fetal problems in brain morphogenesis), examination of ocular fundus, developmental status, neurologic status.

2. *Complete non-CNS examination for major and minor anomalies*

*The combined finding of such a history and physical examination will either provide a specific diagnosis or allow one to assign the patient into one of four clinical groupings, each of which requires a different diagnostic evaluation.*

The accompanying flow sheet illustrates this procedure.

*After Appropriate History and Physical Examination*

| PRENATAL ONSET OF PROBLEM IN MORPHOGENESIS *includes* | PERINATAL ONSET OF INSULT TO BRAIN *includes* | POSTNATAL ONSET *includes* | UNDECIDED AGE AT ONSET *includes* |
|---|---|---|---|
| 1. Single defect of brain development<br>primary microcephaly<br>hydrocephaly<br>hydranencephaly<br>defect of neural tube<br>cerebral dysgenesis<br><br>2. Major and minor malformations in other than CNS as well as chromosomal defects syndromes of nonchromosomal cause unknown patterns of malformation | hypoxic injury<br>kernicterus<br>hypoglycemia<br>neonatal meningitis | trauma<br>meningitis<br>encephalitis<br>hypernatremia<br>water intoxication<br>lead poisoning<br>degenerative disorders<br>metabolic errors | most patients in whom no diagnosis is made |

*Consider Following Diagnostic Procedures*

| | | | |
|---|---|---|---|
| Pneumoencephalogram or CAT scan<br><br>Karyotype<br><br>Viral titers | As indicated from history | Appropriate metabolic studies as provided from clues in history and physical examination<br>Phenylketonuria<br>Mucopolysaccharide disorders<br>Galactosemia<br>Lesch-Nyhan<br>Homocystinuria | If male, get a buccal smear |

| PRENATAL ONSET OF PROBLEM IN MORPHOGENESIS | PERINATAL ONSET OF INSULT TO BRAIN | POSTNATAL ONSET | UNDECIDED AGE AT ONSET |
|---|---|---|---|
| *Relative Frequency* | | | |
| This category makes up 40 to 45% of patients; it is the largest category | Accounts for 15 to 20% of all patients | About 5% of patients fall into this category; normal early development and obstetric history should make you suspect these disorders | Second largest category |

12

Other laboratory studies are rarely indicated. Skull films should be obtained in patients with craniostenosis, cutaneous signs of tuberous sclerosis, or Sturge-Weber syndrome. Long bone films are justified in patients with skeletal abnormalities, and bone age studies are warranted in patients with abnormal growth. EEGs should be reserved for patients with seizures. Other blood chemistries and viral titers are justified only by pertinent findings in the history and physical examination.

Reference: Smith, D.W., and Simons, E.R.: Am. J. Dis. Child., *129*:1285, 1975.

## THE SETTING-SUN SIGN

The setting-sun sign has been said to be a clinical sign of hydrocephalus or kernicterus in infancy. Other conditions that have been associated with the sign are neonatal hyperthyroidism, early myotonia, and congenital abnormalities of the eyelids. The sign has two main components: downward rotation of the eyeballs, elicited by alteration of position; and retraction of the eyelids (sometimes accompanied by raising of the brow), elicited by removal of light. Degree of response depends on the infant's age and alertness and on constitutional factors. A marked response, lasting several seconds, indicates that both main components are functioning.

In a longitudinal study, 19 infants with the setting-sun sign were followed for the first year of life; eight had increased intracranial pressure requiring surgery, two had transient signs of increased pressure that resolved spontaneously, and nine had no evidence of increased intracranial pressure or other illness.

The setting-sun phenomenon can be observed in healthy infants. The response indicates increased intracranial pressure in the following situations:

1. If it can be elicited by alteration of position in infants older than 4 weeks of age.

2. If it is a marked response to removal of light in infants younger than 8 or older than 20 weeks.

3. Especially if the response is combined with constant or intermittent strabismus or undulating eye movements.

The value of the phenomenon in early diagnosis of hydrocephalus is limited because clear clinical signs of intracranial hypertension would have already appeared before the onset of the phenomenon.

Reference: Cernerud, L.: Dev. Med. Child Neurol., *17*:447, 1975.

## CHILDHOOD GLAUCOMA

Childhood glaucoma will be discovered only if you or the patient's mother look for it. It may be discovered at any time from birth through school age, although most cases are found during the first year of life. Presenting symptoms and signs are excessive irritability, clouding of the cornea, tearing, enlargement of the eye, and photophobia. Measurement of the horizontal diameter of the cornea is helpful, and glaucoma should be suspected if this value is greater than 12 mm.

The three types of childhood glaucoma may be associated with other anomalies or diseases as listed below.

| | ASSOCIATED ANOMALIES | |
| --- | --- | --- |
| Form | Intraocular | Extraocular |
| Primary congenital (simple) | Congenital lacrimal duct obstruction (frequent) | Inguinal hernia Pilonidal sinus Tibial torsion Rubella syndrome Hydrocephalus |
| Associated buphthalmos | Microcornea Spherophakia (small, spherical lenses subject to sub-luxation) | Neurofibromatosis Hemangiomatosis |
| Secondary congenital (infantile) | Neoplasm Keratitis Uveitis | None |

Reference: Turner, J.B.: South. Med. J., *64*:1362, 1971.

## OPTIC ATROPHY

Optic nerve atrophy is usually a single manifestation of another disease process. Idiopathic optic atrophy may rarely exist alone. When this idiopathic form occurs, it usually affects children below the age of 3 years. The following findings may be present.

Impaired vision (this may be difficult to detect in the young infant)
Strabismus
Nystagmus
Decreased or attenuated retinal vessels
Pale or white optic discs

Idiopathic optic atrophy may be unilateral or bilateral. The prognosis is relatively good. The majority of those in whom both eyes are affected maintain useful vision, and those with unilateral involvement maintain good vision in the unaffected eye.

Optic atrophy may be a part of a central nervous system disorder. Many patients with optic atrophy have mental retardation, spasticity, microcephaly, hydrocephalus, or seizures. The young infant thought to have idiopathic optic atrophy may later develop one or more of these disorders.

Though systemic or neurologic disease is usually the cause of optic nerve atrophy, there may be no other signs of disease on initial presentation. Diseases that may present with optic atrophy include the following:

Tumors (including glioma, neuroepithelioma, neurofibroma, and any tumor in the region of the optic chiasm)
Fibrous dysplasia
Congenital syphilis
Toxoplasmosis
Osteopetrosis
Neurofibromatosis
Trauma
Congenital glaucoma
Multiple sclerosis

Reference: Schwartz, J.F., Chutorian, A.M., Evans, R.A., et al.: Pediatrics. *34*:670, 1964.

# HEARING DEFICIT IN LATER CHILDHOOD

The severity of the handicap associated with hearing deficit during childhood is a function of several factors in addition to the child's hearing levels, such as:

Age at onset of hearing loss
Characteristics of hearing loss (especially abilities in speech discrimination)
Intelligence
Emotional stability
Presence of associated handicaps

The accompanying table outlines the degree of handicap usually associated with given hearing losses, as well as some potentially useful remedial procedures.

Reference: Goodman, A.C., and Chasin, W.D.: *In* Gellis, S.S., and Kagan, B.M. (Eds.): Current Pediatric Therapy. 7th Ed. Philadelphia, W.B. Saunders Company, 1976, p. 518.

| HEARING LEVEL IN DECIBELS (DB) | PROBABLE HANDICAP | HAS DIFFICULTY HEARING: | SUSTAINED ATTENTION | SPEECH/ LANGUAGE | MAY BENEFIT FROM |
|---|---|---|---|---|---|
| –10 to 26 db normal limits | None for most children; may have some if at upper limits | In classroom for some | May be difficult if at upper limits | Normal | Sitting near front of class or hearing aid, if at upper limits |
| 27–40 db mild loss | Slight for some but significant for many | Faint or distant speech | May be difficult | | All above plus instruction in speech reading |
| 41–55 db moderate loss | Significant for most | Conversation beyond 3 to 5 feet, classroom or group discussion | Very difficult | May be defective | All above plus auditory training speech conversation; speech and language therapy |
| 56–70 db moderately severe loss | Marked | Classroom and group discussion | Very difficult | Defective | All above plus special teaching in language skills and perhaps tutoring in academic subjects |
| 71–90 db severe loss | Severe | Anything but shouted or amplified speech; consonants | Very difficult | Severely defective | All above plus school for or classes for deaf children |
| >90 db profound loss | Extreme | All but some loud sounds | | Severely defective | All above |

12

# EYE SIGNS IN THE COMATOSE PATIENT

Examination of the eyes provides valuable diagnostic information in the patient in coma. Both pupillary signs and eye movements should be noted before examining the ocular fundi.

## PUPILLARY SIGNS IN COMA

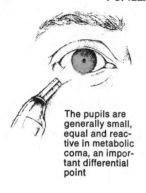

The pupils are generally small, equal and reactive in metabolic coma, an important differential point

Equal, fixed, dilated pupils result from substances like atropine; they also occur in severe anoxia or ischemia and in the terminal state

Pinpoint pupils result from opiates and also occur in patients with pontine lesions (usually hemorrhage or infarct)

*FIG. 12–A*

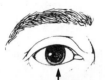

**Dilated ipsilateral pupil due to:**
Compression by herniated uncus
Traction of oculomotor nerve against posterior cerebral artery

A unilaterally widely dilated and fixed pupil results from pressure on the third nerve, often a sign of uncal herniation from a rapidly expanding unilateral lesion, as a rule on the side of the dilated pupil

*FIG. 12–B*

## EYE MOVEMENTS IN COMA

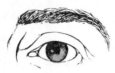

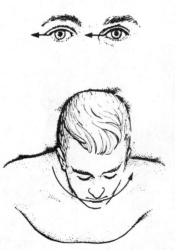

The doll's head maneuver: The head is turned rapidly from side to side and conjugate deviation occurs in the direction opposite the head movement as long as the brain stem centers for eye movement are still intact. Loss of these centers results in absence of doll's head movement. These movements are generally also absent when the patient is not comatose

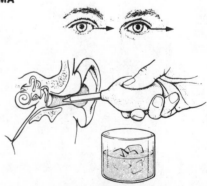

The oculovestibular response: Irrigation of the external auditory canal with ice water results in conjugate motion of the eyes toward the side of stimulation. This response is lost when the pontine centers are compromised

*FIG. 12–C*

Reference: Haerer, A.F.: Hosp. Med., *12*:68, 1976.

# THE DIFFERENTIAL DIAGNOSIS OF NYSTAGMUS

Nystagmus is easily observed. The cause is frequently more difficult to determine. Certain forms of nystagmus suggest an anatomic location of the lesion, while other forms are characteristic of specific disturbances. The direction of the nystagmus is determined by its fast component.

| | |
|---|---|
| *Sustained jerk nystagmus* | indicates impaired vestibular function. This may result from disease in the labyrinth or in its central connection within the brain stem or cerebellum. |
| *Pure vertical nystagmus* | always indicates brain stem dysfunction. |
| *Rotatory nystagmus* | is seen with labyrinthine disease but is also observed when central vestibular mechanisms are affected. In labyrinthine disease, the nystagmus is fine and maximal in a certain direction of gaze. It is often associated with nausea and vomiting. |
| *See-saw nystagmus* | is the term applied to the phenomenon in which eyes rise and fall alternately. It has no localizing value, but has been seen with suprasellar mass lesions. |
| *Wandering nystagmus* | describes the irregular, oscillating, searching eye movements of marked amplitude seen in blind infants and children. It has no rapid jerk component. |
| *To-and-fro nystagmus* | describes the jellylike oscillations of one or both eyes seen characteristically in patients with congenital nystagmus or spasmus nutans. Slow and fast components of the nystagmus are usually not evident. |

**12**

Nystagmus is most commonly caused by defective vision in the pediatric age group. The visual defect may be primarily of optic origin or be a result of a more generalized neurologic process. The causes of nystagmus and some of their associated features are described below.

| CONDITION | ASSOCIATED FEATURES |
|---|---|
| Blindness of optic origin | May be a result of bilateral cataracts, severe chorioretinitis, or retrolental fibroplasia. |
| Congenital nystagmus | Observed at birth or in first weeks of life. Positive family history common. No other neurologic abnormalities. |
| Ingestion of anticonvulsants | May be associated with other cerebellar signs and lethargy. |

| CONDITION | ASSOCIATED FEATURES |
|---|---|
| Spasmus nutans | Head bobbing and head tilting. Head bobbing disappears when patient lies down. Onset at 4 to 18 months. Usually disappears by age 2 years. Cause unknown. Not familial. |
| Albinism | Photophobia. May have platelet abnormality and easy bruising. |
| Chédiak-Higashi syndrome | Large gray-green leukocyte inclusions. Increased incidence of lymphoreticular malignancies. May have seizures, mental retardation, muscle weakness, and neuropathies. |
| Acute cerebellar ataxia | Acute onset with rapid deterioration of gait. Frequently associated with a viral illness (chickenpox most common). Cerebrospinal fluid normal or may have mild lymphocytic pleocytosis. EEG normal. Mild tremor may be present. Approximately two-thirds of children recover completely within 1 week to 12 months. |
| Benign paroxysmal vertigo | Onset usually before age 3 years. Brief attacks of nausea, vertigo, and unsteady gait. All laboratory tests normal. Gradually disappears. |
| Friedreich's ataxia | Ataxia, optic atrophy, vertigo, slowly progressive, family history, cardiac involvement in 50 per cent of patients. |
| Hereditary spinocerebellar ataxia | Familial incidence, stumbling, dizziness, extensor plantar responses, kyphoscoliosis, pes cavus. |
| Hyperpipecolatemia | Onset in first year of life, hepatomegaly, retinal changes, intention tremor, increased plasma pipecolic acid level, progressive demyelinization of brain, and fibrosis of liver. |
| Hypervalinemia | Vomiting, failure to thrive, hepatomegaly, lethargy, poor suck, fever, EEG abnormalities, urine and plasma valine levels increased. |
| Refsum's disease | Chronic polyneuropathy, ataxia, retinitis pigmentosa, ichthyosis, elevated serum phytanic acid. |
| Hypertrophic interstitial polyneuritis | Onset from early childhood to adult life. Weakness and atrophy begin in feet, sharp pains and muscle cramps, sensory loss, absent deep tendon reflexes. |
| Krabbe's disease | Onset 3 to 6 months of age, tonic spasms, rigidity, opisthotonos, loss of vision, optic atrophy. |
| Juvenile cerebral atrophies | A variety of disorders accompanied by progressive cerebral and cerebellar degeneration. Macular degeneration and optic atrophy with blindness. Includes Bielschowsky, Spielmeyer-Vogt, and ceroid lipofuscinoses. |

| Meniere's disease | Rare in children. Acute attacks of vertigo, nausea, and vomiting. Attacks may last several days. Tinnitus persent. Nerve deafness occurs. |
| Posterior fossa tumors | Associated cerebellar signs, evidence of increased intracranial pressure (see page 340). |

# THE DIFFERENTIAL DIAGNOSIS OF COMA IN THE INFANT AND CHILD

The diagnosis of the patient in coma requires a prompt and disciplined approach. Much can be learned from the history and careful attention to the vital signs, neurologic examination, and a few carefully selected laboratory tests.

*Respiration* as a clue to the cause of coma

Cheyne-Stokes respiration indicates bilateral cortical lesions.

Hyperventilation may be a result of:
Central neurogenic origin
Seen in patients with hyperammonemia
Metabolic acidosis
Diabetes
Uremia
Fluid and electrolyte imbalance
Lactic acidosis
Poisoning with acidic substances (acetylsalicylic acid, acetazolamide, methyl alcohol to formic acid, ethylene glycol to oxalic acid, paraldehyde to acetic acid)
Metabolic errors of metabolism
isovaleric acidemia, methylmalonic aciduria, hyperglycinemia, maple syrup urine disease

Periodic breathing, ataxic breathing, and apneusis all suggest brain stem lesions.

*Blood Pressure*

Hypotension suggests that patient is in shock from septicemia, hypovolemia, adrenal insufficiency, or severe hypoxemia.

Hypertension indicates the presence of increased intracranial pressure, severe renal disease, or poisoning with sympathomimetic agents.

*Neurologic Examination*

Positive Kernig and Brudzinski signs suggest central nervous infection, subarachnoid hemorrhage, or posterior fossa tumor.

Eye signs (pupils should be equal and reactive to light).

Unilateral fixed and dilated pupil suggests tentorial herniation or focal lesion in the area of third nerve nucleus.

Bilateral dilated pupils, fixed to light, suggest irreversible brain damage or poisoning with atropine-like agents, barbiturates, or glutethimide. May also be observed with hypothermia or peripheral nerve lesions.

Irregular pupils, unreactive to light, suggest midbrain damage.

Pinpoint pupils indicate metabolic coma, drug intoxication (opiates, barbiturates), or pontine lesions.

Eye Movements

VI nerve palsy — suspect increased intracranial pressure, meningeal inflammatory process, neoplastic invasion of nerve, or pontine lesion.

III nerve palsy (eyes point down and out) suggests a tentorial herniation.

Lumbar puncture should be performed in all instances where central nervous system disease exists as a diagnostic possibility. Always measure opening pressure.

Based on the physical findings and lumbar puncture examination, the following diagnostic categories can be established.

## Differential Diagnosis of Coma

| No Focal Signs | No Focal Signs | Focal Signs | Focal Signs |
|---|---|---|---|
| Normal Spinal Fluid | Abnormal Spinal Fluid (cells, pressure, or protein) | Normal Spinal Fluid | Abnormal Spinal Fluid |
| Poisoning | Infection | Arterial occlusion | Trauma |
| Metabolic disorders | Lead poisoning | Demyelinating disease | Infection brain abscess subdural empyema encephalitis |
| Concussion | Water intoxication | Postictal paralysis | |
| Postictal state | Trauma | | Neoplasm |
| Septicemia | Subarachnoid hemorrhage | | Vascular malformation |
| | Cerebral vein thrombosis | | |
| | Midline tumors | | |
| | Hydrocephalus | | |

Reference: Modified from a lecture by Peter Huttenlocher, M.D., May 1976.

## BENIGN ESSENTIAL TREMOR

Tremor in children may be associated with athetosis, spasticity, cerebellar disease, or generalized metabolic disorders. These conditions must be differentiated from benign essential tremor. Benign essential tremor is inherited as an autosomal dominant trait, but its variable expression is such that only about one-half of the patients exhibiting the tremor have a positive family history. The tremor may be noted first in early childhood, but it tends to become worse with age. It may disappear for years, but recurrence seems inevitable.

The tremor involves the head, hands, and less often the voice and trunk. It is characterized by rhythmic movements of 8 to 10 cycles per second, and the amplitude of the movements may become greater with intentional movements and excitement.

The disorder seems to represent a biochemical defect in which the normal "damping mechanism" of muscle movement does not operate properly. Treatment is usually not totally successful. Diazepam or barbiturates are commonly employed. Propranolol has been used with some success.

Careful guidance may be necessary in advising realistic career goals for affected children.

Reference: Paulson, G.W.: Clin. Pediatr., *15*:67, 1976.

# BREATH-HOLDING SPELL OR IDIOPATHIC EPILEPSY?

About 5 per cent of infants and children will experience at least one breath-holding spell and may lose consciousness. Some features that may be used to distinguish these episodes from idiopathic epilepsy appear in the table below.

|  | GRAND MAL (IDIOPATHIC EPILEPSY) | ANOXIC CONVULSION (BREATH-HOLDING SPELL) |
|---|---|---|
| Age of onset | Rarely in infancy | Often begins in infancy |
| Family history | None or positive for epilepsy | Often positive for breath-holding spell or fainting |
| Precipitating factors | Usually absent (or specific sensory stimuli or nonspecific stresses) | Usually present (specific emotional or nociceptive stimuli) |
| Occurrence during sleep | Common | Never |
| Posture | Variable | Usually erect |
| Sequence and patterns | Single cry (may be absent) with loss of consciousness→tonic→clonic phases, cyanosis may occur later in attack; flushed at first, pale after attack | Long crying or single gasp, cyanosis or pallor→loss of consciousness→limpness→clonic jerks→opisthotonos→clonic jerks |
| Perspiration | Warm sweat | Cold sweat |
| Heart rate | Markedly increased | Decreased, asystole, or slightly increased |
| Duration | Usually >1 minute | Usually 1 minute or less |
| Incontinence and tongue biting | Common | Uncommon (but may occur) |
| Postictal state | Confusion and sleep common | No confusion. Fatigue common |

12

|  | GRAND MAL (IDIOPATHIC EPILEPSY) | ANOXIC CONVULSION (INFANTILE SYNCOPE) |
|---|---|---|
| Interictal EEG | Usually bilateral discharges | Usually normal |
| Oculocardiac activation | No response or bradycardia; 7% may have asystole of less than 4 seconds; asymptomatic | About 50% have asystole $>2$ seconds, usually $>4$ seconds; attack may be precipitated |
| Ictal EEG | Generalized, high-voltage polyspike discharges, gradually subsiding into slow waves and depression for several minutes | Isoelectric pattern preceded and followed by diffuse high-voltage delta waves, promptly reverting to normal pattern upon recovery of consciousness |

Reference: Lombroso, C.T., and Lerman, P.: Pediatrics, *39*:563, 1967.

## FEBRILE SEIZURES—RECURRENCES AND SEQUELAE

Approximately 2 to 5 per cent of all children will develop a febrile seizure during childhood. These seizures can be characterized as to:

*Type:* Most are clonic, generalized seizures. About 15 per cent are focal.
*Precipitating Illness:* Source of fever is always extracranial.
*Age:* Most occur between 6 months and 3 years of age.
*Duration:* Nearly half last less than 5 minutes; 75 per cent are over within 20 minutes.
*Role of Fever:* Fever is always present and is usually greater than 102°F.

Approximately one-third to one-half of these children will have at least one recurrence. Previously normal children who have multiple febrile seizures do not appear to have an increased risk of developing epilepsy.

About 3 per cent of children with febrile seizure will go on to experience seizures without fever by 7 years of age. Seizures without fever are more likely to occur following febrile seizures when the following factors are present: a febrile seizure of more than 15 minutes' duration; more than one febrile seizure in a 24-hour period; a febrile seizure with a focal component; a febrile seizure occurring prior to 1 year of age; the presence of abnormal developmental or neurologic status prior to the first febrile seizure.

The use of phenobarbital, given at the outset of fever, is of no value in preventing a febrile seizure. About one-half of children who will develop seizures without fever following a febrile seizure will do so within a year's time of the first febrile convulsion.

During a febrile seizure, parents should be instructed to place the child on his side to avoid airway obstruction. Hard objects should not be placed in the mouth.

---

References: Wallace, S.J.: Br. Med. J., *1*:333, 1976. Ouellette, E.M.: Pediatr. Clin. North Am., *21*:467, 1974. Nelson, K.B., and Ellenberg, J.H.: N. Engl. J. Med., *295*:1029, 1976.

## CONVULSIONS THAT ARE NOT EPILEPSY

It is well known that convulsions in a child need not represent epilepsy. Breath-holding spells and febrile seizures are the alternatives most frequently thought of; however, there are many other causes of convulsions or convulsive-like behavior that may simulate epilepsy. Some of the conditions that should be considered are listed below.

### Hypoglycemia

Hypoglycemia is a more frequent cause of convulsions in newborns and small infants than in older children. The seizure often occurs in the early morning before the first feeding. Convulsions from hypoglycemia may be differentiated from epileptic seizures because they are preceded by weakness, pallor, and/or sweating.

### Lead Poisoning

This disorder may present with convulsion and is usually associated with increased intracranial pressure.

### Hypocalcemia

In the young infant, hypocalcemia may be brought on by excessive cow's milk feedings. In the older child, hypoparathyroidism should be suspected.

### Heart Disease

Fainting or convulsion may be precipitated by cerebral anoxia. Careful physical examination, blood pressure measurement, chest roentgenogram, and, if there is any question, electrocardiogram should be performed before making the diagnosis of epilspsy.

### Hypertensive Encephalopathy

Blood pressure measurement will rule this out. Acute glomerulonephritis is the most likely cause of severe blood pressure elevation in the young child, and urinalysis should be performed in the child who seizes.

### Vasomotor Syncope

Adolescent girls are the group most likely to faint. This usually occurs in situations of emotional stress.

12

### Orthostatic Hypotension

This is often encountered in the child who has been confined to bed for some time. Dehydration or certain drugs may also precipitate orthostatic changes.

### Hyperventilation

The child who becomes excited may complain of dizziness and tingling of the hands and feet. Fright and confusion may be evident. These symptoms may be reproduced when the child is asked to hyperventilate.

### Hysteria

Recognition of the hysterical seizure is usually not difficult, and accurate history should differentiate this kind of simulated convulsion from true epilepsy.

### Malingering

Children may mimic a seizure they have observed to obtain sympathy or attention. Again, careful history is important.

### Masturbation

Young children may become flushed, appear dazed, and perspire during masturbatory activity. Such children may be felt to be having psychomotor seizures. This activity may be differentiated from the true seizure by the history that the act is voluntary and the child resents being interrupted.

### Shivering on Urination

Some mothers notice a rapid tremorlike shivering while their babies are urinating. The characteristic tremorlike movements may be differentiated from convulsion by the experienced observer.

### Apneic Spells

Cyanosis and limpness may occur during periods of apnea in an infant and suggest seizure activity. It is particularly important to make the correct diagnosis, since treatment with anticonvulsive drugs may further inhibit respiration.

### Labyrinthitis

The child suffering from this disorder is typically a preschool child who is apparently well, except that periodically he cries out, clings to his mother, and sinks to the ground. Vomiting may occur, and if the child is old enough, he may complain of dizziness. The vertigo is brief and may recur at intervals for months or years. There is no effective treatment.

### Paroxysmal Torticollis in Infancy

This is probably the same as the syndrome of labyrinthitis except that the child is too young to complain intelligibly. The infant tilts the head to one side suddenly.

The attack may be heralded by sudden crying, pallor, and vomiting. The attacks last from 15 minutes to several days, and they cease after a few months or years. Caloric testing is abnormal.

### Paroxysmal Dystonia

This occurs in patients who are taking a phenothiazine drug and have an idiosyncratic reaction to it. The attack is accompanied by involuntary extension and twisting of the neck and shoulders and arms. They may be aborted to diphenhydramine (Benadryl) or caffeine, and the attacks cease on withdrawal of phenothiazine drugs.

### Sandifer's Syndrome

Young children with a hiatus hernia or achalasia may have such difficulty swallowing food that they assume bizarre postures. The clue to this diagnosis is that the "convulsions" always occur following meals.

### Inguinal Hernia

Children with inguinal hernia may suffer attacks of pallor and sweating and may vomit and feel faint during exercise. Careful physical examination should reveal this diagnosis.

### Pickwickian Syndrome

Hypoventilation resulting from severe obesity may result in hypercapnia and narcosis. This condition may be mistaken for petit mal attacks. The conditions may be differentiated easily, since hyperventilation exacerbates petit mal seizures and relieves the somnolence of the Pickwickian syndrome.

Reference: Snyder, C.H.: Clin. Pediatr., *11*:487, 1972.

# WHEN TO STOP THE ANTICONVULSANTS IN EPILEPSY

The management of childhood epilepsy is filled with uncertainty. Once a remission has been induced, how long should treatment be continued and when, if ever, should treatment be stopped?

There are no absolute answers, but here are some useful guidelines.

About 25 per cent of children will have a recurrence of seizures once medication is discontinued. About two-thirds of these recurrences will occur within one year of the termination of therapy.

In patients who had their first seizure prior to age 8 years, the chances of recurrence are reduced.

If seizures are controlled within 7 years and, most strikingly, if they are controlled within 2 years of the start of therapy, the likelihood of relapse is small once medication is reduced.

Children with grand mal, petit mal, and simple febrile seizures have the lowest relapse rate.

Absence of neurologic or psychologic defects indicates that relapse will be unlikely.

The EEG, the age of the patient, the sex of the patient, and the onset of puberty are not significant factors.

In conclusion, most children can be expected to do well after seizure medication is discontinued. Be hesitant to stop treatment, even with a four-year remission, if:

1. Seizures began after 9 years of age.
2. Seisures continued for more than six years before being controlled with therapy.
3. Seizures were of Jacksonian or multiple types.
4. The patient had psychologic or neurologic deficits and the seizures began after age 3 years.
5. The electroencephalogram was paroxysmal, severely abnormal, or unchanged over a four-year period of observation.

---

Reference: Holowach, J., Thurston, D.L., and O'Leary, J.: N. Engl. J. Med., *286*:169, 1972.

## THE BULGING FONTANEL

A bulging fontanel in an infant is generally regarded as a sign of serious CNS disease, such as:

| | |
|---|---|
| Meningitis | Subdural hematoma |
| Encephalitis | Lead poisoning |
| Hydrocephalus | Sinus thrombosis |
| Cerebral hemorrhage | Tumor |
| Intracranial abscess | |

The history, however, may suggest a benign cause. A congenital subgaleal cyst over the anterior fontanel may simulate a bulging fontanel. *Benign intracranial hypertension*, a syndrome of increased intracranial pressure, normal ventricular system and CSF composition, and absence of focal neurologic signs can also produce a bulging fontanel.

The causes of benign intracranial hypertension in infancy:

Impaired CSF absorption

Obstructed inferior vena cava secondary to intrathoracic mass or obstructive lung disease

Obstruction of sagittal sinus secondary to skull fracture or other cause

Endocrine/Metabolic

Galactosemia
Addison's disease
Hypophosphatasia
Hypoparathyroidism
Hypothyroidism

Drugs

Hypervitaminosis A
Tetracyclines
Nalidixic acid

Infections

Roseola infantum
Guillain-Barré syndrome

Nutritional

Hypovitaminosis A
Rapid brain growth following starvation

Miscellaneous

Polycythemia vera
Heart disease
Allergic diseases
Anemia (severe)
Wiskott-Aldrich syndrome

References: Hagberg, B., and Silinpää, M.: Acta Paediatr. Scand., 59:328–339, 1970. Barnett, H.L.: Pediatrics. New York, Appleton-Century-Crofts, 1972.

# COMPLICATIONS OF VENTRICULOPERITONEAL SHUNTS

The ventriculoperitoneal shunt has become a popular operation for the diversion of cerebrospinal fluid in patients with hydrocephalus. In many centers it has replaced the ventriculojugular and ventriculoatrial shunt as the procedure of choice. The V-A and V-J shunts were associated with many complications. These complications included septicemia, endocarditis, thromboembolism, superior vena caval obstruction, damage to the tricuspid valve, glomerulonephritis, and a revision rate of close to 40 per cent.

It is now appreciated that the ventriculoperitoneal shunts are also associated with a variety of complications. Approximately 25 per cent of patients demonstrate some complications as a result of the placement of a chronically draining catheter in the peritoneum. These complications are distinctly different from those observed with the V-A and V-J shunts. The physician caring for a child with a V-P shunt should constantly be alerted to these potential problems. The complications include the following:

> Inguinal hernias (75 per cent bilateral)
> Hydroceles
> Perforation of colon
> Perforation of bladder
> Cerebrospinal fluid cyst
> Peritonitis
> Ascites
> Abdominal distention
> Intra-abdominal catheter disconnection
> Catheter knotting
> Intestinal obstruction due to volvulus around the
> catheter

Reference: Grosfeld, J.L., Cooney, D.R., Smith, J., et al.: Pediatrics, *54*:791, 1974.

## ACUTE HEMATOMA—EPIDURAL OR SUBDURAL

Following head injury, an alteration in the state of consciousness always raises the concern of intracranial bleeding. Once bleeding is suspected, a judgment must be made as to whether it is a result of an epidural or subdural bleed. There are no clinical features that are in themselves diagnostic. There are characteristics that tend to occur with greater frequency with bleeding in one location as opposed to the other. The table below provides a guideline to these characteristics.

| FEATURE | EPIDURAL HEMATOMA | SUBDURAL HEMATOMA |
|---|---|---|
| Frequency | Unusual in infants and children | More common in infants and children |
| Skull fracture | In 40–75% of cases | In less than 25% of cases |
| Bleeding | Arterial and venous, usually unilateral | Venous more common, usually bilateral |
| Retinal hemorrhages | Uncommon | Very common |
| Change in consciousness | Unconsciousness following injury; lucid interval followed by neurologic deterioration | Continuous unconsciousness from time of injury |
| Mortality | In 25% | In less than 25% of cases |
| Morbidity in survivors | Low | High |

# CEREBROVASCULAR DISORDERS IN CHILDHOOD

Cerebrovascular disorders are a relatively infrequent problem in children, but they are identified as the cause of death in 17 per cent of pediatric autopsies. Characteristics of the various disorders are delineated in the following table.

| | DURAL SINUS AND CEREBRAL VENOUS THROMBOSIS | ARTERIAL THROMBOSIS | CEREBRAL EMBOLISM | INTRACRANIAL HEMORRHAGE (PRIMARY INTRACEREBRAL AND SUBARACHNOID) |
|---|---|---|---|---|
| Onset | Usually less sudden and clear-cut than in arterial occlusive disease. Usually unrelated to activity. | Sudden, but prodromal episodes may occur. Unrelated to activity. | Sudden onset; no prodrome. Unrelated to activity. | Sudden onset; severe headache, vomiting, loss of consciousness. Related to activity. |
| Underlying conditions | Pyogenic infections of leptomeninges and cranial structures (ear, face, sinuses). Marasmic states and severe dehydration. Congenital heart disease. Blood dyscrasias (sickle cell diseases, polycythemia, thrombotic thrombocytopenia). Lead and other toxic encephalopathies. Trauma. Metastatic tumor. Sturge-Weber disease. | "Idiopathic" (hemiplegia in infancy). Cyanotic congenital heart disease. Inflammatory disease of arteries: "collagen" diseases, granulomatous (Takayasu's), acute infections, syphilis. Trauma or extrinsic compression. Dissecting aneurysm. Arteriosclerosis (progeria). Thrombotic phenomenon: homocystinuria. | Atrial fibrillation and other "arrhythmias": congenital heart disease (R→L shunt), rheumatic heart disease. Acute or subacute bacterial endocarditis. Air: complications of heart, neck, or chest surgery. Fat: complications of fractures of bone, heart surgery. Septic: pneumonia or lung abscess (especially in congenital heart disease). Newborn: infarcted necrotic placental tissue. Tumor. Coronary. | Trauma: birth (intraventricular), subdural hemorrhage, epidural hemorrhage, cavernous sinus fistula. Vascular malformations: arteriovenous, angiomas, aneurysms. Hemorrhagic disorders (leukemia, aplastic anemia, hemophilia, sickle cell anemia, thrombocytopenia/ anaphylactoid purpura, liver disease, vitamin deficiencies [K, C, B₁], anticonvulsants). Hypertensive encephalopathy (renal disease, pheochromocytoma). Toxic or infectious encephalopathy. Intracranial tumors. |
| Neurologic findings | Altered state of consciousness. Increased intracranial pressure. Focal neurologic deficits (leg, arm). Seizures, focal and generalized. | Seizures, frequently focal. Focal neurologic deficits. Behavioral and intellectual changes. Rapid improvement at times. | Transient loss of consciousness common. Seizures, often focal. Focal neurologic deficits (sometimes multiple). Rapid improvement at times. | Consciousness commonly lost; may be regained quickly. Marked meningeal signs (not seen in neonate). Focal neurologic deficits. Seizures, generalized and focal. |

12

| | DURAL SINUS AND CEREBRAL VENOUS THROMBOSIS | ARTERIAL THROMBOSIS | CEREBRAL EMBOLISM | INTRACRANIAL HEMORRHAGE (PRIMARY INTRACEREBRAL AND SUBARACHNOID) |
|---|---|---|---|---|
| Special clinical clues | Lateral dural sinus: mastoiditis. Superior sagittal sinus: caput medusae. Cavernous sinus: homolateral exophthalmos, periorbital edema, palsies of cranial nerves III, IV, VI, and V. | Inflammatory disease: multifocal involvement common. Takayasu's: pulseless upper limbs. Moyamoya syndrome (progressive alternating hemiplegia with basal arterial stenosis and diencephalic telangiectasia). Somatic constitution (progeria, arachnodactyly). Signs of trauma. | Emboli to other organs (spleen, kidneys, lungs). Air embolism: transient blindness. Fat embolism: respiratory distress, bloodtinged sputum in postoperative period, fat droplets in urine, retinal vessels. | Trauma (hemorrhage, subhyaloid hemorrhages, bruises, fractures on x-ray films). Malformations: bruit, heart failure, hydrocephalus, cutaneous stigmas. Previous seizures/neurologic deficit. Coarctation/polycystic kidney. Hemorrhagic diathesis: skin, joints, gastrointestinal tract, newborn. Hypertensive encephalopathy: blood pressure elevated, uremia. |
| Skull films | Signs of increased intracranial pressure within days or a few weeks, depending on age. Sinus involvement or lytic lesion. | Early: usually normal. Later: hypertrophy of skull on atrophic side of brain. Tumor. Dysplasia. Foreign body. | Normal. | Skull fractures. Characteristic calcifications. Signs of increased intracranial pressure/hydrocephalus. Deep groove in inner table from enlarged vein. |
| CSF | Findings vary with primary process. Protein often elevated. Sometimes bloody. If PMNs are present, suspect infection. | Early: usually normal Later: slight monocytic pleocytosis and protein elevation. | Usually normal. Some pleocytosis and protein elevation in bacterial endocarditis. | Bloody CSF all tubes, xanthochromic supernatant. Protein elevated. Sugar may be decreased. Fluid may be clear if hemorrhage is intracerebral only. |
| Neuroradiologic findings | Angiogram on venous phase or sinogram may show obstruction site. Sinogram may be dangerous. | Angiography early may show occlusion or narrowing. (later studies usually negative.) | Angiography usually normal, since emboli commonly lodge in small peripheral vessels. | Angiography usually able to identify subdural and epidural hematoma, site and type of malformation, intracerebral tumor, clot. |

Other studies — Echoencephalography may show midline shift. EEG may show diffuse or focal slowing. Brain scan may show increased uptake. The EMI scan may show the area of infarction. None of these studies is sufficiently specific to obviate the need for other diagnostic — especially angiographic — studies.

Reference: Nelhaus, G.: *In* Kempe, C.H., Silver, H.K., and O'Brien, D. (Eds.): Current Pediatric Diagnosis and Treatment. Los Altos, California, Lange Medical Publications, 1976, p. 550.

*"If I were to choose among all gifts and qualities that which, on the whole, makes life pleasantest, I should select the love of children. No circumstance can render this world wholly a solitude to one who has this possession."*

T. W. Higginson

**12**

# SKULL FILM? SKULL FRACTURE?

It is an unusual day for a pediatrician when he or she is not asked to evaluate an infant or child following head trauma. The knee-jerk response in these situations, all too frequently, is to request x-ray films of the skull. Stop and think, "Does the presence of a skull fracture in a child with a head injury indicate an increased likelihood of an intracranial complication?"

There is an abundance of facts available to answer this question. In a study involving 4465 consecutive head injuries at the Hospital for Sick Children in Toronto, the following was found:

1. 26.6 per cent of the children had skull fractures.
2. The incidence of fracture with head trauma did not vary significantly with age, but 75 per cent of all patients seen were over 2 years of age.
3. A linear fracture occurred in 73 per cent of patients with fracture; a depressed skull fracture occurred in 27 per cent.
4. The parietal bone was involved in 50 per cent of all fractures.
5. In 70 per cent of all patients with a fracture, there was external evidence of trauma. The fracture was present on the same side as the external trauma in 84 per cent of instances, and on the contralateral side in 16 per cent.
6. Cerebrospinal fluid otorrhea was observed in only 22 of 4465 children. In only one patient could a fracture of the petrous bone be demonstrated by routine films.
7. Profuse bleeding from the middle ear was observed in 241 of these 4465 patients, but in only 20 patients could a petrous fracture be demonstrated with conventional skull films.
8. Subdural hematomas occurred in 5 per cent of all children with head trauma. Only 15 per cent of these patients with subdurals had a skull fracture. The overall incidence of subdurals in children without skull fractures was 6 per cent; the incidence in children with skull fractures was 3 per cent.
9. Subdural hematomas were most common in infants 0 to 6 months of age. In this group, 28 per cent of the head injuries had associated subdural hematomas; only 7 per cent of *this group* with subdurals had skull fractures.
10. Bilateral subdural hematomas were observed in 143 children, but only 6 of these patients had bilateral fractures.
11. Extradural hematomas occurred in 1 per cent of the group. They were just as frequent in the nonfracture group as in the fracture group. Extradural hematomas occurred more frequently in children over 5 years of age.
12. Severe brain damage was observed in 3 per cent of the entire group of patients with head trauma. In this group, 65 per cent had a fracture. Of those with a fracture, approximately 80 per cent were depressed fractures.
13. In children with the most severe brain injuries and serious intracranial sequelae, fractures were frequently noted only at operation or at autopsy because clinical condition did not permit time for radiographic studies.

## Conclusions

Presence of skull fracture alone is of little prognostic significance. Presence of skull fracture does not alter management except in patients with a depressed skull fracture. Virtually all depressed skull fractures are associated with a history of injury produced by local trauma by an object and can be anticipated by the findings on physical examination.

Skull films are not an emergency procedure when skull fracture is considered as a diagnostic possibility; in fact, they are rarely necessary at all. The management of an infant or child with a head injury depends on a careful assessment of the patient's neurologic status and requires periodic reevaluation.

The skull roentgenogram is a crutch that does not help you to walk.

Reference: Harwood-Nash, D.C., Hendrick, E.B., and Hudson, A.R.: Radiology, *101*:151, 1971.

## THE BASAL SKULL FRACTURE

These fractures may be hard to diagnose by x-ray examination. When should you suspect them clinically? The clues include:

1. Bleeding from nose, eyes, or ears or discoloration in the mastoid area ("Battle's sign").
2. Blood behind the eardrum.
3. Cerebrospinal rhinorrhea (see below).
4. Cranial nerve palsies. These involve cranial nerves I, III, and VIII.
5. Appearance of "sinusitis."
6. Presence of pneumocephaly.

## CEREBROSPINAL FLUID RHINORRHEA AND GLUCOSE TESTING

It is commonly taught that testing a nasal discharge for the presence of glucose can help to detect the presence of cerebrospinal fluid leak in the patient with head trauma. Unfortunately, this just is not true. Employing a glucose oxidase test strip, approximately 75 to 90 per cent of normal children will give a positive test in their nasal secretions.

Reference: Hull, H.F., and Morrow, G., III: J.A.M.A., *234*:1052, 1975.

## THE POSTCONCUSSION SYNDROME IN CHILDREN

Adults who sustain head injuries typically experience a post-concussion syndrome consisting of headaches, dizziness, and irritability. Children who experience loss of consciousness following head trauma frequently exhibit a very different kind of postconcussion syndrome. The symptoms and behavioral changes noted in 50 children following concussion are noted below in order of decreasing frequency.

12

1. Psychologic changes
   Anxiety
   Withdrawal
   Aggressiveness
   Disobedience
   Sluggishness
   Antisocial behavior
   Temper tantrums
   Other bizarre behavior, such as talking to themselves and wandering around at night
2. Sleep disturbances
3. Headaches
4. Neurologic abnormalities
   Change in deep tendon reflexes
   Central facial palsies
   Strabismus
   Positive plantar responses
   Ataxia
   Decreased hearing
   Intellectual deterioration
   Optic atrophy
   Decreased visual acuity
   Papillary inequality
   Muscular atrophy
5. Ocular symptoms
   Diplopia
   Burning, pain
   Blurring of vision
   Extraorbital puffiness
6. Enuresis (secondary)
7. Signs of regressive behavior
8. Hyperkinesis
9. Dizziness
10. Seizures

Sedation or anticonvulsive medication may be indicated in treatment of a child exhibiting this syndrome, but parents should be reassured that the symptoms are transitory. Following concussions or illness associated with encephalitis, problems with school work, of a temporary nature, may be expected. Both parents and teachers should refrain from being overly critical during this period, or psychologic problems may result that are caused by bad management rather than as a consequence of the injury or illness.

---

Reference: Dillon, H., and Leopold, R.L.: J.A.M.A., *175*:86, 1961.

## BRAIN ABSCESS IN INFANTS AND CHILDREN

A brain abscess is frequently forgotten in the differential diagnosis of infants and children with evidence of neurologic disease. It may often be confused with encephalitis, meningitis, intracerebral tumor, or hematoma.

Middle ear infections are the most commonly found predisposing cause. They also occur with increased frequency in patients with cyanotic heart disease, with chronic lung disease, and following trauma or sepsis, especially pulmonary sepsis.

The abscess is located in the cerebrum about three times more frequently than in the cerebellum.

The significant diagnostic features can be broadly grouped into four large categories:

### 1. Raised Intracranial Pressure

This is manifested by headaches, vomiting, papilledema, and bradycardia. Headache is generally present in every child over 1 year of age. It is most frequent in the early morning or late evening. Careful measurement of head circumference may reveal an enlarging cranium, and skull roentgenograms should be taken to check for splitting of sutures.

### 2. Intracranial Suppuration

Irritability, drowsiness, stupor, weight loss, and signs of meningeal irritation reflect this process. Some degree of mental disturbance is always present.

### 3. General Signs of Infection

Fever, chills, and leukocytosis. The white cell count is elevated in approximately two-thirds of patients.

### 4. Focal Neurologic Signs

Focal or generalized convulsions, cranial nerve palsies, visual field defects, aphasia, ataxia, or paralysis are most common. Convulsions may be observed in 25 to 80 per cent of patients. They are more common in infants.

**Lumbar puncture.** This should not be undertaken lightly in patients with suspected brain abscess if the optic discs are not clearly normal. Brain herniation has been associated with lumbar puncture in patients with brain abscess. Equivalent or superior diagnostic information may be obtained from brain scan, computerized tomographic scan, arteriography, or other procedures suggested by neurosurgical consultation.

Consider brain abscess in:

1. A child with fever, leukocytosis, and bradycardia.
2. A septic infant who has a focal or generalized seizure.
3. A child with recurrent headaches and change in mental status.
4. A child with suspected meningitis who develops signs of herniation after lumbar puncture.

References: Nestadt, A., Lowry, R.B., and Turner, E.: Lancet, *1*:449, 1960. Brewer, N.S., MacCarty, C.S., and Wellman, W.E.: Ann. Intern. Med., *82*:571, 1975.

# BRAIN TUMORS IN CHILDREN

We frequently forget that malignancies within the central nervous system are second only to leukemia as a cause of death from cancer among children. About 31 per cent of all malignancies in children under 15 years of age are due to leukemia, while 18 per cent are central nervous system tumors.

Approximately two-thirds of the intracranial tumors of childhood are beneath the tentorium, in contrast to an incidence of only 10 per cent among adults.

The distribution of intracranial tumors in children is as follows:

| INFRATENTORIAL | PER CENT OF ALL TUMORS |
|---|---|
| Cerebellar astrocytoma | 20 |
| Medulloblastoma | 18 |
| Brain stem glioma | 10 |
| Ependymoma | 8 |
| Other | 10 |
| **SUPRATENTORIAL** | |
| Astrocytoma | 8 |
| Ependymoma | 6 |
| Malignant glioma | 6 |
| Craniopharyngioma | 5 |
| Other | 9 |

## Major Symptoms

**Headache.** Insidious onset, intermittent, most pronounced upon arising.

**Vomiting.** Often occurs after head has been in dependent position, i.e., after sleeping. Not usually associated with nausea.

**Easy Fatigability.** Require long naps. Decrease in normal activity.

**Personality Change.** Irritability. Decline in intellectual function.

**Seizures.** Rare in infratentorial tumors. Occur in about one-third of patients with supratentorial tumors.

## Characteristics of Individual Tumors

### INFRATENTORIAL

| | |
|---|---|
| Cerebellar astrocytoma | Longer duration of symptoms. Ipsilateral incoordination, ataxia with tendency to drift to the side of the lesion, nystagmus with slow component on ipsilateral gaze, and hyporeflexia on side of lesion. |

| Medulloblastoma | More common in infants. Gait disturbances and truncal ataxia. Signs of increased intracranial pressure frequent. |
| --- | --- |
| Brain stem glioma | Insidious onset of cranial nerve dysfunction, long tract involvement, ataxia, gait disturbance. (Seventh nerve, sixth, ninth, tenth, and facial branch of fifth.) |
| Ependymoma | Signs of increased intracranial pressure. |

SUPRATENTORIAL

| Astrocytoma | Signs of increased intracranial pressure, focal seizures, and focal neurologic findings dependent on location. |
| --- | --- |
| Ependymoma | Same as astrocytoma. |
| Craniopharyngioma | Increased intracranial pressure and visual disturbances most common finding. Diabetes insipidus is rare. |

Reference: Walker, M.D.: Pediatr. Clin. North Am., *23*: 131, 1976.

# THE CARDINAL PRESENTING SIGNS OF RETINOBLASTOMA

**12**

A careful examination of the eyes of a struggling and uncooperative infant is often a difficult and frustrating experience. It is quite easy, however, to check the light reflex of the eyes without bothering the infant. This should be a part of every routine physical examination. The absence of the normal red reflex and the presence of a white reflex should be a danger sign that your patient may have a retinoblastoma. More often than not, this sign is first detected by the mother rather than the physician. Retinoblastoma may first present in a variety of ways, but the detection of the white reflex is the most common initial manifestation.

Listed below is a representative example of the presenting signs of retinoblastoma.

| SIGN | PER CENT OF PATIENTS |
| --- | --- |
| White pupillary reflex | 61 |
| Strabismus | 22 |
| Incidental finding during routine examination | 6 |
| Decreased vision | 5 |
| Orbital inflammation and proptosis | 2 |
| Red, painful eye due to secondary glaucoma | 2 |

| SIGN | PER CENT OF PATIENTS |
|------|:---:|
| Unilateral dilated pupil | 1 |
| Spontaneous hyphema | 0.5 |
| Heterochromia iridis | 0.5 |

Reference: Howard, G.M., and Ellsworth, R.M.: Am. J. Ophthalmol., *60*:618, 1965.

## THE FLOPPY INFANT

An infant is considered "floppy" when there is decreased muscular tone. The muscular tone of infants may be assessed in the following manner:

1. Note the head and leg position in prone horizontal suspension.
2. When the infant is lying supine, pull him by the hands to a sitting position, noting resistance of arms, grasping with fingers, and the relationship of the head to the trunk.
3. With the infant supine, pick up each extremity individually, feel the resistance, and note how it falls to the mattress when released.
4. Note resistance to movement of individual joints, paying attention to resistance to rapid abduction of the flexed thighs, a common site for the first evidence of developing spasticity.

Hypotonia in the newborn commonly results from diffuse cerebral dysfunction. Asphyxia, craniocerebral hemorrhage, and congenital abnormalities of the brain are often the cause. Infants destined to develop spastic or athetoid cerebral palsy are often hypotonic during the first six months of life. The generalized conditions listed below may also make themselves manifest by hypotonia.

Chromosomal disorders, especially trisomy 21

Hypothyroidism

Inborn errors of metabolism

Generalized mental retardation syndromes, e.g., Prader-Willi syndrome and Laurence-Moon-Biedl syndrome

Ehlers-Danlos syndrome

The hypotonic infant who has cerebral abnormality or dysfunction typically demonstrates other abnormalities on physical examination, such as microcephaly, macrocephaly, or abnormal level of consciousness. There will often be a history of seizures.

*It is important to remember that hypotonia in the newborn may be the result of excess depressant medication given to the mother.*

In addition to the cerebral lesions mentioned above, hypotonia may result from lesions at any level in the neuromuscular system:

Cerebellum and brain stem

Spinal cord – transecting lesions

Spinal cord – diffuse lesions

Peripheral nerves

Motor end-plate region

Muscle

The table beginning on page 354 lists neuromuscular abnormalities that are characterized by hypotonia according to the site of the basic pathologic change.

Laboratory studies that will aid in making the diagnosis are listed below along with the results to be expected, depending upon the site of the lesion.

*Useful Laboratory Studies in Infantile Hypotonia*

| | BRAIN | SPINAL CORD DIFFUSE (ANTERIOR HORN CELL) | PERIPHERAL NERVE | MUSCLE |
|---|---|---|---|---|
| EEG | Abnormal | Normal | Normal | Normal |
| CSF protein | May be increased | Usually normal | Usually increased | Normal |
| EMG | Normal | Abnormal | Abnormal | Usually Normal |
| Nerve conduction velocity | Normal | Normal or slow | Slow | Normal |
| Muscle biopsy | Normal | Abnormal | Abnormal | Abnormal, frequently diagnostic |

References: Rabe, E.F.: J. Pediatr., *64*:422, 1964. Peterson, H. de C.: Pediatr. Ann., May 1976, p. 300.

12°

| CLINICAL SYNDROME | SITE OF PATHOLOGIC CHANGE | ASSOCIATED MENTAL RETARDATION | HEREDITARY OR FAMILIAL | DIAGNOSTIC AIDS | THERAPY AFFECTING MUSCLE FUNCTION |
|---|---|---|---|---|---|
| Congenital atonic diplegia | Brain | Yes | No | Estimation of developmental level motor and mental, repeatedly | None |
| Congenital cerebellar ataxia | Cerebellum: and occasionally medulla, pons, and cerebrum | Often normal | No | Estimation of developmental level motor and mental, repeatedly | None |
| Congenital chorea | Brain | Yes | No | Estimation of developmental level motor and mental, repeatedly | None |
| Kernicterus | Multiple areas of basal ganglia, pons, medulla, hippocampus | Yes | No | Estimation of developmental level motor and mental, repeatedly | None |
| Tay-Sachs disease | Central nervous system | Yes | Yes | Funduscopic examination | None |
| Infantile spinal muscular atrophy (Werdnig-Hoffmann disease) | Anterior gray horns of spinal cord | No | No | Muscle biopsy | None |
| Myelopathic arthrogryposis multiplex congenita | Anterior gray horns of spinal cord | No | No | Muscle biopsy | Physiotherapy |
| Poliomyelitis | Anterior gray horns of spinal cord | No | No | CSF examination Isolation of agent from stool | Physiotherapy |
| Acute infective polyneuritis (Guillain-Barré disease) | Spinal roots and peripheral nerves | No | No | Nerve conduction time CSF examination | Steroids (?) Physiotherapy |

| Disease | Site | | | Diagnostic tests | Treatment |
|---|---|---|---|---|---|
| Chronic idiopathic polyneuropathy | Peripheral nerve | No | No | Nerve conduction time; EMG; Muscle biopsy | Steroids (?); Physiotherapy |
| Myasthenia gravis — neonatal, transient | Myoneural junction | No | No | Response to neostigmine or edrophonium chloride | Neostigmine |
| Myasthenia gravis — congenital | Myoneural junction | No | No | Response to neostigmine or edrophonium chloride | Pyridostigmine bromide |
| Benign congenital hypotonia | Muscle (?) | No | No | Muscle biopsy; EMG | None |
| Universal hypoplasia of muscle | Muscle (?) | No | Yes | Muscle biopsy | None |
| Infantile congenital myopathy (muscular dystrophy of infancy) | Muscle | No | Yes | Muscle biopsy; Serum enzyme concentrations; Creatine and creatinine coefficients; EMG | Not proved |
| Central core disease | Muscle | No | Yes | Muscle biopsy | None |
| Rod body myopathy | Muscle | No | ? | Muscle biopsy | None |
| Dystrophia myotonica | Muscle, gonads | Yes | Yes | Muscle biopsy; EMG | None |
| Polymyositis | Muscle | No | No | Muscle biopsy | Steroids (?) |
| Glycogen storage disease | Muscle and central nervous system | ? | Probably | Muscle biopsy | None |

12

## ACUTE WERDNIG-HOFFMANN DISEASE (ACUTE INFANTILE SPINAL MUSCULAR ATROPHY)

The mother complains that her infant seems weak and has trouble eating. She also recalls that her infant moved very little in utero. This mother may be describing the symptoms of acute infantile spinal muscular atrophy. It is a familial disease inherited in an autosomal recessive fashion. Approximately one-third of affected infants demonstrate prenatal onset of disease by reduced fetal movements or congenital abnormalities that result from synergist-antagonist imbalance.

Although there are more chronic forms of the disease, 95 per cent of infants with the acute form exhibit symptoms by 4 months of age and are dead by 18 months. The diagnosis is most often suggested by the following presentations:

Weak movements, floppiness

Weak, poor, or prolonged feeding

Failure to progress to specific motor milestones

Combination of orthopedic deformity and weakness

Unusual breathing; usually rapid and diaphragmatic, or periodic apnea

Fasciculation of the tongue and limb muscles

Congenital abnormalities include wrist deformities, orthopedic abnormalities of the hands and feet, chest asymmetry, and discoloration of the radial heads. Birth trauma, especially dislocations or brachial plexus injury, following uncomplicated delivery may suggest the diagnosis in 5 per cent of affected infants.

Appropriate physical and historical findings combined with a normal cerebrospinal fluid examination and electromyography testing may make the diagnosis possible without the need for muscle biopsy. The disease progresses rapidly, and death usually results from repeated aspiration due to bulbar involvement.

Despite delayed or regressive motor development, these infants are mentally normal, and the physician can play an important role in helping parents to cope with their child's need for extra stimulation and affection. Genetic counseling is also the responsibility of the physician. Carrier detection is not possible at this time.

---

Reference: Pearn, J.H., and Wilson, J.: Arch. Dis. Child., *48*:425, 1973.

# ATAXIA, MUSCLE WEAKNESS, EXTRAPYRAMIDAL DISORDERS

The child who presents with ataxia or muscle weakness or extrapyramidal manifestations of disease may pose a difficult diagnostic problem for the pediatrician. The following tables should guide you in the right direction.

*Differential Diagnosis of Chronic Progressive Ataxia*

| CLINICAL DISORDER | PRECEDING HISTORY | USUAL YEAR OF ONSET IN CHILDREN | EXAMINATION | USUAL LABORATORY EXAMINATION | USUAL PROGNOSIS |
|---|---|---|---|---|---|
| Arnold-Chiari malformation | Headache, dysphagia | | Palatal and tongue weakness, pyramidal signs, ataxia | May have hydrocephalus, spina bifida | Slowly progressive; stationary after surgery |
| Hereditary spinocerebellar ataxia | Stumbling, dizziness, familial incidence | 7–10 | Ataxia, loss of position sense, extensor plantar responses, kyphoscoliosis, pes cavus | Frequent associated ECG changes | Progressive, with death usually by 30 years of age |
| Abetalipo-proteinemia | Fatty diarrhea at 6 weeks to 2 years of age | 2–17 | Cerebellar ataxia, posterior column signs, retinitis pigmentosa, scoliosis, pes cavus | Acanthocytosis, lack of β-lipoprotein in serum | Slowly progressive |
| Dentate cerebellar ataxia | Myoclonus, convulsions | 7–17 | Ataxia with severe intention tremor | | Slowly progressive |
| Hereditary cerebellar ataxia | Familial incidence | 3–17 | Ataxia, optic atrophy, occasionally associated posterior column and pyramidal tract signs | Pneumoencephalogram: small cerebellar folia | Slowly progressive |

12

| CLINICAL DISORDER | PRECEDING HISTORY | USUAL YEAR OF ONSET IN CHILDREN | EXAMINATION | USUAL LABORATORY EXAMINATION | USUAL PROGNOSIS |
|---|---|---|---|---|---|
| Ataxia telangiectasia | Recurrent sinopulmonary infections in two-thirds of cases; familial incidence | 1–3 | Oculocutaneous telangiectasia at 4 to 6 years; ataxia, choreoathetosis, dysarthria | Chest roentgenogram: bronchiectasis; absence of IgA in serum | Death before 25 years of age |
| Cerebellar tumors | Headache, vomiting | | Papilledema, ataxia, nystagmus | Skull roentgenogram: separation of sutures | Progressive until operated |
| Heredopathia atactica polyneuritiformis | Anorexia, failing vision, unsteady, familial incidence | 4–7 | Retinitis pigmentosa, ataxia, deafness, polyneuropathy, ichthyosis | Elevated phytanic acid in blood, increased spinal fluid protein | Slowly progressive with death |
| Multiple sclerosis | Preceding neurologic symptoms | 14–17 | Optic neuritis; brain stem, cerebellar, pyramidal, or sensory signs | Spinal fluid may reveal increased cells, protein, or γ-globin | Exacerbations and remissions |
| Spinal cord tumor | May have numbness or bladder disorder | | Ataxia with weakness or sensory loss | Defect on myelography | Progressive until operated |

*Differential Diagnosis of Acute Ataxia*

| DISORDER | PRECEDING HISTORY | EXAMINATION | LABORATORY EXAMINATION | USUAL PROGNOSIS |
|---|---|---|---|---|
| Acute cerebellar ataxia | Half have had a prodromal systemic illness, occasionally exanthems | Cerebellar ataxia | Spinal fluid usually normal | Recovery |
| Dilantin intoxication | Convulsions treated with phenytoin | Cerebellar ataxia, nystagmus | High serum phenytoin level | Recovery |
| Cerebellar tumor or abscess | Headache, vomiting | Papilledema, ataxia, nystagmus | Separation of cranial sutures | Progressive until operated |
| Hartnup syndrome | Skin eruptions on exposure to sun; familial incidence | Skin lesions, ataxia, nystagmus, mental disturbances | Aminoaciduria, increased indole in urine | Recurrent ataxia |
| Multiple sclerosis | Preceding neurologic symptoms | Optic neuritis; brain stem, cerebellar, pyramidal, or sensory signs | Spinal fluid may reveal increased cells, protein, or γ-globulin | Exacerbations and remissions |
| Encephalitides | Headache, stiff neck, fever | Cerebral and brain stem signs; also may have ataxia | Spinal fluid: lymphocytosis; possible virus isolation or rise in antibody titer | May be fatal, or slow recovery with or without residual |
| Spinal cord tumor | May have numbness or bladder disorder | Ataxia with weakness or sensory loss | Defect on myelography | Progressive until operated |
| Infectious polyneuropathy | Half have a prodromal systemic illness | Ataxia with motor and sensory loss | Spinal fluid: normal cells, increased protein | May be fatal, but recovery usually complete |

12

## Differential Diagnosis of Disorders of Muscle, Anterior Horn Cell, and Peripheral Nerves

| CLINICAL AND LABORATORY FEATURES | MUSCLE | ANTERIOR HORN CELL | PERIPHERAL NERVES |
|---|---|---|---|
| Site of predisposition | Usually proximal and axial musculature | Proximal and/or distal extremity musculature | Usually distal extremity musculature |
| Deep tendon reflexes | Preserved until late in course | Reduced to absent early in course | Reduced to absent early in course |
| Sensation deficit | Rarely observed | Not observed | Usually present |
| Fasciculations | Usually absent | Frequently present | Occasionally present |
| CSF protein | Normal | Normal or elevated | Elevated or normal |
| Electromyography Interference pattern | Normal until late in disease | Reduced | Reduced |
| Fibrillation potentials | Not usually present | Usually present | Present |
| Action potentials | Short duration | Prolonged with occasional giant potentials | Prolonged with normal or poly-phasic potentials |
| Evoked sensory and mixed nerve potentials | Normal | Normal | Absent, diminished amplitude, or prolonged con-duction time |

## Differential Diagnosis of Extrapyramidal Disorders

| DISORDER | FAMILIAL | SIGNS | ASSOCIATED FINDINGS |
|---|---|---|---|
| Hepatolenticular degeneration | Autosomal recessive | Rigidity, tremor, dystonia, dementia, corneal ring, jaundice | Increased urinary and hepatic copper, low serum ceruloplasmin |
| Juvenile parkinsonism | Rarely | Resting tremor, rigidity, bradykinesia | Decreased dopamine level in substantia nigra |
| Kernicterus | No | Athetosis, deafness, occasional intellectual impairment | Neonatal hyperbili-rubinemia |
| Huntington's disease | Autosomal dominant | Rigidity, chorea, convulsions, dementia | |
| Torsion dystonia | Autosomal dominant or recessive | Dystonia, involuntary movements, normal intellect | |
| Chorea minor (Sydenham's) | No | Involuntary choreic movements, possibly carditis | Group A streptococcal infections |
| Absence of hypoxanthine-guanine phosphoribosyl transferase (Lesch-Nyhan syndrome) | X-linked recessive | Choreoathetosis, mental retardation, self-mutilation | Increased urinary and blood uric acid |

Reference: Farmer, T.W. (Ed.): Pediatric Neurology. New York, Harper & Row, 1975, pp. 400, 403, 411, and 466.

# OCCULT SPINAL DYSRAPHISM

Spinal dysraphism may quickly enter into the differential diagnosis of the child with awkwardness of the legs and feet who has a tuft of hair in the mid lower back. Occult spinal dysraphism may be associated with a variety of other symptoms and signs, which include the following (in order of frequency):

Back lesion (hair, pigmented macula, etc.)

Incontinence (urinary or fecal)

Foot deformities

Weakness or awkwardness of feet and legs

Diminished reflexes

Numbness of legs

Back stiffness

Pain in the back or leg.

In approximately one-third of patients there is no evidence of the lesion on the skin.

The congenital lesions of occult dysraphism include (1) congenital dermal sinus (Fig. 12–1A), which may convey infection intraspinally; (2) lipomyelomeningocele (Fig. 12–1B), in which the caudal end of the spinal cord is held by fusion to a fibrofatty mass that proceeds through a spinal defect and blends with the skin; (3) aberrant nerve roots or fibrous traction bands (Fig. 12–1C), which adhere to the dura mater or spinal cord and attach to muscle and bone; and (4) abnormal filum terminale caused by improper involution of the distalmost neural tube (Fig. 12–1C).

**12**

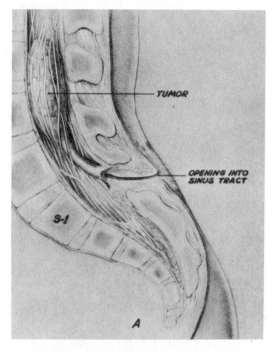

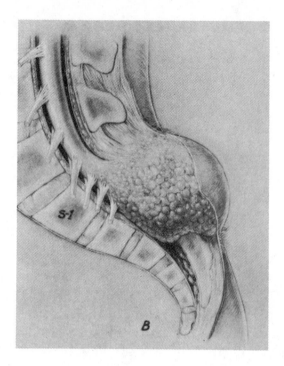

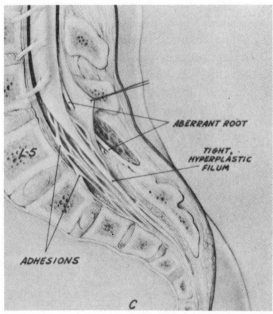

FIG. 12-1

*A*, Congenital dermal sinus. Tract proceeds upward and in this example fuses with epidermal inclusion cyst ("epidermoid," "dermoid"). *B*, Lipoma or lipomyelomeningocele. Low-lying spinal cord is fused to non-neoplastic fibrofatty mass. *C*, Aberrant nerve roots or adherent bands restrict ascent of spinal cord. Maldeveloped filum terminale is short and thick.

Many patients with occult spinal dysraphism have delayed appearance of abnormal findings which then progress. Difficulty is not encountered until the teenage years in some patients.

Radiologic studies are necessary to confirm the diagnosis. Surgical treatment is important to prevent infection where the dermal sinus exists, and surgery frequently leads to improvement of the neurologic condition.

Reference: Anderson, F.M.: Pediatrics, *55*:826, 1975.

## DERMATOMES IN DIAGNOSIS

Knowledge of the cutaneous distribution of the dermatomes plays an important role in determining the level of the lesion in patients with neurologic disorders.

The man in Figure 12–2 with his unusual wrinkles should help you in interpreting your neurologic findings.

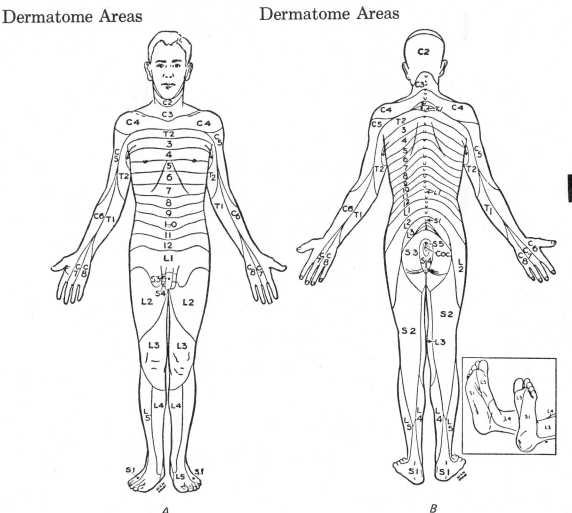

Dermatome Areas

Dermatome Areas

*A*

*B*

The dermatomes from the anterior view.  The dermatomes from the posterior view.

*FIG. 12–2*

# 13
# ENDO-
# CRINOLOGY

# GROWTH HORMONE STIMULATION TESTS

Many provocative tests have been developed to assess the responsiveness of growth hormone. No one test provides proof of growth hormone deficiency. Fasting plasma growth hormone levels are often low or undetectable in normal children.

Screening tests consist of stimulation using glucose, estrogens (diethylstilbestrol), sleep, and exercise. None of these tests is free of a significant percentage of false positives. Probably the best screening procedure in an office or clinic setting is the exercise stimulation test, performed by obtaining plasma growth hormone concentrations following sufficient exercise to make the subjects breathless (e.g., 20 minutes of brisk walking, running, and/or climbing stairs).

More definitive tests include stimulation via insulin-induced hypoglycemia, arginine, glucagon, and L-dopa. Since many patients give discordant responses to these stimulation tests, it is advised that no diagnosis be made until at least two test results are known. Most frequently, sequential testing is done on the same day using both arginine and insulin.

Any growth hormone level less than 3 ng/ml after stimulation is suggestive of growth hormone deficiency. *Any result greater than or equal to 7 ng/ml on any one test precludes the diagnosis of growth hormone deficiency.* Test results between 3 ng/ml and 7 ng/ml may represent a partial deficiency.

Growth hormone response may be affected by some other hormonal influences:

1. Peak growth hormone levels following stimulation may be blunted in the obese child or in the patient with hypothyroidism.
2. Neither physiologic nor pharmacologic glucocorticoid therapy will confuse the results of growth hormone testing.
3. The child with constitutionally delayed puberty may have a decreased or undetectable response to stimulation. The peak growth hormone levels return to normal with the onset of puberty.

---

Reference: Frasier, S.D.: Pediatrics, *53*:929, 1974.

# THYROID FUNCTION STUDIES AND THYROID DISEASE

The availability of new and more sophisticated tests for thyroid function has made the diagnosis of thyroid disease more precise — and more complicated. The tests and the aspect of thyroid function measured by each is listed below.

$T_4$ (Murphy-Pattee) by protein binding assay — measures total thyroxine (bound and unbound). Because of losses in extraction, only about 85 per cent of $T_4$ is actually represented.

$T_4$ by radioimmunoassay — also measures bound and unbound $T_4$. This test is somewhat more accurate than the Murphy-Pattee.

13

$T_3$ — measures the total circulating amount of this more active substance. Patients with thyrotoxicosis may have normal $T_4$ but elevated $T_3$.

PBI (protein-bound iodine) — no longer used except to determine level of circulating iodine.

TBG (thyroid-binding globulin) — this is the most important serum protein that binds thyroid hormone.

$RT_3U$ ($T_3$ resin uptake) results of this test are given as a fraction or percentage relative to the normal value. This fraction, the "resin $T_3$ ratio," has a high correlation to percentage of $T_4$ that is free $T_4$. To correct $T_4$ values for abnormal TBG levels, multiply the resin $T_3$ ratio by the $T_4$.

Free $T_4$ — this value may now be measured directly by determining the dialyzable fraction of $T_4$. It is an expensive test and usually unnecessary.

TRH (thyrotropin-releasing hormone) test — TRH is injected, and measurements are made of TSH response.

RAIU (radioiodine uptake) studies — this is used to access clearance of iodine by the thyroid gland.

RAIU (radioiodine uptake) studies — this is used to assess clearance of iodine by the gland.

Technetium pertechnetate scan — this test localizes thyroid tissue.

Perchlorate discharge test — increased discharge indicates defective metabolism of iodine.

Results of these tests may be correlated with the appropriate diagnosis in the following tables.

---

Reference: Fisher, D.A.: J. Pediatr., *82*:187, 1973.

*Expected Abnormalities of Thyroid Function Tests in Common Disorders of Thyroid Function*

| DISORDER | T₄* | T₃ | TBG | TSH | TRH RESPONSE T₃ | TRH RESPONSE TSH | RADIOIODINE STUDIES |
|---|---|---|---|---|---|---|---|
| **Hypothyroidism** | | | | | | | |
| Primary | D | D | N–I | I | D | I | Decreased or ectopic RAIU |
| Secondary | | | | | | | |
| TSH deficiency | D | D | N–I | D | D | D | Decreased RAIU |
| TRH deficiency | D | D | N–I | D | D | N | Increased 3-day TSH response |
| **Thyrotoxicosis** | | | | | | | |
| Graves' disease | I | I | N–D | D | D | D | Increased RAIU |
| Plummer's disease | N–I† | N–I† | N–D | D | D | D | Increased RAIU in nodule‡ |
| **Chronic lymphocytic thyroiditis** | | | | | | | |
| Euthyroid | N§ | N–I | N | N–I | N–D | N–I | Alerted pattern of uptake |
| Hypothyroid | D§ | N–D | N–I | I | D | I | Perchlorate discharge positive |
| Hyperthyroid | I§ | I | N–D | D | D | D | Reduced TSH response |
| **Adolescent nontoxic diffuse goiter** | N§ | N | N | N | N | N | N |
| **Nontoxic thyroid nodules** | N | N | N | N | N | N | Function of nodules variable |

N = normal, D = decreased, I = increased

*Corrected for alterations in TBG binding.

†Corrected for alterations in TBG binding.

‡Hyperfunctioning nodules may produce $T_4$ and $T_3$ in variable proportions, and occasionally $T_3$ secretion may predominate and produce $T_3$-toxicosis.

‡The remainder of the thyroid gland is suppressed, but will function after TSH administration.

§The PBI often exceeds $T_4$ I by 2 μg/100 ml or more.

13

*Expected Abnormalities of Thyroid Function Tests in Goitrous Hypothyroidism and in Patients with Idiopathic Alterations in TBG Binding*

| DISORDER | $T_4$* | $T_3$* | TBG | TSH | TRH RESPONSE $T_3$ | TRH RESPONSE $TSH$ | ISOTOPE TESTS† |
|---|---|---|---|---|---|---|---|
| **Inborn defects in thyroid metabolism** | | | | | | | |
| TSH-unresponsive | D | D | N | I | D | I | Low RAIU; no response to TSH |
| $T_4$ resistance | I | I | N | N–I | N | N | Increased RAIU |
| Trapping defect | D | N–D? | N | N–I? | D? | N–I? | Low RAIU; no response to TSH; no salivary concentration |
| Peroxidase defect | N–D | N–D | N | N–I? | D? | N–I? | Increased RAIU (2–6 hr. > 24–48 hr.). Perchlorate discharge — positive |
| Iodotyrosine coupling defect‡ | N–D | N–D | N | N–I? | D? | N–I? | Increased RAIU |
| Iodotyrosine dehalogenase defect | N–D | N–D | N | N–I? | D? | N–I? | Increased RAIU; $^{131}$I-DIT excreted intact |
| Iodoprotein-secreting§ | N–D§ | N–D? | N | N–I? | D? | N–I? | Increased RAIU. Circulating non BEI |
| Thyroglobulin defect‖ | N–D | N–D? | N | N | D? | N–I? | Increased RAIU. Circulating non-BEI |
| **Idiopathic alterations in TBG** | | | | | | | |
| Decreased TBG | D | D? | D | N | N | N | N |
| Increased TBG | I | N–I | I | N | N | N | N |

N = normal, D = decreased, I = increased.

*Corrected for alterations in TBG binding except in the case of idiopathic TBG alterations.

†When the increase in early uptake is strikingly out of proportion to the late uptake, the notation 2 to 6 hours > 24 to 48 hours is used.

‡A diagnosis of iodotyrosine coupling defect can be made with certainty only by finding only iodotyrosine (without $T_4$ or $T_3$) during analysis of a gland biopsy.

§The diagnosis of noniodothyronine iodoprotein secretion depends on the finding that the PBI exceeds the $T_4$I by 2 gm/100 ml or more on finding a serum non-butanal-extractable $^{131}$I in excess of 30 per cent after radioiodine administration.

‖The diagnosis of a defect in thyroglobulin synthesis is confirmed by analysis of thyroglobulin in a gland biopsy.

# GYNECOMASTIA IN ADOLESCENT
# AND PREADOLESCENT MALES

Gynecomastia may be defined as the presence of a firm, discoid, occasionally tender nodule or swelling palpable under the areola. It may even extend beyond the areolar area. Gynecomastia is frequently encountered in adolescent males. Some facts concerning its characteristics and natural history can help you in the management of this poorly understood developmental phenomenon.

1.  Between ages 10 and 16, approximately 40 per cent of all males will have gynecomastia.

2.  It is less frequent in black males.

3.  It has a peak occurrence at age 14 to 14.5 years, when its incidence may reach 65 per cent.

4.  It is unilateral in about 25 per cent of cases. When it is unilateral, the right side is affected twice as commonly as the left.

5.  When males are reexamined periodically over a period of three years, the gynecomastia persists in only about 8 per cent of patients.

6.  The occurrence and size of the gynecomastia appears to correlate best with the size of the thyroid, testis, and penis, and the amount of pubic hair.

7.  About 10 per cent of adolescent males will have spider angiomas. In this group, about 60 per cent will have gynecomastia.

8.  It is a benign condition. Surgery is indicated only in those rare situations where extreme prominence of the breasts may produce psychologic problems.

9.  The gynecomastia of Klinefelter's syndrome does not appear until after puberty is reached.

Gynecomastia is much less frequently found in preadolescent boys, although benign, idiopathic breast enlargement may occur at this age as well. Urinary estrogens may be elevated. The gynecomastia may be unilateral or bilateral, and secondary sexual characteristics are those of a prepubertal male. The following table will help in the differential diagnosis of a prepubertal male presenting with gynecomastia.

Persistent elevation of estrogens or gonadotropins or both indicates need for exploratory laparotomy.

Remember, drugs and hormones may produce gynecomastia. These include androgens, estrogens, adrenocorticoids, chorionic gonadotropins, digitalis, isoniazid, amphetamines, and marijuana. It also occurs with increased frequency in males with chronic pulmonary infections.

**13**

| CONDITION | SEXUAL MATURATION | CIRCULATING OR URINARY STEROIDS | | | IVP AND RETROPERITONEAL PNEUMOGRAM |
|---|---|---|---|---|---|
| | | Estrogens | Testosterone | 17-KS and DHA | |
| Idiopathic | Preadolescent | Normal or high | Normal | Normal | Normal |
| Adrenal<br>Feminizing tumor | Accelerated | Elevated | Normal | Elevated | May be normal or tumor may be seen |
| Isosexual tumor | Accelerated | Elevated | Normal or elevated | Elevated | |
| Testicular (tumor usually palpable)<br>Interstitial cell tumor | Accelerated | Elevated | Elevated | Normal | Normal |
| Choriocarcinoma* | Accelerated | Elevated | Normal | Normal | Normal |

*Not yet reported in prepubertal age. Chorionic gonadotropin levels are elevated.

References: Nydick, M., Bustos, J., Dale, J.H., et al.: J.A.M.A., *178*:449, 1961. Latorre, H., and Kenny, F.M.: Am. J. Dis. Child., *126*:771, 1973.

# SEXUAL MATURITY RATING AND
# THE SERUM ALKALINE PHOSPHATASE

Tanner has suggested a rating system using sequential acquisition of secondary sexual characteristics, which provides a logic for the highly variable rates (and ages) at which adolescents mature during puberty. This system is outlined below.

*Boys*

| STAGE | PUBIC HAIR | PENIS | TESTES |
|---|---|---|---|
| 1 | None | Preadolescent | |
| 2 | Scanty, long, slightly pigmented | Slight enlargement | Enlarged scrotum, pink, texture altered |
| 3 | Darker, starts to curl, small amount | Penis longer | Larger |
| 4 | Resembles adult type, but less in quantity; coarse, curly | Larger. Glans penis increased in size | Larger, scrotum dark |
| 5 | Adult distribution, spread to medial surface of thighs | Adult | Adult |

*Girls*

| STAGE | PUBIC HAIR | BREASTS |
|---|---|---|
| 1 | Preadolescent | Preadolescent |
| 2 | Sparse, lightly pigmented, straight, medial border of labia | Breast and papilla elevated as small mound; areolar diameter increased |
| 3 | Darker, beginning to curl, increased amount | Breast and areola enlarged, no contour separation |
| 4 | Coarse, curly, abundant but amount less than in adult | Areola and papilla form secondary mound |
| 5 | Adult feminine triangle, spread to medial surface of thighs | Mature; nipple projects, areola part of general breast contour |

**13**

Among the physiologic measurements shown to correlate with this rating system is the serum alkaline phosphatase (SAP) level. Elevation of SAP may be a perplexing problem in children in this age group. This elevation has been shown to be a normal phenomenon, related to the child's sexual maturity rating. As illustrated in Figure 13–1, SAP values tend to peak at stages 2 and 3, fall during stage 4, and approach adult norms during stage 5.

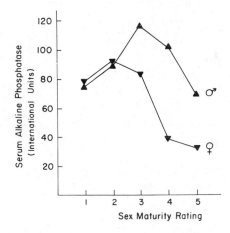

FIG. 13–1

Elevations in SAP seen during normal puberty are due primarily to increases in the bone isoenzyme of alkaline phosphatase. Other causes of elevated SAP, both during puberty and at other times, can be grouped under these broad headings:

Obstructive jaundice
Hepatocellular liver disease
Abnormal bone (calcium/phosphorus) metabolism
Metastatic malignancy in the liver

Reference: Bennett, D.L., Ward, M.S., and Daniel, W.A.: J. Pediatr., *88*:633, 1976.

## PRECOCIOUS SEXUAL DEVELOPMENT (ISOSEXUAL)

Adolescent sexual development may begin in normal children as early as 8 to 10 years of age in girls and 10 to 11 years in boys. Precocious onset of this process may result from the early secretion of gonadotropic hormone (complete sexual precocity) or from secretion of sex hormones by the gonads or adrenals. The following chart lists the types and etiology of sexual precocity in males and females.

| ETIOLOGY | LESION IN MALES | LESION IN FEMALES | CHARACTERISTICS |
|---|---|---|---|
| *Gonadotropin Secretion* | | | |
| Neurogenic | Brain tumor Encephalitis Obscure disorder — hypothalamus | Brain tumor Encephalitis Obscure disorder — hypothalamus Albright's syndrome — (bone dysplasia and pigmentation) | Gonads mature normally Spermatogenesis or ovulation may occur |
| "Idiopathic" activation of pituitary | None found | None found | Sex hormones excreted in normal adolescent or adult amounts |
| Gonadotropin-secreting tumor | Hepatoma Teratoma (?) Other (?) | Hepatoma (?) Teratoma (?) Chorioepithelioma (?) | Leydig cell hyperplasia of testes without spermatogenesis |
| *Sex Hormone Secretion* | | | |
| Gonadal | Interstitial cell tumor of testis | Granulosa cell tumor or (?) cyst Luteoma or thecoma | Tumor usually in one gonad, other gonad may be immature or atrophic Sex hormones *sometimes* excreted in excess amounts |
| Adrenal | Virilizing adrenal hyperplasia Virilizing tumor | Feminizing adrenal tumor (rare) | Gonads usually immature (some exceptions) 17–KS increased |

The cause of sexual precocity must be determined by careful history, physical examination, and laboratory studies. The approach will differ depending upon whether the patient is male or female.

**13**

### Females

Precocious sexual development occurs twice as frequently in females as in males. Approximately 80 to 90 per cent of females with sexual precocity have the idiopathic (constitutional, cryptogenic) form, and the diagnosis must be one of exclusion. Others will have small undiagnosable hamartomas or other small and benign hypothalamic lesions. Exclusion of other causes is essential, however, and the following list includes the conditions to be considered along with the clinical associations of those conditions.

| CONDITION | CLINICAL ASSOCIATIONS |
|---|---|
| Neonatal estrinization | Breast development and vaginal secretion may occur during the newborn period. They are probably due to maternal and placental hormone stimulation during the prenatal period, and vaginal bleeding may result from estrogen withdrawal following birth. |

| CONDITION | CLINICAL ASSOCIATIONS |
|---|---|
| Bleeding due to foreign bodies or lesions in the vagina | Vaginal bleeding without breast development may be due to the presence of a foreign body or a rectovaginal fistula. Vaginal inspection under anesthesia may be necessary. |
| Estrogen ingestion | Breast development and vaginal changes may be a result of accidental ingestion of estrogen or stilbestrol. Cosmetic creams may be an unsuspected source of estrogens. Ingestion of stilbestrol is often accompanied by blackish pigmentation of the areolae. |
| Premature thelarche | Early breast development may occur without accompanying development of the labia minora or changes in the vaginal smear. It may be due to oversensitivity of the breast tissue to low levels of circulating estrogen. This condition is entirely benign. |
| Premature pubarche | Increased sensitivity of sexual hair follicles or early elaboration of adrenal androgens may cause the growth of coarse sexual hair without other sexual changes. These patients eventually mature normally. This condition may suggest the adreno-genital syndrome, but with the latter syndrome there would be rapid progression of sexual maturation and greatly elevated 17-ketosteroids. |
| True sexual precocity due to intracranial lesions | Urinary gonadotropins are not always elevated. Skull roentgen-ogram and careful neurologic evaluation will usually rule out cerebral tumors in girls, because neurologic symptoms are almost always present prior to signs of sexual development. A history of encephalitic disease points to a cerebral origin of precocity. Cerebral lesions causing early puberty may also occur in tuberous sclerosis and neurofibromatosis. |
| Gonadotropin-secreting tumor | Chorioepithelioma, teratoma, or hepatoma may cause precocious puberty. The finding of greatly elevated gonadotropins should suggest this diagnosis. |
| Ovarian neoplasms | Abdominal and rectal examination will usually reveal the presence of a granulosa cell tumor. Urinary estrogens may be elevated in the presence of a granulosa cell tumor. Elevated urinary pregnanediol may accompany a luteoma. In the absence of palpable tumor or elevated hormones, there is little likelihood of feminizing neoplasm. |
| Adrenal tumor | This diagnosis should be suggested by the presence of elevated urinary 17-ketosteroids. |
| Fibrous dysplasia (Albright's syndrome) | History may reveal skeletal fractures, and physical examination may reveal pigmented skin lesion. The entire skeleton and skull should be included in an x-ray search for bone lesions. |
| Hypothyroidism | Sexual precocity has been found along with hypothyroidism in a few cases. The sella turcica may be enlarged. Symptoms and signs abate with treatment of the hypothyroidism. |

## Males

Idiopathic sexual precocity is more unusual in boys than in girls. If the male patient has a family history positive for the condition, he is more likely to have the idiopathic form. Sexual precocity in boys is more likely to be of cerebral origin. Other forms are listed below along with their clinical associations.

| CONDITION | CLINICAL ASSOCIATION |
|---|---|
| Premature pubarche | This is much less frequent in boys than in girls. It includes growth of the penis and testes without accompanying pubic hair. There may be slight elevation of 17-ketosteroids, and epiphyseal development and growth may be slightly accelerated. |
| Iatrogenic virilization | Anabolic steroids and androgens given to promote growth may be virilizing. Careful history should be taken to ascertain accessibility of androgens to a sexually precocious male child. |
| True sexual precocity due to intracranial lesion | Gonadotropins are not always elevated with this condition, and 17-ketosteroids are normal or only slightly elevated. Careful neurologic evaluation should be undertaken, and in the absence of another explanation for precocious sexual development, diagnostic radiologic studies should be carried out. |
| Interstitial cell tumor of the testis | Very high or moderately elevated levels of 17-ketosteroids are present, and they do not decrease with dexamethasone suppression. One testis may be larger than the other. |
| Virilizing adrenal hyperplasia | Elevated 17-ketosteroids suppress with dexamethasone. There is enlargement of the penis without concomitant testicular enlargement. Testicular biopsy shows no spermatogenesis. |
| Virilizing adrenal tumor | Elevated 17-ketosteroids do not suppress with dexamethasone. High levels of dehydroepiandrosterone are almost pathognomonic of adrenal tumor. |
| Teratoma-secreting androgen | Increased levels of chorionic gonadotropin. |
| Hepatoma | There may be elevated 17-ketosteroids that do not suppress with dexamethasone. Levels of chorionic gonadotropin are exceedingly high. Testicular biopsy shows tremendous Leydig cell hyperplasia with underdeveloped or degenerated seminiferous tubules. |
| Chorioepithelioma | Increased chorionic gonadotropin. |

Reference: Wilkins, L.: *In* The Diagnosis and Treatment of Endocrine Disorders in Childhood and Adolescence. Springfield, Illinois, Charles C Thomas, 1965.

**13**

# SOME PROBLEMS WITH OBESITY IN CHILDHOOD

Adult obesity has been associated with many diseases, including diabetes mellitus, hypertension, and coronary artery disease. These problems do not usually manifest themselves in childhood obesity, but the overweight child may present several diagnostic difficulties to the physician. A few clinical problems are listed here.

1. *Hypertension* may be overdiagnosed in the obese child because of use of the usual child's blood pressure cuff. Proper blood pressure measurements may be ascertained only with the cuff usually used to measure blood pressure in the lower extremities.

2. Obese children are often *excessively tall*. This excessive height is accompanied by advanced bone age and may suggest precocious puberty or adrenal

hyperplasia. Careful examination of the genitalia should rule out these possibilities. The genitalia of the obese male child may even appear hypoplastic because of excess pubic fat.

3. The obese female child may present with the puzzling problem of constantly *wet underwear* and smelling of urine. It is felt that the convergence of the thighs against the perineum may lead to reflux of urine into the vagina when voiding, with constant dribbling being the result. These girls should be taught to spread the thighs after voiding.

---

Reference: William H. Dietz, Jr.: Personal communication, 1976.

# 14
# SURGERY/ ORTHOPEDICS

# MANAGEMENT OF RESPIRATORY FOREIGN BODIES

Foreign bodies of the ear or respiratory tract are therapeutic as well as diagnostic problems. These guidelines for removal of foreign bodies of various types may help you and your patient.

| SITE | FOREIGN BODY DESCRIPTION | SUGGESTION FOR REMOVAL |
|------|--------------------------|------------------------|
| Ear | Smaller than external canal | Hartman or alligator forceps |
| | Larger than external canal | Insert loop behind object, then withdraw |
| | Nonvegetable object | Stream of water |
| | Vegetable object | Do *not* irrigate (may cause object to swell) |
| | Attached to drum or associated with perforation | ENT consultation; do not irrigate |
| | Insect | Irrigate with alcohol before removal |
| | Metallic object | Use magnet |

| SITE | SUGGESTIONS FOR REMOVAL |
|------|--------------------------|
| Nose | 1. Explain situation to parents; sedate child p.r.n.<br>2. Spray nasoconstrictor into nostril.<br>3. Examine local area after cleaning with gentle suction.<br>4. Remove soft object with forceps; pass loop behind larger or harder objects.<br>5. If above unsuccessful, try blowing into child's mouth while compressing uninvolved nostril. |
| Pharynx | Foreign body (e.g., fish bone) imbedded in soft palate or tonsil may be removed with tonsil hemostat. Other foreign body in other pharyngeal sites requires ENT consultation. |
| Trachea or bronchial tree | Foreign body here requires ENT and/or surgical consultation. |
| Esophagus | Foreign body at cardioesophageal junction may be observed for 24 to 48 hours. ENT consultation is indicated if no passage by that time. Foreign body at other esophageal sites requires immediate ENT consultation. |

14

Reference: Stool, S.E., and McConnel, C.S., Jr.: Clin. Pediatr., *12*:113, 1973.

## INTUSSUSCEPTION

The pediatrician is usually the first physician to see a child with an intussusception. Prompt recognition of this acute disorder will reduce morbidity and mortality. Remembering the following facts will facilitate early diagnosis and improve management.

| Age of Patients | % Presenting at Given Age |
|---|---|
| Under 12 months | 52% |
| 1 – 2 years | 24% |
| 2 – 3 years | 10% |
| 3 – 7 years | 11% |
| Over 7 years | 3% |

| Signs and Symptoms | % Presenting with Given Sign or Symptom |
|---|---|
| Pain | 94% |
| Vomiting (at least once) | 91% |
| Gross blood with stool | 66% |
| Abdominal mass | 59% |

Patients typically are healthy infants and children with no previous history of gastrointestinal disease. Nearly all infants present with recent onset of abdominal pain and at least one episode of vomiting. The pain is characterized by the child's crying and drawing his legs into his abdomen. Males are affected about twice as often as females. The mass is usually sausage-shaped and is palpable along the course of the colon. On occasion one may elicit Dance's sign — an emptiness in the right lower quadrant that reflects the fact that the intussuscepting bowel has moved out of this portion of the abdomen.

### Etiology of Intussusception

In less than 10 per cent of patients will an etiologic factor be determined. Specific causes include Meckel's diverticulum (most common), ileal polyp, ileal granuloma, inspissated meconium in patients with cystic fibrosis, Henoch-Schönlein purpura, and lymphosarcoma.

Although the barium reduction will successfully reduce approximately 75 per cent of all intussusception, *it is advisable for all patients over 6 years of age to have elective exploratory laparotomy because of the high probability that intussusception at this age has a specific cause; it is frequently produced by an intestinal lymphosarcoma.*

---

Reference: Wayne, E.R., Campbell, J.B., Burrington, J.D., and Davis, W.S.: Radiology, *107*:597, 1973.

# APPENDICITIS IN INFANCY

Less than 2 per cent of children treated for appendicitis are under 2 years of age. It is in the infant, however, that the diagnosis may be the most difficult to make. Common symptoms and signs of infantile appendicitis are listed below in decreasing order of frequency.

*Symptoms*

> Vomiting
> Pain
> Lethargy
> Nausea
> Feeding problems
> Diarrhea

*Signs*

> Tenderness
> Fever
> Spasm
> Guarding
> Positive rectal findings
> Absent bowel sounds
> Mass
> Urinary retention

The clinical findings may often be verified by radiographic abnormalities. Approximately 80 per cent of infants in whom the diagnosis of appendicitis is made at surgery will have one or more of the following x-ray findings if both upright and supine films of the abdomen are obtained preoperatively:

> Abnormal gas pattern (paucity of gas in RLQ, diffuse
>   small bowel dilatation, gas-fluid levels)
> Free peritoneal fluid or air
> Scoliosis
> Obscuration of psoas margin by excessive bowel gas
> Thickened abdominal wall
> Fecalith
> Abscess

14

---

Reference: Wilkinson, R.H., Bartlett, R.H., and Eraklis, A.J.: Am. J. Dis. Child., *118*:687, 1969.

*"Children are like grown people; the experience of others is never of any use to them."*

Daudet

## IMMOBILIZATION AND HYPERCALCEMIA

We often tend to pay little attention to the children on our wards who are in casts recuperating from fractures. It is well recognized that immobilization of previously healthy children can lead to disturbances in calcium metabolism that include osteoporosis, hypercalciuria, urinary calculi formation, and soft tissue calcification. Symptoms of hypercalcemia are often ignored. They include:

Anorexia
Nausea
Vomiting
Irritability
Constipation
Muscular weakness
Weight loss
Tachycardia
Excessive thirst

Remember that the irritable and anorexic child in the cast may not be merely expressing his boredom and unhappiness with prolonged hospitalization. Four weeks of immobilization appears to be the peak time for both hypercalcemia and "cabin fever."

Reference:  Henke, J.A., Thompson, N.W., and Kaufer, H.: Arch. Surg., *110*:321, 1975.

## TORTICOLLIS

Torticollis, or wryneck, is a sign of a disorder in and around the cervical spine. Pediatricians, all too often, are aware of congenital muscular torticollis but are unfamiliar with a variety of other disorders that may also produce wryneck. The table below describes the types of torticollis and their features.

*Types of Torticollis*

| BASIC PATHOLOGIC PROCESS | UNDERLYING ABNORMALITY | SPECIAL FEATURES |
|---|---|---|
| Osseous | Congenital defect of the odontoid process. Hypoplastic odontoid process may result in posterior dislocation of anterior ring of axis | |
| | Failure of odontoid process to fuse with body of axis | Seen in a variety of forms of dwarfism and in mucopolysaccharidosis. |
| | Rotary subluxations | May follow "horseplay," upper respiratory infections, sleeping in a draft, a blow to the mandible, and infections in the pharynx. |
| | Congenital anomalies of the cervical vertebrae, e.g., hemivertebrae | Look for in patients with Klippel-Feil syndrome or Sprengel's deformity. |
| Ligamentous | Seen rarely in patients with congenital absence of transverse ligament. Results in subluxations or dislocations | Ligamentous laxity observed in patients on high-dosage, long-term steroids. |
| Muscular | Congenital form appears within 10 days of birth. Fibrous mass present at base of sternocleidomastoid muscle | Head tilts toward affected muscle-face, rotated to the opposite side. Uncorrected may produce underdevelopment of face on involved side. |
| | Traumatic injury to muscle | |
| Neurologic | Posterior fossa tumor | |
| | Phenothiazine intoxication | May be accompanied by trismus and opisthotonos. |
| | Syringomyelia | |
| | Myasthenia gravis | |
| Ocular | Vertical strabismus as a result of fourth nerve palsy | Patching eye corrects torticollis. |
| | Congenital nystagmus | |
| Functional | Rare in children | Disappears with sleep. |

Reference: Clark, R.N.: Pediatr. Ann., 5:231, 1976.

14

# JOINT FLUID ANALYSIS IN DIFFERENTIAL DIAGNOSIS OF ARTHRITIS

A joint aspirate is often the most rapid and accurate way to establish a diagnosis in a child with arthritis. Listed below are the usual findings in patients with juvenile rheumatoid arthritis, septic arthritis, and traumatic arthritis.

| DIAGNOSTIC TEST | JUVENILE RHEUMATOID ARTHRITIS | SEPTIC ARTHRITIS | TRAUMATIC ARTHRITIS |
|---|---|---|---|
| Appearance | Clear to opalescent | Cloudy or turbid | Clear to blood-tinged |
| Mucin clot (add a few drops of joint aspirate to a beaker containing 10 to 20 ml of 5% acetic acid; let stand for one minute, then shake) | Good to poor | Poor (clot flakes and shreds) | Good (remains a firm and ropelike mass) |
| White cell count | 15,000–25,000/mm$^3$ (50–90% neutrophils) | 50,000–100,000/mm$^3$ (90% neutrophils) | Less than 5000/mm$^3$ (20–50% neutrophils) |
| Blood glucose/joint fluid glucose difference | 10–25 mg/100 ml | Greater than 50 mg/100 ml | Less than 10 mg/100 ml |

# THE THREE MODES OF ONSET OF JUVENILE RHEUMATOID ARTHRITIS

The onset of juvenile rheumatoid arthritis (JRA) takes three general forms: the acute febrile onset, the monoarticular onset, and polyarticular onset. All three forms may be confused with other diseases, and the diagnosis is often difficult. Awareness of the clinical characteristics of the three presentations of this disease may help avoid the devastating effects of misdiagnosis.

| | ACUTE FEBRILE ONSET | MONOARTICULAR ONSET | POLYARTICULAR ONSET |
|---|---|---|---|
| Per cent | 20 | 30 | 50 |
| Joint manifestations | One-half have no joint swelling at onset. The other one-half have only arthralgia. Pain may be inferred from the flexed-knee position in which these children tend to lie. | The knee is most common site of onset. Other sites are ankle, elbow, wrist and finger joints. Swelling, stiffness, and pain are usually minimal. Painful tendinitis or bursitis, especially of the heel, may be the presenting symptom.<br><br>In early stages, the arthritis may be asymmetrical and migrating. | Four or more joints are involved. May have abrupt onset with painful swelling of knees, ankles, feet, and hands. May have insidious onset with no complaint of pain. Joint involvement must be inferred from guarding movements and knee-flexed position. Arthritis may be migratory at first. Cervical spine may be involved. Subcutaneous nodules are not present. |
| Fever | Daily spikes to 105° F or higher with temperature falling sometimes to subnormal levels. Fever may precede arthritis by weeks, months, or years. | There may be low-grade daily fever spikes. | Low-grade fever with daily spikes. |
| Rash | 90% have macular or slightly maculopapular rash usually on the trunk and extremities, occasionally on the neck and face. Rash is rarely pruritic, is usually fleeting with macules appearing for a few hours during the day or week, usually in conjunction with fever. Rash is more florid when the skin is rubbed or scratched (Köbner phenomenon). | Rash is sometimes present, but is rarely of diagnostic help. | Maculopapular rash is sometimes present. |

14

| | ACUTE FEBRILE ONSET | MONOARTICULAR ONSET | POLYARTICULAR ONSET |
|---|---|---|---|
| Iridocyclitis | Rarely occurs in patients presenting in this way. | This group is most susceptible to ocular disease. It is often asymptomatic and may smolder for weeks or months. It may be the first manifestation of the disease. If undetected and untreated, it may lead to blindness from band keratopathy and cataracts. Diagnosis may be made only by slit lamp examination. | Rarely occurs in patients presenting in this way. |
| Lymphadenopathy | May be generalized. Splenomegaly may be present. Enlarged mesenteric nodes may lead to abdominal pain and vomiting. Lymphadenopathy may suggest lymphoma or leukemia. | Infrequent. | Infrequent. |
| Cardiac manifestations | 10% have pericarditis clinically. Pericarditis may last 2 to 12 weeks and may recur years later.<br><br>Myocarditis and resulting heart failure may occur. | — | Infrequent. |
| General appearance | Patient is usually irritable, listless, anorectic, and suffers from weight loss. | May have generalized symptoms. | Patient is usually listless, anorectic, and underweight. |
| Laboratory | Neutrophilic leukocytosis with WBC of 15,000 to 50,000/mm$^3$.<br><br>There may be a moderate normocytic, normochromic anemia. | CBC and ESR may be normal. X-ray examination may reveal accelerated maturation or early closure of epiphyses, periosteal proliferation, metaphyseal | WBC may be elevated, but is rarely higher than 20,000. ESR is elevated, usually corresponding roughly to the intensity of the arthritis. |

The ESR is usually elevated.

overgrowth of long bones, especially about the knee.

Synovial fluid aspiration reveals clear to opalescent fluid with good to poor mucin clot, 15,000 to 25,000 WBC/mm$^3$ with 50 to 90% neutrophils. Glucose of synovial fluid is about 25 mg/100 ml less than the serum glucose.

Differential diagnosis

Must be differentiated from other connective tissue diseases by absence of antinuclear antibody, difference in the nature of the rash, and age of onset (peak onset of JRA is 1 to 3 years of age, while SLE is rare in children under 5 years of age).

Must be differentiated from traumatic injury and from infectious arthritis by synovial fluid analysis. (Onset of symptoms commonly follows trauma.)

Must be differentiated from rheumatic fever by difference in fever pattern (fever of rheumatic fever is remittent or sustained), by x-ray findings, and by arthritis persisting longer than a few weeks.

Differentiation from the arthritis sometimes accompanying rubella is made by detection of an increase in the HI antibody to rubella in acute and convalescent sera. The synovial fluid of rubella arthritis has a predominance of mononuclear cells.

Reference: Calabro, J.J.: Hospital Practice, February 1974, p. 61.

## BONE TUMORS IN CHILDREN AND ADOLESCENTS—THE DIFFERENTIAL DIAGNOSIS

Malignant tumors of bone are rare in the experience of most pediatricians and thus one frequently forgets their diagnostic features. Unwarranted pessimism accompanies their diagnosis. Recent advances in treatment have dramatically improved the prognosis in some of these tumors. Early and precise diagnosis is now more critical than ever for appropriate treatment. The accompanying table describes the salient features of the more common malignant tumors encountered in children and adolescents.

14

| EWING'S SARCOMA | OSTEOGENIC SARCOMA | METASTATIC NEUROBLASTOMA | NON-HODGKIN'S LYMPHOMA | EMBRYONAL RHABDOMYOSARCOMA |
|---|---|---|---|---|
| Most common in second decade — occurs below age 10 | Most common of the bone tumors. Peak incidence in early teens | Usually in children under age 5 | No age predilection | Systemic symptoms are rare |
| Rare in blacks | | Long bones symmetrically involved | Long bones most common site | Soft tissue swelling usually initial complaint |
| Pain most common presenting symptom | Pain most common presenting complaint. Often follows trivial trauma | | | |
| Flat bones common site (ribs, scapula, pelvis) | Occurs most commonly in long bones (distal femur, proximal tibia, proximal humerus) | Lytic lesions can be extensive without soft tissue masses | Diffuse metaphyseal lesions | Lesions of trunk or extremely frequently involve bone as a result of invasion |
| Femur most common site | | Bone marrow often displays tumor cells | Lymphadenopathy and splenomegaly often present | |
| Diaphyseal lesions in long bones | X-ray films show both lytic and sclerotic changes | Presence of primary tumor. Paraspinal or suprarenal mass most common | Diffuse bone marrow involvement may be seen | Lesions in head and neck usually primary, not metastatic |
| Diffuse osteolytic lesion | Involves metaphysis of bone | Urine positive for VMA and/or catecholamines | | |
| Large soft tissue mass often present — originating in bone | Tissues mass late sign | | | |

Reference: Rosen, G.: Pediatr. Clin. North Am., 23:183, 1976.

# GROWING PAINS

"Growing pains" are a frequent complaint in children, and knowledge of their usual characteristics may help in differentiating these pains from those associated with other illnesses. Notable features of growing pains are as follows:

*Frequency* — intermittent.

*Intensity* — generally mild; however, a few children complain of severe pain that provokes crying.

*Location* — muscular, *not articular*. The legs are more frequently affected.

*Onset* — usually in late afternoon or evening. Not provoked by walking. The gait is always normal.

*Other findings* — pain is occasionally accompanied by restlessness, but never by tenderness, erythema, or local swelling.

*Outcome* — pain is usually gone by the following morning. It is not associated with organic disease.

Growing pains occur in approximately 15 per cent of children. They are more frequent in girls (18 per cent of girls; 13 per cent of boys). There is a decreasing incidence in boys after age 13, but they may persist in both boys and girls until young adulthood.

Children who have growing pains are more likely to complain of periodic headache and/or abdominal pain as well.

There is no relationship between the rate of growth and the occurrence of growing pains.

Reference: Oster, J., and Nielsen, A.: Acta Paediatr. Scand., *61*:329, 1972.

# THE UNKINDEST CUT—UNNECESSARY SURGERY

**14**

An important aspect of preventive pediatrics is the protection of children from unnecessary surgery. There are "traditional" surgical procedures whose almost routine performance obscures the fact that they have yet to be shown to be effective in the treatment for which they are advocated.

The following procedures should be reserved for situations where valid indications exist.

## Tympanostomy Placement

This procedure is commonly performed in children with chronic serous otitis media because of anxiety about hearing loss and delay in acquisition of language skills.

Although tympanostomy tubes improve hearing when in place in children with serous otitis media, the hearing deficits frequently recur when the tubes are spontaneously extruded, removed, or plugged with cerumen. There are no controlled studies to substantiate claims that hearing loss associated with serous otitis media is correctable over the long term by the use of tympanostomy tubes.

Indications for tube placement (keeping in mind the lack of controlled studies) include the following: persistent middle ear effusions unresponsive to adequate medical treatment or myringotomy; recurrent otitis media; persistent tympanic membrane retraction with impending cholesteatoma; and persistent negative pressure in the middle ear associated with significant hearing loss.

Reference: Mortimer, E.A., Jr.: Pediatrics, *58*:151, 1976.

## Clipping the Frenulum

Contrary to popular opinion, the presence of "tongue-tie," high attachment of an otherwise normal lingual frenulum, is not felt to interfere with either nursing or speech.

The indication for surgery is the rare instance of true ankyloglossia, in which the frenulum is replaced by a short thick fibrous band.

## Umbilical Herniorrhaphy

Umbilical hernias usually close spontaneously by 3 to 4 years of age. During this period of life, they virtually never become incarcerated.

The indication for surgery is persistence of this defect beyond age 3 to 4 years.

## Correction of Pectus Excavatum

Correction of pectus excavatum has been recommended both for cosmetic reasons and for correction of impaired cardiopulmonary function. There is no evidence to suggest that the surgery improves either problem.

A recent study of 75 patients, followed for more than 10 years, revealed that the 37 operated patients had poorer pulmonary function than did the 38 nonoperated patients. Operated and nonoperated patients were similar in their work capacity, frequency of lower respiratory tract infections, and frequency of psychological problems.

There appears to be no indication for such surgery at present.

Reference: Gyllensward, A., Irness, L., Michaelson, M., et al.: Acta Paediatr. Scand., Suppl., 225, 1975.

## Correction of Craniostenosis

It has been proposed that correction of craniostenosis will produce a good cosmetic result and decrease the possibility of restricting brain growth. Opponents of the procedure argue that the small risk does not justify surgery for cosmetic reasons alone and that there is no evidence that a single closed suture carries any risk of impaired neurologic function. Children with multiple fused sutures do have an increased risk of increased intracranial pressure, and in these children cosmetic deformities can be severe.

Indications for surgery in this condition include intracranial hypertension; involvement of multiple sutures with progressive exophthalmos; or visual, auditory, or neurologic dysfunction.

### Tonsillectomy

This is the most abused pediatric surgical procedure. There is no evidence to support continued performance of this procedure in most instances. It must be remembered that it carries a mortality rate of 0.1 per cent.

Indications for tonsillectomy and adenoidectomy include:

**Absolute**

1. Upper respiratory obstruction by tonsils and adenoids producing cor pulmonale.
2. Chronic or recurrent peritonsillar abscess.
3. Suspected or proved tonsillar malignancy.

**Relative**

1. Severe adenoidal nasopharyngeal obstruction.
2. Recurrent or chronic otitis media unresponsive to medical therapy.
3. Chronic or recurrent cervical adenitis.
4. Multiple culture-proven group A streptococcal tonsillar infections.

These two sets of lymphoid organs should be considered independently of each other. A decision to remove one (i.e., either tonsils or adenoids) should not automatically lead to removal of the other.

**14**

Reference: Sharkh, W., Vayda, E., Feldman, W., et al.: Pediatrics 57:401, 1976.

# 15
# DERMATOLOGY

# DIFFERENTIAL DIAGNOSIS OF EXANTHEMATOUS DISEASES

Differentiation of the various viral exanthems may be difficult. The chart below points out the importance of accurate history taking and the complete physical examination.

| DISEASE | PRODROME | RASH | OTHER DIAGNOSTIC SIGNS |
|---|---|---|---|
| Measles | 3–4 days Fever, conjunctivitis, coryza, cough | Reddish brown maculopapular rash appearing first on face and neck and spreading to trunk and extremities. Duration 5 or 6 days. Brawny desquamation (hands and feet do not desquamate). | Koplik's spots |
| Rubella | Children — none Adults — 1–4 days Malaise, fever | Discrete pink maculopapular rash appearing first on face and neck and spreading to trunk and extremities. Disappears after 3 days in same order it appeared. Does not usually desquamate. | Lymphadenopathy |
| Enteroviral infections (echovirus and coxsackievirus) | ECHO 16 – 3–4 days Fever, irritability Others — none usually | Maculopapular, discrete, nonpruritic, and generalized – rubella-like. | Aseptic meningitis Summer and fall |
| Erythema infectiosum (fifth disease) | None | 1. Red flushed cheeks with circumoral pallor 2. Maculopapular eruption over upper and lower extremities 3. Evanescent stage with recurrences | Slapped cheek appearance of "well" child |
| Rocky Mountain spotted fever | 3–4 days Fever, chills, malaise, anorexia, severe headache, and myalgia | Maculopapular and petechial eruptions with centrifugal distribution. First appears on wrists and ankles, more marked on extremities, regular occurrence on palms and soles. | Tick bite Centrifugal eruption |

15

| DISEASE | PRODROME | RASH | OTHER DIAGNOSTIC SIGNS |
|---|---|---|---|
| Scarlet fever | 12–48 hours<br>Fever, sore throat, vomiting | Erythematous punctiform eruption appearing first on flexural surfaces before becoming generalized. Most intense on neck, axillary, inguinal, and popliteal skin folds. Desquamates as large, thick flakes. | Strawberry tongue<br>Exudative or membranous tonsillitis |
| Meningococcemia | 24 hours<br>Fever | Petechiae develop in areas subject to pressure — axillary folds and belt line. Purplish ecchymoses and maculopapular nodules develop first on trunk and then on extensor surfaces of thighs and forearms. | (?) Meningeal signs<br>(?) History of sore throat |
| Exanthem subitum (roseola) | 3–4 days<br>High fever, irritability | Rose-pink maculopapules on trunk and neck which spread to face and extremities. Duration several hours to 2 days. Rarely desquamates. Appears with disappearance of fever. | Younger age group<br>Age 1 to 4 years |

# ATOPIC DERMATITIS OR SEBORRHEIC DERMATITIS

Do you have trouble distinguishing these two common entities? The following facts may help you in remembering the differences.

|  | SEBORRHEIC DERMATITIS | ATOPIC DERMATITIS |
|---|---|---|
| Family history of allergy | 15–25% | 40–60% |
| Character of individual lesions | Dry, scaly, "potato chip" lesion which may or may not appear greasy | Erythema, papules, vesicles, weeping, scales, lichenification, or a combination. May have superimposed pyoderma |
| Color of lesion | Only slightly erythematous, but more often of a salmon, yellow, or brown color | In acute phase, always red and often of an intense redness |
| Feature of lesion | More intense color at periphery — clearing at center. Appears sharply demarcated | More red at center. Gradually tapers out at periphery, fading into normal skin |
| Vesicles | Never present | Present in acute phase |
| Weeping and edema | Absent | Always present at some time in evolution of disease |
| Lichenification | Absent | Characteristic of late stage |
| Pruritus | Mild or moderate | Paroxysmal and severe |

Reference: Perlman, H.H.: Ann. Allergy, *23*:583, 1965.

**15**

# MILIARIA AND ITS COMPLICATIONS

Although sweating is a natural phenomenon, complications can occur. The miliarias are caused by retention of sweat in a functional sweat gland. The naturally occurring lesions involve the covered parts of the body. They rarely involve the face and lower extremities and never appear on the palms and soles. The lesions are accentuated by agents that provoke sweating. In infants and children they are commonly caused by overdressing or overheating of the home.

Depending on the number of glands involved and chronicity of the lesions, various degrees of anhidrosis are produced. Two common forms of miliaria are encountered in infants and children. They are:

Miliaria crystallina

An asymptomatic, noninflammatory eruption of small discrete vesicles of short duration. The vesicles are located in the stratum corneum. Slight abrasion will rupture them and cause the discharge of translucent or clear and colorless sweat.

Miliaria rubra
(prickly heat)

The lesion is a papulovesicular rash that is usually bilateral and symmetrical. The papules are surrounded by an erythematous halo and may be surmounted with a vesicle or pustule. It produces a tingling, burning, or pricking sensation.

The application of common sense can prevent most miliaria. Principles of prevention include:

Avoid overheating
Avoid overdressing
Clothing should be loose fitting and well ventilated
Use cotton underwear in the summer
Never place the child in the direct rays of the sun for periods in
    excess of 10 to 15 minutes at a time
Sponge or wash frequently with plain water

Treatment of prickly heat includes:

Institution of preventive measures
Avoid the use of soaps and ointments
Aveeno soap is useful or shake lotions containing zinc oxide
    and talc

Complications of miliaria include:

Impetigo bullosa
Multiple boils
Fungal infections
Periporitis

---

Reference: Sargent, F., II, and Slutsky, H.L.: N. Engl. J. Med., *256*:401, 1957.

# THE AMPICILLIN RASH

The child who develops a rash while or just after being treated with ampicillin presents a diagnostic problem. Here are some characteristics of ampicillin rash that should help clarify such a situation.

1. Seven to 10 per cent of children who receive ampicillin develop a rash. Children who have infectious mononucleosis and are treated with ampicillin will develop a rash 70 to 95 per cent of the time. There is also an increased incidence of rash in patients who have cytomegalovirus infection or acute lymphocytic leukemia who are given ampicillin.

2. The rash is likely to be maculopapular, mildly pruritic, and unaccompanied by systemic symptoms. In this case it is safe to continue with therapy. If the rash is of the florid or urticarial type, discontinue therapy immediately. This type of rash may also be accompanied by fever, periarticular swelling, and/or lymphadenopathy.

3. Truncal involvement almost always occurs first in the ampicillin rash. The face and extremities are involved more than one-half the time. There is usually sparing of palms, soles, and mucosal surfaces.

4. The onset of the rash may be any time from 24 hours to 16 days after beginning treatment with ampicillin.

5. The patient with a personal history of atopic manifestations is *not* more likely to develop a rash when given ampicillin.

6. Lack of response to penicillin skin testing is no assurance that the patient will not develop an ampicillin rash. The mild, maculopapular rash described above is not thought to be related to penicillin allergy; however, the patient who develops an urticarial reaction to ampicillin may have a true penicillin sensitivity.

Reference: Kerns, D.L., Shira, J.E., Go, S., et al.: Am. J. Dis. Child., *125*:187, 1973.

## THE DERMOID CYST IN CHILDREN

The child who presents with a mass that has appeared suddenly may have a benign dermoid cyst. Dermoids are epithelial-lined cavities that contain skin appendages such as hair follicles, sweat glands, or sebaceous glands. They are probably present from birth, but may manifest themselves at any time in childhood or adulthood. In adults they are primarily located in the genital and anal area, while in children most dermoids are located around the head and neck. The following table gives the usual distribution in children.

15

| LOCATION | PER CENT |
|---|---|
| Scalp | 11.0 |
| Eye (eyelid, eyebrow, and orbit) | 36.6 |
| Nose | 2.6 |
| Ear | 9.9 |
| Neck | 17 |
| Anterior chest wall | 13 |
| Post anal | <1 |
| Genital | 1 |
| Generalized skin | 7.3 |

Interestingly, dermoids seem to occur on the left side of the face twice as often as they occur on the right.

Orbital dermoids may present as proptosis and may involve deep orbital structures. Preoperative radiologic studies should be performed to determine the extent of the cyst.

Dermoid cysts are almost never malignant.

---

Reference: Pollard, Z.F., Robinson, D.H., and Calhoun, J.: Pediatrics, 57:379, 1976.

*"An infallible way to make your child miserable is to satisfy all of his demands. Passion swells by gratification; and the impossibility of satisfying every one of his demands will oblige you to stop short at last, after he has become a little headstrong."*

Henry Home

# BENIGN RHEUMATOID NODULES

Benign rheumatoid nodules resemble the nodules of rheumatoid disease clinically and histologically. They occur in healthy children. Awareness of this benign but somewhat alarming entity may prevent anxiety and many unnecessary laboratory tests. Characteristics of benign rheumatoid nodules are as follows:

## Age at Onset

Usually occurs in infancy or childhood (less than 1 year to 10 years of age), but cases have been reported in adults.

## Characteristics of Lesions

The nodules are firm and vary in diameter from less than 1 cm to several centimeters. They may increase in size very rapidly. There is no associated tenderness, pain, or erythema. The nodules are often immobile. They are fixed to deeper tissues, but not to the overlying skin. Figure 15–1 illustrates a typical lesion.

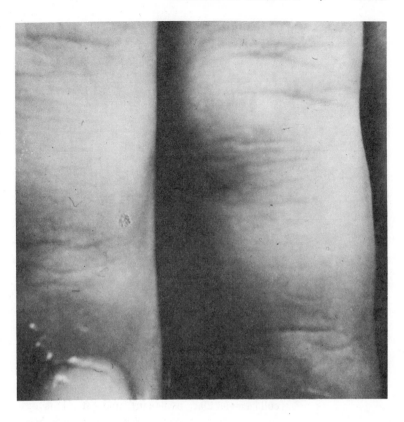

FIG. 15-1

### Location of Lesions

Nodules may be multiple or solitary. They are most frequently found in the pretibial area or on the dorsum of the foot; however, nodules have been found on the fingers, the cervicothoracic spine, and the scalp. Underlying lytic lesions may accompany scalp lesions.

### Laboratory Data

Blood counts, latex agglutination tests, lupus erythematosus cell preparations, antinuclear antibody tests, sedimentation rates; and electrocardiograms are within normal limits.

### Prognosis

All lesions recede spontaneously within months to years. Some patients experience recurrences. There is no evidence that patients with benign rheumatoid nodules later develop rheumatic disease.

### Association

These nodules are histologically similar to rheumatoid nodules and to the nodules of granuloma annulare. Patients with benign rheumatoid nodules may develop the lesions of granuloma annulare. (Granuloma annulare lesions are cutaneous nodules usually distributed in a raised annular fashion and sometimes accompanied by a redness of the overlying skin. These lesions also occur in healthy individuals and regress spontaneously. They may recur.) Figure 15-2 shows the lesion of granuloma annulare.

15

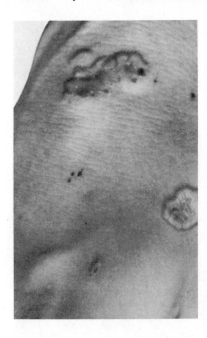

*FIG. 15-2*

### Differential Diagnosis

Benign rheumatoid nodules may be mistaken for a variety of rheumatoid, collagen-vascular, malignant, and infectious diseases. Many of these entities are ruled out by a normal physical examination. Normal laboratory studies along with a biopsy showing histology typical of a rheumatoid nodule should clinch the diagnosis.

### Treatment

Reassurance.

Reference: Simons, F.E.R., and Schaller, J.G.: Pediatrics, *56*:29, 1975.

## KAWASAKI DISEASE (THE MUCOCUTANEOUS LYMPH NODE SYNDROME)

This syndrome, first described in 1967 by Kawasaki in Japan, is now being recognized with increasing frequency all over the world. Familiarity with its features will help you to make the diagnosis.

### Major Manifestations

Fever in excess of 38.5° C for five days
Redness and induration of palms and soles
Desquamation of skin over fingers during convalescence
Polymorphous exanthem over trunk; no vesicles
Conjunctivitis
Redness and fissuring of the lips

Strawberry tongue
Diffuse redness of oropharynx
Acute, nonpurulent swelling of cervical lymph nodes

*Other features of the disease* may include tachycardia, gallop rhythm, distant heart sounds, heart murmurs, EKG changes, diarrhea, proteinuria, pyuria, leukocytosis, mild anemia, elevated platelet count, increased erythrocyte sedimentation rate, and increasing level of IgE during period of illness.

*Less frequent manifestations* include arthralgia, arthritis, aseptic meningitis, and mild jaundice.

*Mortality* is approximately 1 to 2 per cent. Deaths are due primarily to coronary artery thrombosis and resultant myocardial infarction, and occur late in the course of the disease. Coronary angiography during the illness may reveal abnormalities in as many as 60 per cent of patients. These include aneurysms, dilatation, stenosis, tortuosity, and irregularity of arterial vessel walls. These appear to regress with recovery, but at present, the long-term prognosis is unknown.

*Age Incidence:* The incidence is highest in children of 1 year of age and approximately 80 per cent of all patients are under 4 years of age.

*Etiology:* Unknown.

*Treatment:* None that is effective.

*May mimic* some of the features of scarlet fever, measles, atypical measles, rubella, Stevens-Johnson syndrome, juvenile rheumatoid arthritis, staphylococcal scalded-skin syndrome, and acrodynia (mercury poisoning).

---

References: Kawasaki, T., Kosaki, F., Okawa, S., et al.: Pediatrics, *54*:271, 1974. Lancet, *1*:675, 1976.

# ERYTHEMA NODOSUM

Erythema nodosum is an inflammatory cutaneous manifestation of certain systemic or local inflammatory diseases. These painful lesions are most commonly found on the legs between the knees and the ankles. They also may be found over the elbows, forearms, wrists, or anterior thighs. Although in the past tuberculosis and streptococcal infections were their most frequent cause, other diseases now are also recognized to be associated with these lesions. Remembering them may provide an early clue to diagnosis.

*Infection*
  Bacterial
    *Streptococcus*
    *Neisseria gonorrhoeae*
    *Neisseria meningitidis*
    *Streptococcus pneumoniae*
    *Yersinia*
  Mycobacterial
    Tuberculosis
    Leprosy
  Fungal
    Coccidioidomycosis
    Histoplasmosis

15

Blastomycosis
*Monilia*
Other Infectious Agents
Psittacosis
Lymphogranuloma venereum
Influenza

*Systemic*
Ulcerative colitis and regional ileitis
Sarcoidosis
Systemic lupus erythematosus
Glomerulonephritis

*Drugs*
Iodides
Bromides
Sulfa drugs, including acetazolamide and tolbutamide
Birth control pills

*Miscellaneous*
Behçet's syndrome
Secondary to positive skin test
Pancreatitis

---

References: Blomgren, S.E.: N.Y. State J. Med., *72*:230, 1974.  Beachler, K.J.: Brooke Army Medical Center Progress Notes, *18*:13, 1974.

# SKIN MANIFESTATIONS OF SYSTEMIC DISEASE

A variety of systemic diseases may be suspected by dermatologic findings. This table below lists a number of these cutaneous signs along with the disease they suggest.

| SIGN | DISEASE |
| --- | --- |
| Acnelike erythematous papules in midface and white ash-leaf macules on trunk, shiny thickened patch on back, subungual fibromas | Tuberous sclerosis |
| Pruritic blisters on buttocks, elbows, knees, and scapula | Dermatitis herpetiformis (celiac disease) |
| Café au lait macules | Neurofibromatosis, Albright's disease |
| "Chicken skin" — yellow rows of soft papules with wrinkled valleys in between in neck, axilla, groin | Pseudoxanthoma elasticum |

| | |
|---|---|
| "Dirty" neck and axillae (hyperpigmented, velvety flexural papules) | Acanthosis nigricans and obesity (endocrinopathies) |
| Eczematous erosions around the mouth, eyes, perineum, fingers, and toes; alopecia and diarrhea | Acrodermatitis enteropathica (zinc deficiency) |
| Erythematous, isolated papules on elbows, knees, buttocks, face | Papular acrodermatitis (antigen-positive hepatitis) |
| Erythematous, truncal macules with central pallor | Juvenile rheumatoid arthritis |
| Erythematous, flat-topped papules over knuckles | Dermatomyositis |
| Hemorrhagic (1 to 2 mm) macules on lips, tongue, palms (epistaxis, gastrointestinal bleeding) | Hereditary hemorrhagic telangiectasia (Osler-Weber-Rendu syndrome) |
| Hyperpigmentation in palmar creases, knuckles, scars, buccal mucosa, linea alba, scrotum | Addison's disease |
| Linear or oval vesicles on hands or feet, erosions on soft palate, tonsillar pillars | Hand, foot, and mouth syndrome (coxsackie A16 and others) |
| Palpable purpura | Vasculitis |
| Pigmented macules on oral mucosa | Peutz-Jeghers disease (benign small intestinal polyps) |
| Purpuric lakes | Purpura fulminans — disseminated intravascular coagulation |
| Purpuric pustules on hands and feet | Gonococcemia |
| Purpuric (petechiae) seborrheic dermatitis | Histiocytosis X |
| Sebaceous (multiple) cysts on face and trunk | Gardner's syndrome (premalignant polyps of colon and rectum) |
| Stretchy skin; healing with large purple scars | Ehlers-Danlos syndrome |
| Tight, hard skin, telangiectases, hypo- and hyperpigmentation | Scleroderma |
| Ulcers with undermined, liquefying borders | Pyoderma gangrenosum (ulcerative colitis, regional enteritis, rheumatoid arthritis) |
| Vitiligo (completely depigmented macules with hyperpigmented borders) | Pernicious anemia, Hashimoto's thyroiditis, Addison's disease, diabetes mellitus |
| Yellow papules (lower eyelids, joints, palms) | Xanthomas, hyperlipidemias |

**15**

Reference: Weston, W.L., Philpott, J.A., and Osgoode, S.P.: *In* Kempe, C.H., Silver, H.K., and O'Brien, D. (Eds.): Current Pediatric Diagnosis and Treatment. Los Altos, California, Lange Medical Publications, 1976, p. 195.

# 16

# GENETICS AND CONGENITAL ANOMALIES

# THE RISK OF PRODUCING A CHILD WITH CYSTIC FIBROSIS

At the present time there is no convenient, reliable method for detecting either the heterozygote for cystic fibrosis or the homozygote in utero.

Genetic counseling, at present, is limited to providing risk calculations. The table below should assist you in such counseling. It is based on the assumption that the prevalence of cystic fibrosis is 1 in 1600 in the Caucasian population, and its mode of inheritance is autosomal recessive with complete penetrance. The risk in blacks and Orientals is very much lower.

| ONE PARENT | THE OTHER PARENT | RISK OF CYSTIC FIBROSIS IN EACH PREGNANCY |
|---|---|---|
| No CF history | No CF history | 1 in 1600 |
| No CF history | With first cousin with CF | 1 in 320 |
| No CF history | With aunt or uncle with CF | 1 in 240 |
| No CF history | With sib with CF | 1 in 120 |
| No CF history | With CF child by previous marriage | 1 in 80 |
| No CF history | With parent having CF | 1 in 80 |
| No CF history | Has CF | 1 in 40 |
| With sib with CF | With sib having CF | 1 in 9 |
| With CF child | With CF child | 1 in 4 |

Reference: Bowman, B.A., and Mangos, J.A.: N. Engl. J. Med., *294*:937, 1976.

*"Man, discontented with the present, imagines for the past a perfection that never existed. He praises the dead out of contempt for the living, and beats the children with the bones of their ancestors."*

Comte de Volney, Constantin
François de Chasseboeuf

**16**

# THE THREE COMMON AUTOSOMAL TRISOMIES

Trisomy for chromosomes 13, 18, or 21 occurs with sufficient frequency that one should be familiar with their distinguishing characteristics. The following tables provide the information necessary to make a clinical diagnosis.

*Major Clinical Features of the Three Most Common Autosomal Trisomies*

| CHARACTERISTIC FEATURES | 21-TRISOMY | 18-TRISOMY | 13-TRISOMY |
|---|---|---|---|
| General | Mental retardation; hypotonia | Mental retardation; hypertonia; failure to thrive; preponderance of females; low birth weight | Mental retardation; failure to thrive; capillary hemangiomas; increased nuclear projections in neutrophils; persistent fetal hemoglobin; seizures |
| Craniofacies | Flat occiput; oblique palpebral fissures; epicanthic folds; speckled irides (Brushfield spots); protruding tongue; prominent, malformed ears; flat nasal bridge | Prominent occiput; small features; micrognathia; low-set, malformed ears | Microcephaly; cleft lip ± palate; midline scalp defects; microphthalmia, colobomas; low-set malformed ears; apparent deafness |
| Thorax | Congenital heart disease; mainly septal defects, especially of the endocardial cushion | Congenital heart disease, mainly VSD and PDA;* short sternum | Congenital heart disease, mainly septal defects, PDA |
| Abdomen and pelvis | Decreased acetabular and iliac angles; small penis; cryptorchidism | Horseshoe kidney; small pelvis; cryptorchidism; limited hip abduction; inguinal or umbilical hernia | Polycystic kidneys; bicornuate uterus; cryptorchidism |

| | | | |
|---|---|---|---|
| Hands and feet | Simian crease; short broad hands; hypoplasia of middle phalanx of fifth finger; gap between first and second toes | Flexion deformity of fingers; short, dorsiflexed big toes; rockerbottom feet or equinovarus | Polydactyly; hyperconvex fingernails; simian crease |
| Other features observed with significant frequency | High-arched palate; strabismus; broad, short neck; small teeth; furrowed tongue; intestinal atresia; imperforate anus | Cleft lip ± palate; ocular anomalies; simian crease; hypoplasia of fingernails; widely spaced nipples; webbed neck; single umbilical artery | Flexion deformity of fingers; single umbilical artery; shallow supraorbital ridges; micrognathia; retroflexible thumb; rockerbottom feet |

*VSD = ventricular septal defect; PDA = patent ductus arteriosus.

*Important Dermatoglyphic Patterns and Flexion Creases Found in the Three Common Autosomal Trisomy Syndromes*

| AREAS | 21-TRISOMY | 18-TRISOMY | 13-TRISOMY |
|---|---|---|---|
| Digits | Ulnar loops on most fingers; radial loops on fourth and fifth fingers | Arches on fingers and toes | — |
| Palms | Distal axial triradius or large *atd* angle | — | Distal axial triradius or large *atd* angle |
| Soles | Arch tibial or small loop distal in hallucal area | — | Arch fibular or arch fibular-S in hallucal area |
| Flexion creases | Simian crease; single crease on fifth finger | Single crease on fifth finger or on all fingers | Simian crease |

16

Reference: Uchida, I.: *In* Vaughan, V.C., and McKay, R.J. (Eds.): Nelson Textbook of Pediatrics. 10th Ed. Philadelphia, W.B. Saunders Company, 1975, p. 305.

## MULIBREY NANISM

Mulibrey (*mu*scle, *li*ver, *br*ain, and *ey*e) nanism (Fig. 16–1) is an unusual disorder inherited as an autosomal recessive. Growth failure is generally evident at birth. The patients have a triangular face and a large head. The patients exhibit muscular hypotonia, a peculiar voice, an enlarged liver, a raised venous pressure, and yellow dots dispersed throughout their ocular fundus. Constrictive pericarditis appears to be a regular feature of this syndrome. Two-thirds of patients also demonstrate cutaneous nevi flammei, and approximately one-third have cystic dysplasia of the tibia.

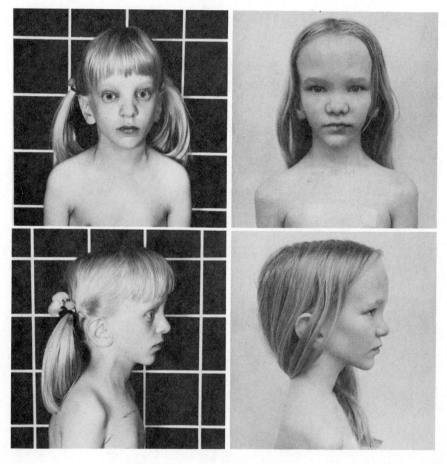

*FIG. 16–1*

When you see children who look like this, think of this syndrome and quickly look for evidence of constrictive pericarditis.

Reference: Perheentupa, J., Autio, S., Leisti, S., et al.: Lancet, 2:351, 1973.

*"Any system of religion that has anything in it that shocks the mind of a child cannot be a true system."*

Thomas Paine

# THE FETAL ALCOHOL SYNDROME

It is now quite clear that infants born to mothers with severe chronic alcoholism display a recognizable pattern of malformations as well as abnormalities of growth and development. It is important to be aware of these abnormalities. When they are present, a careful and nonthreatening discussion should be held with the parents in an attempt to determine if alcohol abuse might be responsible for the patient's problems.

The more common abnormalities include the following.

| ABNORMALITY | PER CENT OF PATIENTS |
|---|---|
| *Growth and Performance* | |
| Prenatal growth disturbance | 97 |
| Postnatal growth deficiency | 97 |
| Microcephaly | 93 |
| Developmental delay or mental deficiency | 89 |
| Fine-motor dysfunction | 80 |
| *Craniofacial* | |
| Short palpebral fissures | 92 |
| Midfacial hypoplasia | 65 |
| Epicanthic folds | 49 |
| *Limb* | |
| Abnormal palmar creases | 49 |
| Minor joint anomalies | 41 |
| *Other* | |
| Cardiac defects | 49 |
| Minor anomalies of external genitalia | 32 |
| Hemangiomas | 29 |
| Minor ear anomalies | 22 |

Other defects that may be present include microphthalmos, intraocular defects, strabismus, ptosis of eyelids, cleft palate, pectus excavatum, diaphragmatic anomalies, hypoplastic nails, pigmented nevi, and hirsutism.

These abnormalities can be recognized at birth. Be suspicious of the fetal alcohol syndrome in infants who are born small for gestational age or who fail to thrive. Two examples of patients with characteristic facies are shown in Figure 16–2.

**16**

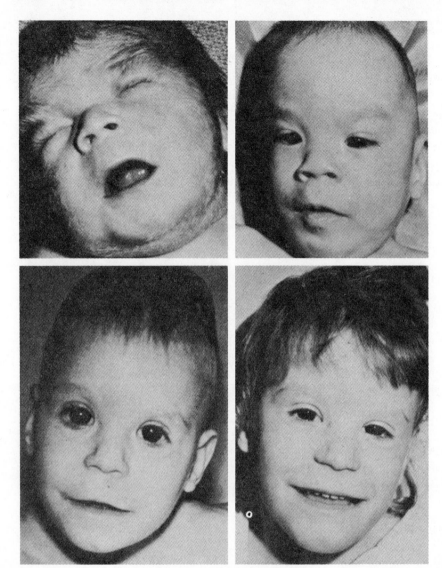

FIG. 16–2

Reference: Hanson, J.W., Jones, K.L., and Smith, D.W.: J.A.M.A., *235*:1458, 1976.

## TERATOGENIC EFFECTS OF ANTICONVULSANTS

Infants born to mothers who were treated with hydantoin anticonvulsants during pregnancy have a two to three times greater chance of congenital malformation than the general population of newborn infants. Congenital anomalies and retarded development have been noted for some time in children whose mothers are epileptic. A particular pattern of malformation has been traced to prenatal exposure to hydantoin drugs. Children affected by the fetal hydantoin syndrome exhibit some or all of the following anomalies.

Growth and performance
    Motor and/or mental deficiency
    Microcephaly
    Prenatal growth deficiency
    Postnatal growth deficiency

Craniofacial anomalies
    Short nose and low nasal bridge
    Hypertelorism
    Epicanthal folds
    Ptosis of eyelid
    Strabismus
    Low-set and/or abnormal ears
    Wide mouth
    Prominent lips
    Cleft palate
    Metopic suture ridging
    Wide fontanel

Limb
    Hypoplasia of nails and distal phalanges
    Fingerlike thumb
    Abnormal palmar creases
    Five or more digital arches

Other
    Short or webbed neck with or without low hairline
    Coarse hair
    Widely spaced, hypoplastic nipples
    Rib, sternal, or spinal anomalies
    Hernias
    Undescended testes

Figures 16–3 and 16–4 demonstrate the facial and limb anomalies of four children affected by the fetal hydantoin syndrome.

**16**

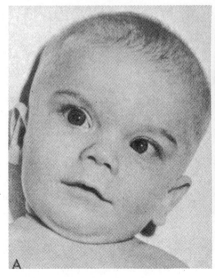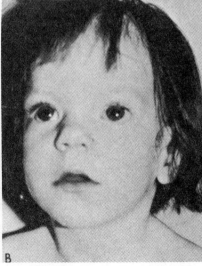

*FIG. 16–3*  A    B

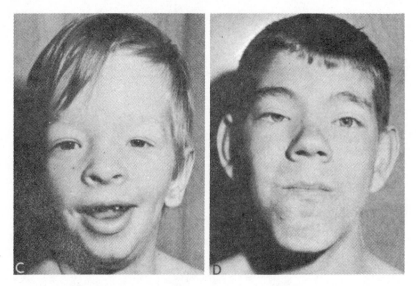

FIG. 16–3

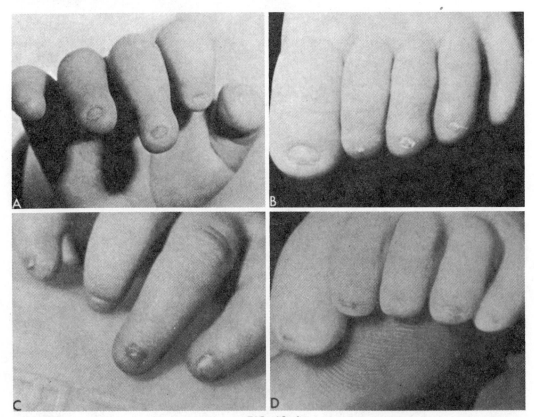

FIG. 16–4

Trimethadione is a drug used to treat petit mal epilepsy. Because petit mal attacks decrease in frequency as children grow older and usually disappear in adulthood, trimethadione is rarely administered to women of child-bearing age. A pattern of congenital anomalies has been identified, however, in infants born to mothers treated with trimethadione during pregnancy. The common and less common features of the fetal trimethadione syndrome are:

| COMMON FEATURES | LESS COMMON FEATURES |
|---|---|
| Mild mental retardation | Intrauterine growth retardation |
| Speech difficulty | Short stature |
| V-shaped eyebrows | Microcephaly |
| Epicanthus | Cardiac anomalies (septal defect, tetralogy of Fallot, and others) |
| Low-set, backward sloped ears with anteriorly folded helix | Ocular anomaly (strabismus, myopia) |
| Palatal anomaly (high-arched and/or cleft) | Hypospadias |
| | Inguinal hernias |
| | Simian crease |
| | Genitourinary anomalies |
| | Gastrointestinal anomalies, including tracheoesophageal irregularities |

Children exhibiting some of these anomalies are pictured in Figure 16–5.

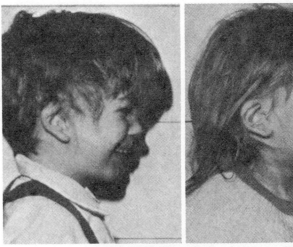

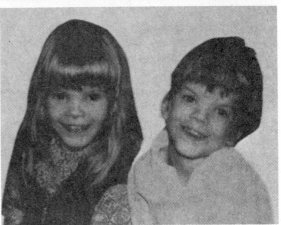

FIG. 16–5

References: Hanson, J.W., and Smith, D.W.: J. Pediatr., 87:285, 1975. Zackai, E.H., Mellman, W.J., Neiderer, B., et al.: J. Pediatr., 87:280, 1975.

# 17

# THERAPEUTICS/ TOXICOLOGY

# POISONING—FERRIC CHLORIDE

A possible aid to diagnosis in potentially poisoned children is 10 per cent ferric chloride solution. A few drops of this material in 5 ml of urine (or serum) may provide an additional clue to diagnosis.

*Conditions and Drugs Associated with Color Reaction of Ferric Chloride*

| CONDITION OR DRUG | COLOR WITH FERRIC CHLORIDE | REACTING MATERIAL |
|---|---|---|
| Phenylketonuria | Blue-green | Phenylpyruvic acid |
| Oasthouse urine disease (methionine mal-absorption) | Purple to red-brown | Alpha-ketobutyrate |
| Odor of rancid butter syndrome (tyrosinemia) | Transient blue-green | Para-hydroxyphenyl-pyruvate |
| Maple syrup urine disease | Greenish gray | Branched chain keto acids |
| Histidinemia | Blue-green | Imidazole pyruvic acid |
| Alkaptonuria | Blue or green transient | Homogentisic acid |
| Ketosis | Reddish brown | Acetoacetic acid |
| Pyruvic acid | Deep yellow | |
| Xanthurenic acid | Dark green | |
| 3-Hydroxyanthranilic acid | Dark brown | |
| Bilirubin | Blue-green | |
| Melanin | Gray precipitate | |
| Alpha-ketobutyric acid | Purple | Faint purple |
| Salicylates | Purple | Purple salicylate |
| Para-aminosalicylic acid | Purplish brown | PAS |
| Isonicotinic hydrazide | Gray | INH |
| Phenothiazines | Purple-brown | |
| Lysol ingestion | Green | |
| Antipyrine or acetophenetidin | Cherry red | |
| Normal urine | Brown-white precipitate | Phosphates, other anions |

Reference: Snyderman, S.: Pediatr. Clin. North Am., *18*:199, 1971.

# POISONING—UNKNOWN POISON

Situations sometimes arise where a possible poisoning has occurred but the amount and nature of the ingested substance are unknown. Features that should suggest poisoning in an ill child include:

1. Abrupt onset of illness
2. Child's age 1 to 4 years
3. History of previous ingestion
4. Multiple organ system involvement that does not fit single disease

Sometimes a combination of symptoms will suggest the drug or poison involved:

| SYMPTOMS AND SIGNS | POSSIBLE POISON |
|---|---|
| Agitation, hallucinations, dilated pupils, bright red color to the skin, dry skin, and fever | Atropine-like agents LSD |
| Marked activity, tremors, headache, diarrhea, dry mouth with foul odor, sweating, tachycardia, arrhythmia, dilated pupils | Amphetamines |
| Slow respirations, pinpoint pupils, euphoria, or coma | Opiates |
| Salivation, lacrimation, urination, defecation, miosis, and pulmonary congestion | Organic phosphates or poison mushrooms |
| Sleepiness, slurred speech, nystagmus, ataxia | Barbiturates or tranquilizers |
| Hypernea, fever, and vomiting | Salicylates |
| Oculogyric crisis, ataxia, and unusual posturing of head and neck | Phenothiazines |
| Nausea, vomiting, sweatiness, and pallor are early manifestations; late manifestations include stupor and signs of liver failure | Acetaminophen |

# POISONING—ACTIVATED CHARCOAL

Initial treatment of poisoning usually calls for removal and/or neutralization of any unabsorbed substance yet remaining in the gastrointestinal tract. The table lists those substances for which activated charcoal (by mouth or by nasogastric tube) is felt to be a useful adjunct to therapy. A slurry of this material suspended, for example, in Hawaiian Punch is tolerated surprisingly well by children when a positive approach is used.

## Inorganic Substances or Their Salts

Arsenic
Silver
Mercury
Potassium permanganate
Iodine or iodides
Phosphorus
Lead
Tin
Titanium
Antimony

## Organic Substances

Acetaminophen
Aconite
Alcohol
Antipyrene
Atropine
Barbiturates
Camphor
Cantharides
Chloroquine
Chlorpheniramine
Chlorpromazine
Cocaine
Delphinium
Digitalis
Elaterin
Ethchlorvynol
Glutethimide
Hemlock
Imipramine
Ipecac
Isoniazid
Kerosene

Mefenamic acid
Methylene blue
Morphine
Muscarine
Nicotine
Nortriptyline
Opium
Oxalates
Paracetamol
Parathione
Penicillins
Phenol
Phenolphthalein
Phenylpropanolamine
Pispantheline
Propoxyphene
Quinine
Salicylates
Stramonium
Strychnine
Sulfonamides
Veratrum

References: Corby, D.G., and Decker, W.J.: Pediatrics, *54*:324, 1974. Harriet Lane Handbook. 6th Ed. Chicago, Year Book Medical Publishers, 1972. p. 175.

**17**

*"Alas! regardless of their doom,
The little victims play;
No sense have they of ills to come,
Nor care beyond today."*

Gray

## INGESTIONS OF LOW TOXICITY

Knowledge of substances that cause little or no toxicity when ingested can be helpful both in immediately allaying parental (and your own) anxiety as well as in preventing iatrogenic problems associated with unnecessary hospitalization, induced emesis, gastric lavage, or other measures used in treatment of ingestions. The table lists those substances that are nontoxic or toxic only in large amounts.

| NO TREATMENT REQUIRED | REMOVAL NECESSARY ONLY IF LARGE AMOUNTS INGESTED |
|---|---|
| Ball-point inks | After-shave lotion |
| Bar soap | Body conditioners |
| Bathtub floating toys | Colognes |
| Battery (dry cell) | Deodorants |
| Bubble bath soap | Fabric softeners |
| Candles | Hair dyes |
| Chalk | Hair sprays |
| Clay (modeling) | Hair tonic |
| Crayons with AP, CP or CS 130–46 designation | Indelible markers |
| Dehumidifying packets | Matches (greater than 20 wooden matches or two books of paper matches) |
| Detergents (anionic) | No Doz |
| Eye makeup | Oral contraceptives |
| Fish bowl additives | Perfumes |
| Golf balls | Suntan preparations |
| Hand lotion and cream | Toilet water |
| Ink (blue, black, red) | |
| Lipstick | |
| Newspaper | |
| Pencils (lead and coloring) | |
| Putty and Silly Putty | |
| Sachets | |
| Shampoo | |
| Shaving cream and shaving lotions | |
| Shoe polish (occasionally aniline dyes present) | |
| Striking surface materials of matchboxes | |
| Sweetening agents (saccharin, cyclamate) | |
| Teething rings | |
| Thermometers | |
| Toothpaste | |

The minimal toxicity associated with these substances should not preclude investigation of the circumstances of the ingestion or advice regarding future preventive measures.

Reference: Mathies, A.W.: *In* Gellis, S.S. and Kagan, B.M. (Eds.): Current Pediatric Therapy. 6th Ed. Philadelphia, W.B. Saunders Company, 1973, p. 730.

# THE ANATOMY OF POISONING

The ingestion of drugs or toxins by children is frequently not an "accident." The physician should always gather all the facts surrounding an ingestion because it may indicate the presence of chronic stress in a household. If efforts are not directed to correct such circumstances, a repeat ingestion can occur.

A study of 94 episodes of aspirin poisoning in children 1 to 5 years of age revealed the following three patterns of ingestion.

## Transient Unusual Episode in Home

In such circumstances, the normal family routine was disrupted by a nonfamily visitor or the presence of illness in a member of the family. In this setting, the aspirin was unusually available because it had been used to treat a member of the family.

## Unusual Resourcefulness by Child

In these instances, the majority of incidents were social in nature, with several children sharing the drug as "play medicine" or candy. Children often displayed unusual skill and curiosity in obtaining the medicine.

## Serious Chronic Family Situations

These instances were characterized by one-parent homes, marital discord, working mothers, inadequate play space, and other signs of strife.

Try to categorize the circumstances of ingestion in your patients so that appropriate advice and guidance can be offered.

---

Reference: Meyer, R.J.: Am. J. Dis. Child., *102*:47, 1961.

# SUBSTANCES SECRETED IN HUMAN MILK

Fortunately, an increasing number of mothers are choosing to breast-feed their infants. The following list will enable you to advise mothers properly concerning the drugs that may appear in their milk if ingested while nursing. The concentrations present in milk are indicated in parentheses where that information is known.

Alcohol
Anthraquinone, 1, 8-dihydroxy (Dorbane, Dorbantyl)
Atropine (less than 0.1 mg/100 ml of milk when mother takes
  600 mg daily)
Bromide (0 to 6.6 mg/100 ml of milk when mother takes 1 gm
  5 times daily for 3 days)
Caffeine (1 per cent of that ingested)

**17**

Chloral hydrate (0 to 1.5 mg/100 ml of milk when mother receives 1.33 gm suppository)

Chloramphenicol (2.5 mg/100 ml of milk when mother takes 250 mg 4 times daily by mouth)

Chlorpromazine (tested only in dogs)

Cortisone (tested only in rats)

DDT (tested only in dogs and goats)

Diphenhydramine (Benadryl)

Diphtheria antibodies (less than 0.30 per cent of dose administered)

Ergot

Erythromycin (tested only in cows and goats)

Estrogen (tested only in cows)

Ethyl biscoumacetate (Tromexan) (0 to 0.17 mg/100 ml of milk — no correlation with dosage)

Folic acid (0.7 micrograms/liter of milk)

Heroin

Hexachlorobenzene

Hydroxypropylcarbamate (Robaxin) ("small amounts")

$^{131}$I (total in 48-hour sample of milk = 1.3 microcuries)

Isoniazid (0.6 to 1.2 mg/100 ml of milk when mother taking 5 to 10 mg/kg every 10 hours)

Mandelic acid (0.3 gm/24 hours when mother taking 12 gm daily)

Nicotine (trace present in milk when mother smoking 10 to 20 cigarettes per day)

Novobiocin (0.3 to 0.5 mg/100 ml of milk when mother receiving 250 mg every 6 hours)

Penethamate hydriodide (Leocillin) (tested only in cows and goats)

Penicillin (2 to 6 units/100 ml of milk when sample taken 2 hours after mother received 100,000 units)

Pentothal ("small amounts" present in milk)

Phenylbutazone (Butazolidin) (0.63 mg/100 ml of milk when mother taking 750 mg intramuscularly every 1½ hours)

Phenytoin (Dilantin)

Prochlorperazine (Compazine) (tested only in dogs)

Propoxyphene (Darvon) (tested only in rats)

Pyrazolone (Isopyrin) (2.3 mg/100 ml of milk when mother received 1200 mg)

Pyrimethamine (Daraprim)

Quinine sulfate (0 to 0.1 mg/100 ml of milk when mother taking 300 to 600 mg 3 times daily)

Rh antibodies

Senna (Senokot)

Sodium salicylate (1.0 to 3.0 mg/100 ml of milk when mother taking 4 gm every 4 hours)

Sulfanilamide (9 mg/100 ml of milk when mother taking 2 to 4 gm daily)

Sulfapyridine (3 to 13 mg/100 ml of milk when mother taking 3 gm daily)

Sulfathiazole (0.5 mg/100 ml of milk when mother taking 3 gm daily)

Tetracycline (0.5 to 2.6 micrograms/ml of milk when mother taking 500 mg 4 times daily per os for 3 days)

Thiouracil (9 to 12 mg/100 ml of milk when mother took 1 gm 2
   hours before sampling)
Trifluoperazine (Stelazine) (tested only in dogs)
Vitamin $B_1$ (1.0 to 13 micrograms/liter of milk)
Vitamin $B_{12}$ (0.1 to 0.4 micrograms/liter of milk)

The following drugs have been found not to be secreted in human milk.

Barbital
Codeine
Imipramine (Tofranil)
Morphine
Oxacillin
Potassium iodide
Phenolphthalein

Some general principles should be kept in mind when advising a nursing mother.

1. Most drugs a woman takes will be excreted in her milk. The amount is usually small and has no effect on the infant. It is rarely necessary to advise the mother to discontinue nursing because of medications she is taking.
2. When the drug the mother must take is potent enough to suspect that minute quantities may be harmful to the infant, cessation or temporary discontinuation of nursing may be necessary. Such drugs are anticoagulants, antineoplastic drugs, and radioactive products.
3. Drugs with significant antigenic properties, such as penicillin, may require temporary discontinuation of nursing.
4. If the mother has ingested a toxic substance, such as heavy metals or benzene, nursing should cease.
5. If the mother is significantly ill and in negative calcium or nitrogen balance or is vitamin deficient, continuation of nursing is potentially dangerous for both mother and child.

References: Avery, G.B.: Neonatology: Pathophysiology and Management of the Newborn. Toronto, J.B. Lippincott Company, 1975, p. 1092. Knowles, J.A.: Drug Therapy, May 1973, p. 57.

## THE ANTIPYRETIC EFFECTS OF ASPIRIN AND ACETAMINOPHEN

**17**

Is aspirin any better than acetaminophen (Tylenol) for reducing fever? Studies indicate that used in equivalent doses, they do the same job.

The table on page 430 gives you some indication as to how fast these agents act and how much reduction in temperature you can expect.

*Fall in Temperature (C°) After Treatment*

| DRUG | TIME (HR) | | | |
|---|---|---|---|---|
| | ½ | 1 | 1½ | 2 |
| Aspirin | 0.4 | 0.8 | 1.2 | 1.5 |
| Acetaminophen | 0.6 | 1.1 | 1.5 | 1.6 |

Maximum temperature depression occurs 2 to 3 hours after ingestion. The effect of the drug begins to disappear within 3 to 4 hours and is totally gone by 6 hours.

Reference: Hunter, J.: Arch. Dis. Child., *48*:313, 1973.

## THE "DONE NOMOGRAM" FOR SALICYLATE INTOXICATION

The nomogram in Figure 17–1 has proved extremely useful as a rough guide to the severity of salicylate intoxication in previously well patients. In order to use the nomogram appropriately, you must know the approximate time of ingestion as well as make the assumption that the salicylate was all taken over a brief period. The nomogram helps to identify rapidly those patients who are not likely to recover with conventional treatment alone.

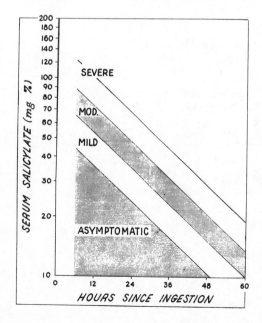

*FIG. 17–1*

Nomogram relating serum salicylate concentration and expected severity of intoxication at varying intervals following the ingestion of a single dose of salicylate.

Reference: Done, A.K.: Pediatrics, *26*:800, 1960.

# ASPIRIN SENSITIVITY IN CHILDREN WITH ASTHMA

Intrinsic asthma, nasal polyps, and aspirin intolerance form a constellation that has been well recognized in adults. Aspirin sensitivity has recently been detected in 14 (28 per cent) of a group of 50 children with atopic asthma. This sensitivity was manifested by a 30 per cent reduction in FEP (maximal midexpiratory flow rate) lasting four hours or more. Characteristics of the children who demonstrated aspirin sensitivity included the following:

Most were female
Most had experienced onset of asthma before the age of 2 years
They had more frequent episodes of sinusitis than other
  children with asthma

None of these children were aware of their aspirin sensitivity, although all of them had taken aspirin in the past. This failure to detect sensitivity may be due to the delay in onset of manifestations by 30 minutes to one hour. Another reason for failure to identify aspirin as a cause for worsening symptoms may be the presence of salicylates in a wide variety of preparations that the asthmatic child may ingest. In addition to many pain relievers not identified as "aspirin," salicylates are also contained in indomethacin and tartrazine (a yellow coloring material found in soft drinks, canned vegetables, and, until recently, in Marax, a drug used frequently in the treatment of asthma).

There is little evidence for the genetic transmission of aspirin sensitivity, and the mechanism for the sensitivity is not known.

It seems reasonable to avoid aspirin administration in any child who suffers from asthma.

Reference: Rachelefsky, G.S., Coulson, A., Siegel, S.C., et al.: Pediatrics, 56:443, 1975.

# "BLACK TONGUE FEVER"

Pepto-Bismol is used frequently in the treatment of gastroenteritis. It is well recognized that this medication may cause black stools (pseudomelena), which results from the oxidation of bismuth, possibly

**17**

enhanced by fever. Patients taking Pepto-Bismol for the treatment of gastroenteritis may also develop a black discoloration of the tongue and buccal mucosa. If the cause of this finding is unrecognized, it may be quite alarming to both patient and physician.

---

Reference: William H. Dietz, Jr.: Personal communication, 1976.

# DRUG DOSAGE IN PATIENTS WITH RENAL DISEASE

The administration of drugs to patients with renal disease is a complicated process. Careful attention to rational physiological principles can simplify this task and safeguard the patient.

The following tables and nomograms have been developed to facilitate the process of computing dosage schedules.

The table below provides overall elimination rate constants for a variety of drugs in patients with normal kidney function ($k_n$) and in anuric patients ($k_{nr}$). Patients with normal renal function are assumed to have a creatinine clearance of 100 ml/min, while anuric patients are assumed to have a creatinine clearance of 0 ml/min.

*Overall Elimination Rate Constants of 31 Drugs in Anuric Patients ($k_{nr}$) and in Patients with Normal Kidney Function ($k_n$)*

|  | $k_{nr}$ (per hour) | $k_n$ (per hour) |
|---|---|---|
| Penicillin G | 0.03 | 1.4 |
| Ampicillin | 0.1 | 0.8 |
| Methicillin | 0.17 | 1.4 |
| Oxacillin | 0.35 | 1.4 |
| Carbenicillin | 0.06 | 0.6 |
| Cephalothin | 0.03 (?) | 1.4 |
| Cephalexin | 0.03 | 0.7 |
| Cephazolin | 0.02 | 0.36 |
| Tetracycline | 0.01 | 0.08 |
| Chlortetracycline | 0.1 | 0.1 |
| Doxycycline | 0.03 | 0.03 |
| Minocycline | 0.04 | 0.06 |
| Chloramphenicol | 0.3 | 0.3 |
| Rifampin | 0.25 | 0.25 |
| Isoniazid (fast inactivators) | 0.3 | 0.5 |
| Isoniazid (slow inactivators) | 0.1 | 0.2 |
| Streptomycin | 0.01 | 0.27 |
| Kanamycin | 0.01 | 0.35 |
| Vancomycin | 0.003 | 0.12 |
| Gentamicin | 0.007 | 0.3 |
| Tobramycin | 0.005 | 0.35 |
| Colistin | 0.02 | 0.3 |

| | | |
|---|---|---|
| Polymyxin | 0.02 | 0.16 |
| Erythromycin | 0.13 | 0.5 |
| 5-Fluorocytosine | 0.007 | 0.25 |
| Sulfamethoxazole | 0.7 | 0.7 |
| Sulfadiazine | 0.03 | 0.08 |
| Trimethoprim | 0.02 | 0.06 |
| Procainamide | 0.007 | 0.21 |
| | *(per day)* | *(per day)* |
| Digoxin | 0.17 | 0.45 |
| Digitoxin | 0.24 | 0.72 |

The values listed in the table are used in conjunction with the nomogram in Figure 17–2 for computing dosage schedules.

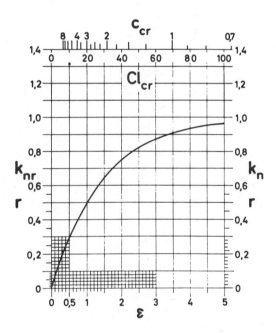

*FIG. 17–2*

*Steps in Calculation*

1. Locate in table the drug to be administered and record values for $k_n$ and $k_{nr}$.

2. Enter these points on nomogram at appropriate points on left- and right-hand columns of the nomogram. Draw a line connecting these points. This is the dosing line.

3. Next, locate the point at the upper margin of the nomogram that corresponds to the patient's creatinine clearance. The serum creatinine ($C_{cr}$) may also be employed if the patient is in a stable state, is not undergoing dialysis, or does not have a significant muscle disease, and if the serum creatinine value is not greater than 8 mg/100 ml.

**17**

4. Draw a line from the value for creatinine clearance that intercepts the dosing line. This will give you the "r" value or elimination rate constant for the patient. The "r" values are indicated on the left and right ordinates of the nomogram.

5. The drug half-life (t½) for the drug in the patient is then equal to:

$$\frac{0.7}{\text{elimination rate constant (r)}}$$

Example:

What is the drug half-life for penicillin G in a patient with a creatinine clearance of 55 ml/min?

Solution (depicted in nomogram in Figure 17–3):

1. The $k_n$ value for penicillin is 1.4 and the $k_{nr}$ is 0.03.
2. A straight line is drawn between these points on the nomogram.
3. The creatinine clearance is 55 ml/min.
4. A line intercepting the creatinine clearance and the dosing line gives an r value of 0.75.
5. The half-life of penicillin in this patient is:

$$\frac{0.7}{0.75} \quad \text{or} \quad 0.93 \text{ hours}$$

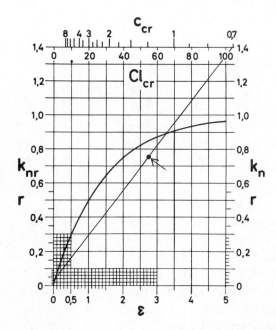

FIG. 17–3

The loading dose employed in the patient with renal disease should be no different from that used in the normal patient. Adjustments should be made in the dosing interval *or* the maintenance dose. If the calculated $t_{1/2}$ is shorter than the usual dosing interval, adjustment should be made in the amount of drug given per dose. The usual dosing interval for penicillin is three hours; therefore, the patient described in the example may be given penicillin every three hours.

One must also determine the relative dosage interval ($\epsilon$). This value is used to determine the percentage reduction of the maintenance dose. It is calculated in the following way:

$$\epsilon = \frac{\text{normal dosage interval}}{t_{1/2} \text{ in patient}}$$

In our example, this value would be $\dfrac{3 \text{ hours}}{1 \text{ hour}} = 3$.

Once $\epsilon$ has been calculated, return to the nomogram and find the point on the solid curved line at which $\epsilon$ intercepts the line (Fig. 17–4).

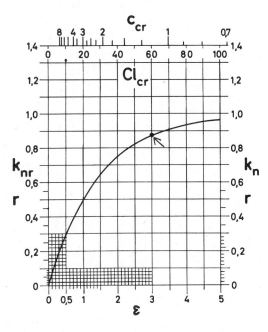

*FIG. 17–4*

When $\epsilon$ is 3, the line intercepts the curve at a point that corresponds to 0.88 on the ordinate. Thus, the patient in the example should receive 88 per cent of the usual penicillin maintenance dose every three hours, following the normal loading dose.

Let us try another example.

Assume that the patient to whom you want to give penicillin has a creatinine clearance of only 8 ml/min. According to the dosing line drawn on the nomogram previously, the r value for this patient (the point where a creatinine clearance intersects the dosing line) is 0.14.

The half-life of penicillin in this patient is then $\frac{0.7}{0.14}$, or five hours. The loading dose should remain the same as that for the patient without renal disease. Since the half-life of five hours is longer than the normal dosing interval of three hours, adjustment must be made in both the dosing interval and the maintenance dose. For this patient, the maintenance dose should be one-half the loading dose. This maintenance dose should be administered at five-hour intervals, since the half-life of the drug is five hours in this patient.

*Summary*

1. Draw on the nomogram the dosing line for the drug you wish to use.

2. Find the r value, using the dosing line and the creatinine clearance of the patient.

3. Calculate the half-life of the drug: $\frac{0.7}{r}$

4. If the half-life is shorter than the usual dosing interval, give the patient the normal loading dose, and then calculate $\epsilon = \frac{\text{(normal dosage interval)}}{\text{half-life in patient}}$. The percentage of normal maintenance dose to be given is determined by the point on the ordinate corresponding to the intersection of $\epsilon$ and the solid curved line.

5. If the half-life of the drug is greater than the normal dosage interval, give the normal loading dose, then give a maintenance dose of one-half the loading dose, and give it at intervals equal to the $t_{1/2}$ of the drug for the patient.

# A SIMPLETON'S GUIDE TO DIURETICS

| AGENT | MECHANISM OF ACTION | SIDE-EFFECTS |
|---|---|---|
| Sulfonamide derivatives Thiazide diuretics and their congeners | Inhibit sodium reabsorption in the cortical portion of the ascending tubule and the distal convoluted tubule (site of 10% of all sodium reabsorption). Possess a flat dose-response curve beyond the upper limits of dosage. | Hypokalemia and hypochloremic alkalosis Hyperuricemia Hyperglycemia Azotemia (avoid in patients with impaired renal function) Hypercalcemia Hyponatremia (Gastrointestinal upset, weakness, dry mouth, bad taste in mouth, leukopenia, thrombocytopenia, pancreatitis, skin rash, photosensitivity.) |
| Loop diuretics Furosemide (Lasix) Ethacrynic acid (Edecrin) | Inhibit sodium reabsorption in the ascending limb of the loop of Henle, where almost 20% of all sodium is reabsorbed. More potent than the "thiazide" diuretics. Possess an infinite dose-response curve, therefore more dangerous. Will work in volume-depleted patient. Should be used only in refractory edema or in presence of renal failure. | Similar to side-effects listed above. Exceptions are: Do not cause hypercalcemia. Ethacrynic acid unlikely to produce photosensitivity but produces more gastrointestinal upset. May produce temporary nerve deafness when given intravenously and rapidly to azotemic patients. |
| Distal tubular diuretics Spironolactone (Aldactone) Triamterene (Dyrenium) | Prevent exchange of sodium for potassium in distal tubule. Only 5% of sodium reabsorption occurs here. Spironolactone is a specific inhibitor of aldosterone. | Hyperkalemia (drug contraindicated in patients with renal failure). Gastrointestinal side-effects. Spironolactone may produce gynecomastia, hirsutism, and menstrual irregularities. |

17

*The Diuretic of Choice in Patients without Edema*

| DIAGNOSIS | DIURETIC |
| --- | --- |
| Primary (essential) hypertension | |
|    Normal renal function | Thiazide class |
|    Impaired renal function | Loop class |
| Primary aldosteronism | Spironolactone |
| Hypercalcemia | Loop class |
| Idiopathic hypercalciuria | Thiazide class |
| Nephrogenic diabetes insipidus | Thiazide class |

*The Diuretic of Choice in Patients with Edema*

| DIAGNOSIS | DIURETIC |
| --- | --- |
| Congestive heart failure | Thiazide class (take precautions to avoid hypokalemia if patient receiving digitalis) |
| Nephrotic syndrome | Thiazide and spironolactone |
| Cirrhosis and ascites | Thiazide and spironolactone |
| Acute and chronic renal failure | Loop class |
| Chronic lymphedema | Thiazide class |

# THE USE OF GLUCOCORTICOSTEROIDS

The multiple clinical uses of glucocorticosteroids reflect the many modes of action of these drugs. The effects of glucocorticoids may be divided into two general categories: the anti-inflammatory effects and the immunosuppressive effects. The mechanisms by which these effects are attained are outlined below.

*Anti-inflammatory Effects*

Vascular stabilization
   Maintenance of vascular tone
   Reduction of capillary permeability and resulting edema
Decreased leukocyte accumulation
   Decreased adherence of leukocytes to endothelium of
     small blood vessels
   Decreased neutrophil and monocyte chemotaxis

Transient monocytopenia and eosinopenia
Decreased bactericidal effect of monocytes
Decreased level of complement components

## Immunosuppressive Effects

Decreased circulatory lymphocytes and monocytes
Decreased lymphocytes, monocytes, and macrophage function
Decreased clearance of opsonized and nonopsonized materials
by the reticuloendothelial system
Decreased levels of serum immunoglobulins and complement
Interference with passage of immune complexes across the
basement membranes
Inhibition of immune clearance of sensitized erythrocytes

The mechanisms by which lymphocyte function is decreased are listed in the following table.

| PROCESS | RECOGNIZED EFFECTS | CONTROVERSIAL EFFECTS |
|---|---|---|
| Delayed hypersensitivity | Decreased expression of lymphocyte function | |
| Antigen processing | Decreased lymphoid cell access to antigen in inflammatory sites | Macrophage processing per se |
| Lymphocyte activity | Normal lymphocyte sensitization | |
| Lymphocyte proliferation | Decreased antigen-induced blastogenesis | Mitogen blastogenesis |
| Mediator production | Normal release of MIF, MAF and SRF | Release of LT and MCTF |
| Response to mediators | Decreased effect of MIF and MAF on macrophage | Effect on activity of LT and MCTF |
| Cell-mediated cytotoxicity | Target cell protection | Killer lymphocyte function |

MIF = macrophage migration inhibitory factor; MAF = macrophage aggregating factor; SRF = skin-reactive factor; LT = lymphotoxin; MCTF = monocyte chemotactic factor.

The use of corticosteroid medications may be clarified by reference to the following table, which compares equivalent potency, sodium-retaining potency, and half-life in plasma of the commonly used glucocorticosteroids.

**17**

| COMPOUND | EQUIVALENT POTENCY (mg) | SODIUM-RETAINING POTENCY | PLASMA T½ (min) |
|---|---|---|---|
| Cortisone | 25 | 2+ | 30 |
| Cortisol | 20 | 2+ | 90 |
| Prednisone | 5 | 1+ | 60 |
| Prednisolone | 5 | 1+ | 200 |
| Methylprednisolone | 4 | 0 | 180 |
| Triamcinolone | 4 | 0 | 300 |
| Dexamethasone | 0.75 | 0 | 200 |

The dangers of glucocorticoid therapy are almost as numerous as the clinical uses. Many of these dangers may be allayed by alternate-day rather than daily divided dosage. The advantages of alternate-day therapy are as follows:

1. Manifestations of Cushing's syndrome, retardation of linear growth, and suppression of delayed hypersensitivity may be ameliorated or prevented.
2. Urinary excretion of nitrogen and potassium is not increased over controls.
3. Susceptibility to infection is not increased.
4. There is little or no hypothalamic-pituitary-adrenal (HPA) suppression.
5. Effectiveness is equivalent to daily divided doses in all conditions tested except in giant cell arteritis.

Pitfalls that may be encountered with the use of alternate-day therapy are listed below.

1. Alternate-day doses are beneficial in the initial treatment of some disorders, but not in others. Initial therapy for acute fulminant cases of ulcerative colitis or pemphigus vulgaris may be unsuccessful unless daily doses are used. Treatment has been successful with alternate-day doses from the outset in patients with the nephrotic syndrome, lupus, nephritis, rheumatoid arthritis, myasthenia gravis, asthma, sarcoidosis, rheumatic fever, and a variety of ocular diseases.
2. There is no reason to use alternate-day therapy if treatment is anticipated for several weeks or less.
3. Institution of alternate-day therapy instead of daily doses must be gradual to prevent symptoms of adrenal insufficiency.
4. Side-effects may not be prevented if a long-acting form is used or if frequent doses are given on alternating days.
5. Supplemental, nonsteroid medication should not be neglected. For example, symptoms of rheumatoid arthritis or asthma may be worse on the day-off therapy, but on these days use of antiinflammatory medication or bronchodilators may be encouraged.
6. Patients who do not understand the advantages to alternate-day treatment may enjoy the daily euphoria they had been used to on daily medication. The benefits of alternate-day therapy must be carefully explained to patients so that compliance will be optimal.

When alternate-day therapy is impossible, single, daily doses have been shown to prevent HPA suppression and are as effective in controlling disease as daily divided doses. Cushing's syndrome is not prevented with single daily doses, however.

Patients being treated with pharmacologic doses of glucocorticoids for longer than one to four weeks should be assumed to have HPA suppression. This should be taken into consideration during anesthesia or any other metabolically stressful experiences.

---

References: Fauci, A.S., Dale, D.C., and Balow, J.E.: Ann. Intern. Med., *84*:304, 1976. Axelrod, L.: Medicine, *55*:39, 1976.

# CALCULATING THE DOSE OF PARENTERAL IRON

The use of intramuscular iron to correct anemia in iron-deficient infants and children is rarely indicated. The indications include the following.

    1. Demonstrated noncompliance by parents in the administration of oral iron.
    2. Anticipated noncompliance.
    3. Presence of disease involving the stomach and upper small bowel.
    4. Rare instances of demonstrated iron malabsorption.

It should be remembered that the administration of parenteral iron will not raise the hemoglobin level any more quickly than oral iron therapy. When intramuscular iron therapy is indicated, the following procedure should be followed in determining the appropriate dose of medication.

*Principles*

    1. Each gram of hemoglobin requires 3.4 mg of iron.
    2. Must supply enough iron to synthesize hemoglobin deficit and replenish body iron stores.
    3. Assume a blood volume of 75 ml/kg.

*Steps in Procedure*

    1. Calculate hemoglobin deficit.
    2. Multiply deficit by 3.4.
    3. Give an additional 50 per cent to restore iron stores.

*Example*

A 10 kg infant has a hemoglobin of 6 gm/100 ml. He will require Imferon. What is his required dose?

**17**

1. Blood volume is

$$(10 \text{ kg} \times 75 \text{ ml/kg}) = 750 \text{ ml}$$

2. Hemoglobin deficit is

(desired Hb – observed Hb)
$$12.0 - 6.0 = 6.0 \text{ g/100 ml}$$

Body hemoglobin deficit is

$$6.0 \times 7.5 = 45 \text{ g}$$

3. Iron for hemoglobin deficit is

$$45 \times 3.4 = 153 \text{ mg}$$

4. Body iron stores require an additional 50 per cent

$$0.50 \times 153 = 76 \text{ mg}$$

5. Total iron required is $153 + 76 = 229$ mg

6. Patient will require 4.5 ml of Imferon (Imferon contains 50 mg/ml)

7. Formula can be reduced to the following:

*ml* of Imferon = Wt (kg) $\times$ desired Hb rise (gm/100 ml)
required $\times$ 0.076

in previous example
$$= 10 \times 6 \times 0.076$$
$$= 4.5 \text{ ml}$$

8. Children under 1 year of age should not receive more than 2 ml at one time. Between ages 1 and 2 years, 3 ml at one time should be maximal dose. Give Imferon on alternate days if more than one dose is required. Do not give more than 2 ml in one site.

## PITFALLS IN ANTICONVULSANT DRUG THERAPY

Seizures are a common and often difficult management problem for the pediatrician. Careful attention to detail in the treatment of the child with seizures will often eliminate mistakes in management that make intervention by the physician part of the problem instead of part of the solution. The common treatment errors are listed below.

1. Incomplete evaluation prior to the institution of treatment: Every child with seizures should have a fasting blood sugar, serum calcium and phosphorus, and BUN determinations before the institution of anticonvulsant therapy. Seizures resulting from metabolic disorders are not controlled by anticonvulsants.

2. Making the wrong drug choice: Correct treatment of seizure disorders varies, depending upon the classification of the seizures. Grand mal, focal motor, myoclonic, and psychomotor seizures should be treated with barbiturates and/or phenytoin; however, treatment for petit mal seizures should include ethosuccimide, acetazolamide, or methsuximide.

3. Prescribing an insufficient dose: Accurate dosage is important, and careful attention should be paid to the need to increase dosage as the child grows.

4. Institution of therapy with two drugs at once: One drug is usually sufficient in the treatment of a seizure disorder if appropriate doses are employed and if measurement of blood levels ensures optimal concentration is present. Side-effects are more frequent with two drugs, and it is difficult to determine which drug is the cause of the side-effect if a combination of drugs is being used. If seizures persist and side-effects are encountered with increasing doses of one drug, the dose of that drug should be lowered, and therapy with a second drug should be instituted.

5. Use of liquid medication: Liquid medication, especially if mixed with food or other liquid, may be incompletely swallowed, spit out, or lost by dribbling or drooling. Particles in suspensions may be incompletely dissolved, and the child may receive too little medication on one day and too much on another day. Tablet medication provides more uniform dosage, and the tablet may be made palatable by crushing it and mixing it with a variety of foods.

6. Misinterpretation of blood levels: Noncompliance is perhaps the most common cause of lack of control of seizures, and the determination of blood levels of the drug prescribed helps to detect failure to receive adequate doses. Blood levels also help to determine which drug is responsible for toxic symptoms in a child who is taking more than one medication. It should not be assumed that noncompliance is the only reason for low blood levels, however. Phenytoin may be incompletely absorbed from the gastrointestinal tract, and increasing oral dosage may be necessary to bring about therapeutic levels of this drug. Patients being treated with phenytoin may have optimal levels of circulating drug for the first few months of treatment, but subsequent measurement reveals suboptimal concentrations despite compliance and maintenance of the same drug dosage. These decreasing concentrations may precipitate seizure episodes.

Therefore, blood levels of anticonvulsant drugs should be used to achieve optimal dosage at the institution of therapy and to ensure the maintenance of adequate drug concentration.

7. Failure to recognize behavioral side-effects: Behavioral alterations in children being treated with anticonvulsant medication may include hyperactivity, agitation, irritability, insomnia, and general irascibility, as well as the oversedation seen in adults. Phenobarbital and primidone are usually responsible for the "paradoxical response" seen in children. Children who respond in this way should be treated with another barbiturate or a nonbarbiturate anticonvulsant.

8. Early termination of treatment: Parents and children may exert pressure on the physician to terminate medication after a long seizure-free period. The physician should not succumb to such pressure, but rather should follow the current guidelines for length of anticonvulsant treatment for the particular type of seizures to which the child is subject (see p. 339).

9. Excessive restrictions on the child's activity: Children with seizure disorders should not be unduly restricted, and their parents should be made aware of their normal capabilities.

10. Inadequate counseling: Parents should be made fully aware of known facts about seizure disorders and the plan for treatment. Emotional reactions to the

**17**

diagnosis should be expected and should be dealt with by the physician. Counseling should include specific suggestions about information to be given to the child's school, to the parents of the child's friends, and to any others whose attitudes toward the child may change.

Reference:  Ferry, P.C.: Drug Therapy, August 1974, p. 37.

# PROPHYLAXIS FOR CONTACTS IN MENINGOCOCCAL DISEASE

A diagnosis of meningococcal disease often precipitates unnecessary anxiety among those who have been in contact with the patient. Who requires prophylactic treatment? The following facts should provide guidelines in making a decision.

1.  In nonepidemic situations, close contacts are the only ones at significant risk of acquiring meningococcal disease. Close contacts are defined as "those individuals who slept and ate in the same dwelling as the index case" and include household and day care nursery contacts. The attack rate for all household contacts is approximately 6 per cent; for 1 to 4 year olds, the rate is nearly 12 per cent.

Other school or kindergarten contacts, casual contacts on buses or airplanes, and hospital contacts are *not* considered close contacts and are *not* candidates for prophylactic antibiotics. One important exception is anyone who has given mouth-to-mouth resuscitation to a patient with meningococcal disease.

2.  Throat cultures are *not* helpful in deciding which contacts are at risk. Those with negative cultures for meningococci may be at the same risk as those with positive cultures.

3.  Sulfonamides are no longer used for prophylaxis because a large proportion of strains are resistant to this drug. Current recommendations for close contacts include either close observation with no antibiotics, or rifampin twice a day for two days. Both recommendations have their adherents among infectious disease experts.

No matter which course is chosen, the approach to contacts who develop any objective symptoms (e.g., exanthem, pharyngitis, fever, or meningeal signs) is the same. They are hospitalized and, after blood and cerebrospinal fluid are obtained, they are treated for 36 to 48 hours with intravenous penicillin G (or chloramphenicol, if penicillin-allergic) as if they had meningococcal disease. Decision to continue therapy at the end of this period is based on culture results.

References: Artenstein, M.: J.A.M.A., *231*:1035, 1975. McCormick, J.B., and Bennett, J.V.: Ann. Intern. Med., *83*:883, 1975.

# SIDE-EFFECTS OF ANTICONVULSANTS

Awareness of potential side-effects of anticonvulsants is important for their safe long-term use. The following two tables describe specific side-effects and include comments on detection and management of the more common side-effects.

| GENERIC NAME | TRADE NAME | DROWSINESS | NYSTAGMUS, DIPLOPIA, AND/OR ATAXIA | HYPERACTIVITY, BEHAVIOR CHANGE | HEPATITIS | RENAL INVOLVE-MENT | RASH | BLOOD DYSCRASIA | GASTRO-INTESTINAL UPSET | LUPUS-LIKE SYNDROME | OSTEO-MALACIA | MISCELLANEOUS |
|---|---|---|---|---|---|---|---|---|---|---|---|---|
| Phenobarbital | Many | X | X | X | | | X | | | | X | Rash uncommon |
| Phenytoin | Dilantin | X | X | | X | | X | X | X | X | X | Drowsiness uncommon; hypertrichosis and/or gingival hyperplasia |
| Mephenytoin | Mesantoin | X | | | X | | | X | | X | | |
| Ethosuccimide | Zarontin | X | | X | | | X | X | X | X | | |
| Carbamazepine | Tegretol | X | X | | X | X | X | X | X | X | | Neuropathy or cardiac problems may be seen |
| Trimethadione | Tridione | X | | | X | X | X | X | | X | | Visual problems (hemeralopia) |
| Primidone | Mysoline | X | X | | | X | X | X | X | X | X | |
| Mephobarbital | Mebaral | | | Similar to phenobarbital. | | | | | | | | |
| Paramethadione | Paradione | | | Similar to trimethadione. | | | | | | | | |

## Side Effects of Anticonvulsants

| SIDE-EFFECT | COMMENT |
|---|---|
| Drowsiness | Usually dose-related; try dosage adjustment. |
| Nystagmus, diplopia, and/or ataxia | Frequently encountered with phenytoin; usually dose-related; often manageable by dose reduction. |
| Hyperactivity and/or behavioral changes | Most often encountered with phenobarbital; an idiosyncratic reaction; dosage adjustment *not* helpful. |
| Gingival hyperplasia | Most common with phenytoin; maximal after 9 to 12 months of therapy; can be minimized — but *not* eliminated — by fastidious oral hygiene; gingivectomy may be indicated. |
| Hepatic involvement | Periodic liver function studies indicated when using drug associated with hepatitis; parents should be asked to notify you of any symptoms (e.g., jaundice, malaise, fever, dark urine) possibly referable to the liver; stop drug immediately if hepatic involvement found. |
| Renal involvement | Periodic urinalyses and renal function studies indicated if drug associated with renal problems (e.g., trimethadione). |
| Skin rash | May be accompanied by lymphadenopathy, fever, and hematopoietic disorders (particularly leukopenia); anticonvulsants should be stopped immediately upon noting rash (remember to substitute another drug); if the rash is mild and disappears completely, is not associated with the above, or other systemic signs, *and* is not hemorrhagic, exfoliative or bulbous in character, a cautious trial of the same drug may be tried. |
| Hematologic involvement | May affect platelets, neutrophils, or red cells; periodic CBC indicated when using drug known to be associated with this problem. |
| Lupus-like syndrome | Usually resolves some time after drug discontinued; antinuclear antibodies may persist for months or years. |
| Gastrointestinal upsets | Usually dose-related; often manageable by dividing dose or giving with meals. *Rule out hepatic involvement.* |
| Osteomalacia | *May* be related to duration of therapy; serum calcium and phosphorus usually normal; alkaline phosphatase may be elevated. |

References: Livingston, S.: *In* Gellis, S.S., and Kagan, B.M. (Eds.): Current Pediatric Therapy. 6th Ed. Philadelphia, W.B. Saunders Company, 1973. Guinane, J.E.: *In* Gellis, S.S., and Kagan, B.M. (Eds.): Current Pediatric Therapy. 7th Ed. Philadelphia, W.B. Saunders Company, 1976.

# DRUG ALLERGY

Both immunologic (allergic) and nonimmunologic reactions to drugs may occur. Nonimmune reactions, sometimes difficult to distinguish from allergic reactions, include intolerance, overdose, side-effects, idiosyncrasy, and secondary effects.

The following aphorisms relating to drug allergy may be useful in preventing or treating such problems.

1. Patients who react to one drug are more likely to react to others.

2. Before prescribing any drug, obtain as precise a history as possible of the patient's prior experience with the drug.

3. If a choice is available between an oral or a systemically administered drug, always choose the oral route.

4. Always check the exact composition of a drug, particularly if the prescription is a combination of drugs; e.g., many combinations contain varying amounts of aspirin, which can cause severe responses in the aspirin-sensitive patient.

5. The incidence of drug allergy is greater in adults than in children.

6. Always stop a drug at the first sign of an adverse reaction. Patients and/or parents should be given such instructions before the medication is prescribed.

7. Intermittent administration of drugs is more likely to result in an allergic reaction.

8. Reactions generally do not occur on initial exposure. Usually a latent period exists prior to reaction. An exception to this is illustrated by reactions provoked by chemically related drugs. For example, a patient with known sensitivity to procaine received a sulfa preparation, which is biologically related to procaine, and promptly developed a urticarial reaction.

9. Patients with proved drug sensitivity should wear a bracelet or other conspicuous emblem detailing their specific sensitivities. Medic Alert Foundation, P.O. Box 1009, Turlock, California, 95380, provides this type of emblem.

10. Aspirin is probably the most widely used and abused medication in the United States. Aspirin sensitivity, probably not mediated by immune mechanisms, is a source of concern because it is seen with increasing frequency. Acetaminophen, available as Dularin, Tylenol, Datril, and Valadol, is a suitable substitute and should be used in preference to aspirin, unless the latter is clearly needed.

11. Corticosteroid hormones are not useful for immediate effect in severe drug-allergic reactions. Epinephrine and antihistaminics are needed for immediate effect, and corticosteroid hormones should be included only if it is anticipated that a beneficial response is required 4 to 24 hours later.

---

Reference: Berman, B.A.: *In* Gellis, S.S., and Kagan, B.M. (Eds.): Current Pediatric Therapy. 6th Ed. Philadelphia, W.B. Saunders Company, 1973. p. 716.

**17**

# PENICILLIN ALLERGY

What should be done about the patient with a history of penicillin allergy and a problem for which penicillin or its synthetic derivatives is clearly the best therapy? How reliable is a history of penicillin allergy?

Patients with a history of penicillin allergy should be skin tested with both penicillin G and penicilloyl polylysine (PPL) before administering penicillin in situations in which doubt exists and therapy with this group of antibiotics is necessary. With this approach, many patients with a false-positive history of penicillin allergy, or patients who have lost their hypersensitivity, can be identified and treated if necessary.

Here are some statistics that may help you place the problem in perspective.

| | |
|---|---|
| Incidence of positive skin tests | |
| History of penicillin allergy | 19% |
| No history of penicillin allergy | 7% |
| | |
| Incidence of positive skin tests as related to allergic symptoms | |
| Previous anaphylactic reactions | 45% |
| Previous maculopapular eruption | 7% |
| | |
| Reactions with penicillin challenge | |
| With positive history and skin test | 67% |
| With positive history alone | 6% |
| With negative history | 2% |

No test presently available can detect 100 per cent of patients at risk from penicillin therapy. When penicillin hypersensitivity is highly suspected, and the drug is necessary for treatment, skin testing should be performed. Initial testing should be done by the scratch technique; if this is negative, intradermal testing should be employed. If testing is negative, then penicillin can be administered with careful observation.

---

Reference: Greene, G.R.: Hospital Practice, June 1976, p. 28.

# GASTROGRAFIN AS THERAPY

Gastrografin (E.R. Squibb) is a 76 per cent aqueous solution of sodium methylglucamine diatrizoate with 0.1 per cent Tween 80, a wetting agent. The solution also contains 37 per cent of finely bound iodine, which makes it radiopaque.

The undiluted Gastrografin has an osmolarity of 1900 milliosmols per liter. As a result of its high osmolarity, when introduced in the gastrointestinal tract, it draws fluid into the bowel. This can be a dangerous side-effect of its use for diagnostic purposes or it can be capitalized on for therapy.

## Meconium Ileus

The use of the Gastrografin enema has been demonstrated to be extremely effective in relieving intestinal obstruction produced by thick meconium in infants with *meconium ileus*.

## Procedure

1. Prepare infant as if he were to have a surgical procedure. Correct pre-existing dehydration. Continue nasogastric suction.

2. Maintain intravenous fluids during procedure at a rate of 120 ml/$M^2$/hour. Intravenous fluid should consist of 5 per cent glucose and 0.2 normal saline.

3. *Enema technique.* Under fluoroscopic control, inject 60 to 90 ml of undiluted Gastrografin into the high colon, using a 30 ml syringe with a soft rubber No. 8 French catheter. Tape the catheter into position in the anal canal and tape buttocks together to prevent leakage. Terminate enema when dye reaches the involved ileal segment. Do not palpate abdomen during procedure.

4. The first stools of green-black meconium are passed within minutes to an hour from the termination of the enema. Loose stools may continue for a day.

5. When stooling has abated, commence oral feedings.

### Congestive Heart Failure

We have found that the use of Gastrografin, either by mouth or by enema, is a rapid, effective means of removing excess fluid in patients with pulmonary edema and congestive heart failure. Its use should be reserved for patients with transient or chronic renal insufficiency in whom conventional diuretics would not be expected to work.

Undiluted Gastrografin is given in a dose of 5 ml/kg. The patient's serum electrolytes should be monitored frequently in view of the unpredictable losses of sodium, potassium, and bicarbonate that may accompany this form of diuresis. The treatment may be repeated as necessary.

References: Wagget, J., Johnson, D.G., Borns, P., et al.: J. Pediatr., 77:407, 1970. Rowe, M.I., Furst, A.J., Altman, D.H., et al.: Pediatrics, *48*:29, 1971.

# DO NOT DROWN YOUR PATIENTS

Most physicians are aware of the fact that excess fluid retention and hyponatremia may occur as a result of inappropriate antidiuretic hormone (ADH) secretion in patients with either central nervous system or pulmonary disease.

It is less well appreciated that water intoxication can be produced by therapeutic procedures, such as the tap water enema, or the use of a mist tent or isolette.

**17**

### The Tap Water Enema

The administration of tap water by enema can produce a rapid drop in serum sodium concentration in patients who have an enlarged absorptive surface or have prolonged retention of the enema. Tap water enemas should never be given to:

1. Patients with a history of chronic constipation.
2. Patients who are unconscious.
3. Patients receiving hypotonic fluids intravenously.

Even in normal children, the volume of a tap water enema should not exceed 3.5 per cent of the patient's weight.

### The Mist Tent

When infants are placed in a high humidity atmosphere, normal insensible water losses are markedly diminished. Insensible water loss accounts for approximately 40 per cent of daily maintenance fluid requirements. Adjustment of intravenous intake should be appropriately modified in patients in whom prolonged exposure to a high humidity atmosphere is anticipated. This is particularly true in patients with cardiac, respiratory, or renal disease. These patients must be weighed daily.

In addition, patients in a high humidity atmosphere are receiving unsuspectedly large quantities of water by mouth. Approximately 90 per cent of the water vapor is deposited in the nose, and with condensation is eventually swallowed.

Being aware of these facts can allow you to avoid problems of overhydration.

---

References: Ziskind, A., and Gellis, S.S.: Am. J. Dis. Child., *96*:699, 1958. Bau, S.K., Asken, N., Wood, D.E., et al.: Pediatrics, *48*:605, 1971. Rossiter, M.A., Borzyskowski, M., and Bower, B.D.: Lancet, *1*:935, 1974.

# TOXICITY OF CANCER CHEMOTHERAPY

Longer survival of children with malignancies and an ever increasing number of chemotherapeutic agents given to these children mean that pediatricians will need to be alert to both the early and the late side-effects of these agents. The following list suggests the possible side-effects that could be anticipated for each agent. (L) = late effect only.

*Adriamycin.* Nausea, vomiting, stomatitis, alopecia, cardiac toxicity, red urine, bone marrow depressions, hyperpigmentation of dermal creases and nails, and cellulitis at injection site (total dose–related).

*Arabinosylcytosine (Ara-C, Cytarabine).* Nausea, vomiting, abdominal pain, diarrhea, hepatic toxicity (rarely), fever, alopecia, conjunctivitis, epithelial ulceration, keratitis, megaloblastosis, and bone marrow depression (leukopenia and thrombocytopenia).

*Asparaginase (Elspar).* Nausea, vomiting, fever, anaphylactic reaction, hepatotoxicity, pancreatitis, lethargy, confusion, azotemia, urticaria, hyperglucosemia, hypoproteinemia, hypolipidemia and hyperlipidemia, fatty metamorphosis of the liver, decreased levels of coagulation factors, and pancytopenia.

*Bischloroethyl nitrosourea (BCNU).* Nausea and vomiting, hepatic toxicity, and bone marrow depression (leukopenia and thrombocytopenia).

*Bleomycin.* Nausea and vomiting, stomatitis, fever, chills, edema and dermatitis of hands, hyperpigmentation, nail changes, alopecia, pneumonitis, and pulmonary fibrosis. There is no evidence for bone marrow or immunologic depression.

*Busulfan (Myleran).* Bulbous eruption of the skin, cataracts, glossitis, adrenal insufficiency–like syndrome, skin pigmentation, diffuse pulmonary fibrosis and ossification, and bone marrow depression; menstrual dysfunction (L).

*Chlorambucil (Leukeran).* Bone marrow depression; menstrual dysfunction (L); azoospermia (L).

*Corticosteroids.* Cushingoid features, osteoporosis, growth retardation, hypertension, psychosis, peptic ulcers, hyperglucosemia, fluid retention, hypokalemia, myopathy, cataracts, and thromboembolic phenomena.

*Cyclohexylchloroethyl nitrosourea (CCNU).* Nausea and vomiting, hepatic toxicity, and bone marrow depression (leukopenia and thrombocytopenia).

*Cyclophosphamide (Cytoxan).* Nausea and vomiting, alopecia, transverse ridging of nails, skin pigmentation, hemorrhagic cystitis, fibrosis of urinary bladder, possibly interstitial pneumonitis, and bone marrow depression (leukopenia, thrombocytopenia, and anemia); primary ovarian failure (L); azoospermia (L).

*Dactinomycin (Actinomycin D).* Nausea and vomiting, stomatitis, diarrhea, alopecia, irritant at infusion site, and bone marrow depression.

*Daunomycin.* Nausea and vomiting, alopecia, cardiac toxicity, red urine, irritant at infusion site, and bone marrow depression (leukopenia and thrombocytopenia).

*Fluorouracil (5-FU).* Nausea, ulcerations of mouth and gastrointestinal tract, maculopapular rash, photophobia, diarrhea, acute cerebellar syndrome, and bone marrow depression.

*Hydroxyurea (Hydrea).* Nausea, vomiting, stomatitis, maculopapular rash, facial erythema, and bone marrow depression.

*Mechlorethamine (Nitrogen mustard).* Nausea, vomiting, leukopenia, thrombocytopenia, and strong vesicating effect on skin and veins.

*Methotrexate (Amethopterin).* Ulcerations of mouth and gastrointestinal tract, diarrhea, hepatic necrosis, cirrhosis, perifolliculitis, acne, pneumonitis, megaloblastosis from folate deficiency, and bone marrow depression; hepatic fibrosis (L); diffuse pulmonary disease (L); osteoporosis with pathologic fractures (L).

*Procarbazine (Natulan).* Nausea, vomiting, mental depression, stomatitis, constipation, diarrhea, myalgia, and arthralgia, chills and fever, dermatitis, paresthesia, ataxia, and bone marrow depression (leukopenia and thrombocytopenia).

*Thioguanine (6-TG).* Nausea, vomiting, and bone marrow depression.

*Triethylenemelamine (TEM).* Nausea, vomiting, abdominal pain, alopecia, cystitis, and bone marrow depression.

*Triethylenethiophosphoramide (Thio-Tepa).* Nausea, vomiting, headache, and bone marrow depression.

*Vinblastine (Velban).* Nausea, vomiting, irritant at infusion site, alopecia, areflexia, constipation, stomatitis, and bone marrow depression; menstrual dysfunction (L).

*Vincristine (Oncovin).* Alopecia, irritant at infusion site, constipation, paralytic ileus, abdominal pain, oral ulcers, bladder atonia, dysuria, muscular weakness, joint pain, jaw pain, fever, hypertension, inappropriate antidiuretic

**17**

hormone secretion, vocal cord paralysis, peripheral neuritis, ataxia, foot drop, neuralgia, paresthesia of fingers and toes, sensory loss, neuralgia, cranial nerve palsies, depressed to absent deep tendon reflexes, patchy liver necrosis, and mild depression of the bone marrow.

References: Hughes, W.T.: Pediatr. Clin. North Am., *23*:225, 1976. Jaffe, N.: Pediatr. Clin. North Am., *23*:233, 1976.

# 18
# TUMORS

# TIP-OFFS TO MALIGNANT DISEASE

A significant number of both congenital malformations and acquired diseases are now recognized to be associated with an increased incidence of malignancy. Detection of a condition listed below should occasion a high index of suspicion, regular observation, and appropriate studies for early detection of malignancy.

| CONDITION | ASSOCIATED MALIGNANCY |
|---|---|
| Agammaglobulinemia | Lymphoma, lymphosarcoma |
| Albinism | Basal cell carcinoma, squamous cell carcinoma |
| Aniridia (non-familial) | Wilms' tumor |
| Ataxia telangiectasia | Leukemia, lymphoma, lymphosarcoma |
| Beckwith's syndrome | Wilms' tumor, liver carcinoma, adrenal cortical carcinoma, nesidioblastosis of pancreas |
| Bloom's syndrome | Leukemia |
| Chédiak-Higashi syndrome | Lymphoma, lymphosarcoma, leukemia |
| D-trisomy | Leukemia |
| Down's syndrome | Leukemia |
| Familial polyposis of colon | Colonic carcinoma |
| Family history (first degree) of malignancy | Same or other malignancy |
| Genitourinary anomalies | Wilms' tumor |
| Giant cell hepatitis | Carcinoma of liver |
| Hemihypertrophy | Wilms' tumor, adrenal cortical carcinoma, liver carcinoma, hepatoblastoma |
| Hippel-Lindau disease | Pheochromocytoma |
| Horner syndrome | Neuroblastoma |
| Irradiation: | |
|   in utero | Leukemia |
|   of head and neck in early life | Thyroid carcinoma, brain and parotid tumors |
|   for retinoblastoma | Osteosarcoma |
|   for Wilms' tumor | Osteosarcoma, osteochondroma |
|   for neuroblastoma | Osteosarcoma, osteochondroma |
| Klinefelter's syndrome | Leukemia |
| Multiple mucosal neuromas | Medullary thyroid carcinoma |
| Maternal stilbestrol during pregnancy | Vaginal adenocarcinoma |
| Neurofibromatosis | Pheochromocytoma, sarcoma, schwannoma, leukemia |

18

| CONDITION | ASSOCIATED MALIGNANCY |
|---|---|
| Nevus sebaceous | Basal cell carcinoma |
| Poland's syndrome | Leukemia |
| Thyroid cancer (medullary) | Pheochromocytoma |
| Ulcerative colitis/regional ileitis | Colonic carcinoma |
| Wiskott-Aldrich syndrome | Lymphoma, lymphosarcoma |
| Xeroderma pigmentosa | Basal cell or squamous cell carcinoma |

References: Craven, E.M.: J.A.M.A., *215*:795, 1971. Feman, S.S., and Apt, L.: J. Pediatr. Ophthalmol., *9*:224, 1972.

## MEDIASTINAL MASSES IN CHILDREN

The finding of a mediastinal mass is always a cause for alarm. The age of the patient and the location of the mass can provide valuable clues as to its probable cause. The mediastinum can be divided into three areas, based on easily recognizable structures that are visible on the lateral film of the chest. These areas are the anterior mediastinum, the middle mediastinum, and the paravertebral sulcus. The anterior mediastinum is bounded by the sternum, the thoracic inlet, and the anterior border of the heart. The middle mediastinum is located between the anterior border of the heart and the anterior border of the vertebral bodies. The paravertebral sulcus, not truly part of the mediastinum, is located posterior to the anterior border of the vertebral bodies. About 40 per cent of all masses in children up to 16 years of age occur in the middle mediastinum, and another 40 per cent occur in the paravertebral sulcus. The specific masses in each area are:

| ANTERIOR MEDIASTINUM | MIDDLE MEDIASTINUM | PARAVERTEBRAL SULCUS |
|---|---|---|
| *Common* | *Common* | *Common* |
| Thymic "hyperplasia" | Lymphoma | Neuroblastoma |
| Teratoma | Lymphosarcoma | Ganglioneuroblastoma |
| Malignant thymoma | Hodgkin's disease | Ganglioneuroma |
| | Duplication cyst Bronchogenic Esophageal | |
| *Unusual* | *Unusual* | *Unusual* |
| Lipoma | Granuloma | Plexiform neurofibroma |
| Undifferentiated sarcoma | Esophageal adenoma | Undifferentiated sarcoma |
| | | Hydatid cyst |

Cystic hygromas, hemangiomas, and undifferentiated sarcomas may involve more than one compartment.

The distribution of mediastinal masses by age, as shown below in one study, illustrates that neuroblastoma is the most common mass in children under 2 years of age, while lymphomas are the most common cause of mediastinal masses in the older child.

| MASS | TOTAL NUMBER | NUMBER OF PATIENTS | |
|---|---|---|---|
| | | *0–2 years* | *2–16 years* |
| Neuroblastoma | 18 | 13 | 5 |
| Ganglioneuroblastoma | 8 | 2 | 6 |
| Ganglioneuroma | 6 | 0 | 6 |
| Plexiform neuroma | 3 | 1 | 2 |
| Duplication cyst | 14 | 4 | 10 |
| Angiomatous malformation | 7 | 4 | 3 |
| Lymphoma | 27 | 0 | 27 |
| Thymic hyperplasia | 7 | 6 | 1 |
| Sarcoma | 6 | 1 | 5 |
| Teratoma | 4 | 2 | 2 |

Reference: Pokorny, W.J., and Sherman, J.O.: J. Thorac. Cardiovasc. Surg., *68*:869, 1974.

18

# 19
# PATIENT CARE

# HINTS IN CARING FOR THE HOSPITALIZED CHILD

Children are particularly susceptible to emotional trauma during hospitalization. Painful procedures and separation from home and family cannot be avoided, but the physician can do a great deal to diminish fear and gain the trust of patients. Some useful hints are listed below.

Inform parents of hospital mealtimes, and encourage them to visit during that time.

Establish an area where several children may sit together during mealtime.

Provide opportunities for the parents and child to talk to the dietician so that the child's likes and dislikes may be noted. This is also the time to point out particular touches that the dietary department may provide to make meals more appealing; for instance, a straw for milk, extra ketchup, or smaller portions that do not overwhelm the child.

Permit parents to bring food to children, even if they are not on regular diets. Parents may be advised to tell the nurse what their child ate from home.

Encourage parents to provide a doll, blanket, or other favorite object from home in order to have some familiar object in the unfamiliar environment.

If the child is used to falling asleep with a bottle, this is no time to change that practice. The parents may be instructed about the danger of producing caries at the time of discharge.

Avoid performing procedures in the middle of the night. Children may fear night in a strange place, and fear of painful procedures may make relaxation and sleep impossible.

Whenever possible, the child's room and the playroom should be safe havens for the child. Procedures should be reserved for the treatment room.

If procedures must be performed within sight and sound of another child, they should be carefully explained to both children, and the observing child should be reassured that he will not be involved.

The patient should be asked what he knows about an impending procedure. Gaps in his understanding of what will be done should be filled in so that what is actually done will be no more or less than what is expected.

Keep pleasant, inexpensive trinkets with you to provide a surprise for the child.

Find some way to express interest in patients, such as brief participation in a game they were playing when you entered the room, before beginning a procedure or examination.

Encourage parents to visit at any time, even if this means writing special orders for unlimited visiting hours.

If a child is to be examined on the parent's lap, explain what is to be expected of the parent; that is, is the child to be restrained, comforted, or just supported?

Supply a roll-away cot for parents who wish to spend the night with a child who is under 5 years old or in pain.

Explain to parents the need for children to talk about the hospitalization and play out their strong feelings about it. Help them guide their children to draw pictures, pound clay, hammer nails, and engage in any activity that will help the child express emotion.

Excessively loud or long outbursts of crying, throwing objects, hurting others, and other frightening behavior are obvious calls for help. They should be responded to with comfort and explanation of what the child may expect during the rest of the hospital stay.

19

---

Reference: Azarnoff, P.: Resident and Staff Physician, May 1976, p. 153.

# THE CHILD WITH A CHRONIC HANDICAP

The care of a child with a chronic, severe, physical or mental handicap provides the pediatrician with the greatest challenge. It is the real test of a physician's compassion, humanity, patience and understanding, and capacity to give to others. These qualities must be combined with a firm knowledge of the science of medicine in order to provide the patient, and his family, the best of care and caring that medicine has to offer.

In addition to the competence and concern of the professional staff, other factors significantly improve the ability of the family to cope with a child's chronic illness. These factors include:

1. A good relationship between the mother and maternal grandmother.
2. A strong marital relationship.
3. A birth order other than the first.
4. An opportunity for recreation both with and without the other family members.
5. Access to a circle of understanding friends.
6. An ability to plan and prepare household management matters ahead of time.
7. A dwelling location that is convenient to shopping, schools, and transportation.
8. A deep religious faith.
9. An opportunity to help others, especially other families with the same problem.
10. Being told of the child's disability as early as possible.

For the physician to be of most benefit, he must understand how the parents feel and deal with the problems created by their child's illness. The physician should not fear that he will produce damage by gentle questioning. Included among the things a physician should ask are:

Was this child a planned baby?

When did you first find out that there was something wrong?

What did the doctor say at first? Did you understand what the doctor said at the beginning?

How long after the birth of the baby did you see your child? (if there is a birth defect)

What do you think about your child's problem?

How did your husband/wife feel about it?

What did your mother say?

Did anyone suggest institutionalizing your child?

Did you ever think it would have been better if the baby had died?

Did you feel uneasy about showing your baby to relatives and friends?

Were your friends helpful? Do they stay away?

Was the baby difficult to care for in early infancy?

Do you and your husband/wife feel the same way about your child's condition? What do you disagree about?

Do you feel comfortable now about taking your child out in public?

Do you and your husband/wife share in the care of the child?

Do you ever get an opportunity to be away from home to do something you would like for yourself?

Does anyone ever babysit for your child?

How often do you and your husband/wife go out together?

Do you feel that this child takes up most of your time?

Do you think that your normal children resent the time you spend with your child?

What worries you about the future of your child? What are your plans for the future of your child?

(Tell me Doctor, how do *you* feel about this child?)

Reference: Battle, C.U.: Pediatr. Clin. North Am., *22*:525, 1975.

## "REASONS WHY YOU SHOULD SEND ME HOME"

We sometimes forget the loneliness and the sadness of the hospitalized child. This is particularly true when the child is in the hospital for extended periods of time and may be taken care of by ever-changing medical and nursing personnel.

Several years ago one of us received a letter that poignantly illustrates these problems. Reading it from time to time can improve the lot of other hospitalized children.

The following are excerpts from this letter.

Dear Doctor:

Richard was a 10 year old leukemic child who died in April or May this year at the _____ hospital. I am estimating when I say that Richard lived one year after diagnosis and, again estimating, spent six months of that year hospitalized.

Richard was in a private room and everyone entering the room used masking precautions. His parents visited daily for most of the day. As far as I know there were no conversations with Richard or his parents and the nursing staff concerning his diagnosis or prognosis.

When Richard died, the nursing staff found the enclosed composition in his bedside stand. It has been very inspirational for the pediatric staff at our hospital.

*Reasons Why You Should Send Me Home*

1. I could get some sleep.
2. I could exercise more.
3. I would eat better.
4. I could go outside when I want to.
5. I'd be a lot happier.
6. I wouldn't be stuffed up in one room.
7. I could get better quicker.

**19**

8. I'd be comfortable.
9. I could help around the house.
10. I wouldn't be bored.
11. I'd make my mother happier by showing her I'm eating.
12. I'd be with my family.
13. I could get more fresh air.
14. It would be peaceful and quiet.
15. I wouldn't get any shots.
16. I could talk and see my mother and father before 11:00 A.M.
17. I could stay up later in the night.
18. I wouldn't be such a grouch.
19. I wouldn't be laying down all day.
20. I could go to sleep in *my own bed*.
21. I could build up my muscles.
22. I could get out of bed when I want to.
23. I wouldn't be in the hospital.
24. I could play all different games and stuff.
25. I could watch color TV instead of black and white TV.

Ricky

26. It's Spring.


# THE PRESCRIPTION

The sequence of events that starts with a decision to prescribe a medication and ends with the patient receiving the drug is fraught with many possible errors. Among these errors can be included:

1. Inappropriate drug selection. Never write for a medication whose mechanism of action is unknown to you; be familiar with indications, contraindications, and common side-effects; remember that many drugs have multiple ingredients.
2. Errors in writing and illegible writing.
3. Failure to take prescription to be filled because of transportation or financial reasons.
4. Error in filling of prescription by pharmacist.
5. Noncompliance on part of the parent or patient because of misunderstanding directions for taking the medicine or because of stopping the medicine prematurely.

The important aspects of prescription writing include the following.

| | |
|---|---|
| Name of drug | Generic names are preferred. Trade name may be added, although when trade name is specified a comment should be included as to whether a substitution can be made by the pharmacist if item is not in stock. For some multiple component medications, such as Lomotil, a trade name alone is adequate. |
| Form of drug | Always specify; e.g., 500 mg capsules, 125 mg/5 ml. |

| | |
|---|---|
| Amount of drug | Whenever possible, prescribe the precise amount of medication to treat the current illness. Always make a notation in your record as to the amount prescribed, thereby providing yourself with a convenient means of detecting compliance. If, for example, a child is seen after a ten-day course of treatment for otitis media, you may ask the mother casually, "How much medicine is left?" The response may vary from "Doctor, I just ran out" to "Doctor, I don't need any more because the bottle is half-full." When prescribing medications that may be abused, such as narcotics or tranquilizers, it is a good practice to write out the amount of drug, i.e., fifteen rather than 15. Numbers can be easily altered unless written in full. |
| Directions | Specify amount and time of dose, as well as route when appropriate. When writing for more than one drug, try to give them simultaneously. Do not merely write, "Take as directed." Specify the duration of treatment or state, "Until the bottle is empty." Remember that school children may have difficulty with medicines to be taken four times daily or every six hours. |
| Label notation | Always request that the pharmacist place the name of the drug on the label. |
| Refill notation | A statement concerning refills should always be provided, even if only to say "no refills." |
| Daily maximum | If a drug is to be taken "prn," always specify the indications for its use and the maximum quantity to be taken in a 24-hour period. |
| Signature | Make it legible. |
| BNDD number | Must be included where required. |

To encourage compliance, verbal instructions should accompany the written prescription. Areas to discuss include the following.

1. An explanation of the purpose of the medicine. This explanation should include the name of the drug, the amount and duration of the treatment, and instructions about refills, if appropriate.

2. An explanation of side-effects. This should include those predictable side-effects that should cause no concern, e.g., darkening of stools with iron, as well as those side-effects that require notification of the physician, e.g., staggering or rash while taking phenytoin (Dilantin).

3. An explanation, when a child is receiving multiple drugs, of which drugs should or should not be taken together.

4. Suggestions on how best to give the drug. This is particularly useful for new mothers.

5. Instructions on where to store the medicine in terms of need for refrigeration. Warnings, when necessary, about the drug's potential dangers if ingested by other children.

6. Instructions not to use the medicine for illness in other children.

**19**

7. An inquiry as to whether the parents may have problems reaching a drugstore or paying for the medicine.

8. A request that you be called if the parents find it difficult to get or give the medication or have noted unanticipated side-effects.

## THE PATIENT MANAGEMENT PLAN (WRITING HOSPITAL ORDERS)

In order to facilitate nursing care and to insure against omissions in the management of your patients, it is important to develop a routine method of writing hospital orders. Each individual, or institution, should develop such a routine and use it continually. A suggested sequence and its components is described below.

| AREA OF MANAGEMENT | DETAILS OF MANAGEMENT |
|---|---|
| Vital signs | Request the specific signs you wish monitored and the frequency of such measurements. Do not request more than is useful — it consumes a great amount of nursing time. Always specify what should be done when certain limits are exceeded. For example: Notify physician if pulse is greater than 160 or less than 80; notify physician if respirations are greater than 60 or less than 20; notify physician if temperature exceeds 39° C. These instructions should be tailor-made to the patient's disease and your therapeutic plans. |
| How frequently is the patient to be weighed? | All patients receiving intravenous fluids should be weighed at least daily. All patients under 2 years of age should be weighed daily. All hospitalized patients should be weighed at least weekly. |
| Are intake and output to be recorded? | All patients receiving intravenous fluids will require such measurements. All patients with diarrhea or vomiting require such information. |
| Patient's environment and activity | Items to be considered in this category include: croup tent, isolation precautions, crib, bed, bed with side rails, bathroom privileges, playroom privileges, bedtime hour, parents and friends' visiting privileges. |
| Diet | Specify caloric goals. Do not write "diet for age" in patients under 2 years of age. Specify type and frequency of feedings. Are fluids to be from bottle or cup? Any dietary exclusions. |
| Is calorie count required? | |

| | |
|---|---|
| Nutritional supplements | Patients receiving intravenous medications will require vitamin supplements. Patients receiving less than optimal diets will require supplements as well. Infants not receiving the equivalent of a reconstituted quart of a commercial formula are not receiving daily vitamin requirement. |
| Therapy | Intravenous fluids — composition, amount, rate. Medications — dose, route, frequency, duration. |
| Special treatments | Eye care, skin care, respiratory care, physical therapy, pulmonary toilet, occupational therapy, school teacher. |
| Diagnostic procedures and preparations for procedures | May include stools for occult blood, urine testing, and other ward procedures as well. |
| Special nursing | Observe mother-child interaction; child-to-child interactions; child's understanding of disease process. |

When orders are written, they should be accompanied with both the date and the *time* the entry was made. Unfortunately, in some instances, hours may go by without the order being translated into action.

When changes in therapy are instituted, they should be accompanied by a progress note in the patient's record so that your colleagues, sharing in the care of the patient, will understand the reasons for change in the patient's management.

## BOOKS THAT PREPARE A CHILD FOR A MEDICAL ENCOUNTER

A hospitalization, or even a visit to a hospital clinic or a doctor's office, can create fear and anxiety for a child. Thoughtful preparation for such experiences can reduce its potential unpleasantness. One means of preparation is by the use of books. Ideally, the book should be read by the child and parents together.

The following is an annotated bibliography of books that are considered best suited for this purpose.

Bemelmans, Ludwig: *Madeline.* New York, Viking Press, 1939, 27 pp. Full-color illustrations by the author. Ages 3 to 9. $3.50. Paperback, $1.25. Also available in Little Golden Books edition from Simon & Schuster, 1954, 25 cents. Very good.

Children's Hospital of Philadelphia: *Michael's Heart Test.* Philadelphia, Pa., Children's Hospital, 1967, 14 pp. Illustrated with black and white photos. Ages 3 to 12. Paperback, 15 cents. Excellent.

**19**

Children's Hospital of Philadelphia: *Margaret's Heart Operation*. Philadelphia, Pa., Children's Hospital, 1969, 14 pp. Illustrated with black and white photos. Ages 3 to 12. Paperback, 15 cents. Excellent.

Deegan, Paul J: *A Hospital: Life in a Medical Center*. Mankato, Minn., Amecus Street, Inc., 1971, 79 pp. Illustrated with black and white photos by B.C. Ross-Larson. Grades 4 to 7. $5.95. Excellent.

Falk, Ann Mari: *The Ambulance*. Toronto, Burke Publishing Company, Ltd., 1966, 22 pp. Translated by Irene D. Morris. Full-color illustrations by Tord Nygren. Ages 3 to 9. $3.95 (Canadian). Excellent.

Froman, Robert: *Let's Find Out About the Clinic*. New York, Franklin Watts, Inc., 1968, 47 pp. Two-color illustrations by Joseph Veno. Grades k to 3. $3.75. Good to very good.

Haas, Barbara Schuyler: *The Hospital Book*. Baltimore, Md., The John Street Press, 1970, 48 pp. Coloring book illustrated in black and white by Lun Harris. Ages 4 to 10. $1.50. Very good to excellent.

Kay, Eleanor: *The Clinic*. New York, Franklin Watts, Inc., 1971, 51 pp. Illustrated with black and white photos. Grades 4 to 6. $3.75. Good to very good.

Pope, Billy N. and Emmons, Ramona Ware: *Let's Go to the Doctor's Office*. Dallas, Texas, Taylor Publishing Company, 1967, 32 pp. Illustrated with full-color photos. Ages 3 to 7. $3.00. Very good.

Rey, H.A., and Rey, Margret: *Curious George Goes to the Hospital*. Boston, Mass., Houghton Mifflin Company, 1966, 48 pp. Illustrated in red, black and white drawings. Ages 3 to 8. $3.75. Also available in paperback from Scholastic Book Services, 75 cents. Excellent.

Stein, Sara Bonnett: *A Hospital Story*. New York, Walker and Company, 1974, 47 pp. Black and white and color photographs by Dick Frank and Doris Pinney. Ages 3 to 10. $4.50. Excellent.

Tamburine, Jean: *I Think I Will Go to the Hospital*. Nashville, Tenn., Abingdon Press, 1965, 48 pp. Illustrated in four-color drawings by the author. Ages 3 to 10. $3.50. Excellent.

Watson, Jane Werner, Switzer, Robert E. and Hirschberg, J. Cotter: *My Friend the Doctor*. New York, Golden Press, 1972, 24 pp. Illustrated in three colors by Hilde Hoffman. Ages 2 to 5. $1.95. Excellent.

Weber, Alfons: *Elizabeth Gets Well*. New York, Thomas Y. Crowell Company, 1970, 28 pp. Full-color illustrations by Jacqueline Blass. Ages 5 to 9. $4.50. Excellent.

Wolde, Gunilla: *Tommy Goes to the Doctor*. Boston, Houghton Mifflin Company, 1972, 23 pp. Full-color illustrations by the author. Ages 2 to 5. $1.65. Excellent.

Wolff, Angelika: *Mom! I Broke My Arm!* New York, The Lion Press, Inc., 1969, 45 pp. Three-color illustrations by Leo Glueckselig. Grades k to 4. $3.95. Excellent.

---

Reference: Altshuler, A.: Department of Health, Education, and Welfare, Publication No. 74–5402 (Health Services Administration), 1974.

## MEDICAL CARE OF THE YOUNG ATHLETE

The pediatrician becomes involved in medical care of the young athlete on two occasions: during preseason examination to determine the child's fitness to participate, and when injury has occurred. The physical examination of the child should be thorough and should be directed toward the child's physical ability to participate in competitive sports. Important aspects of the athlete's examination include the following.

*Laboratory procedures:* Urine analysis for sugar, acetone, and protein. Hemoglobin and hematocrit.

*Determination of* height, weight, visual acuity, chest and waist measurements, blood pressure, and vital capacity.

*Muscle strength testing exercises:* These are especially important for determination of muscular support of the knee. The child who is to be participating in contact sports such as football, hockey, soccer, or lacrosse should be able to sit on a table and extend his knee from 90 to 180 degrees with a 50 pound weight fastened to his foot 10 times in 40 seconds.

*Skin:* Infections, contagious and chronic infections, and fungal infections should be noted.

*Head:*

> Eyes — if visual acuity is less than 20/30, corrective lenses may be needed.
>
> Nose — deformity may limit endurance because of inadequate breathing space.
>
> Mouth — impacted third molars should be removed before participating in contact sports, since their presence is often associated with severe injuries to the mandible.

*Neck:* Any limitation of normal motion should be noted for future reference in case of some injury to this part.

*Chest:* Murmurs and wheezing are obviously important and may suggest the need for further testing or restriction of some kind.

*Abdomen:* Careful examination should be made of organ size. Look carefully for inguinal hernias.

*Genitalia:* Absence of one or failure of descent of one or both testes is a contraindication to participation. Hydrocele should be corrected before contact sports are allowed. Varicocele may be aggravated by strenuous physical exercise. Female pelvic examination should be performed if indicated by history.

*Extremities:* Any abnormal mobility requires special individual consideration. Important muscles in the athlete's body from the standpoint of protection against injury are those on the anterior and posterior surfaces of the thigh, and the quadriceps and biceps femoris groups. Although the ankle can be reasonably well protected against injury by wrapping, the knee cannot. When deficiencies in muscle strength are sufficient to restrict a child from athletic competition, recommendation should be made for appropriate weight training to strengthen those muscles if the child desires such training.

When serious injury occurs on the playing field and the physician is called to examine the patient, the six situations that may immediately threaten the life of the athlete should be kept in mind.

*Airway obstruction:* This is of greatest threat to the unconscious athlete. Immediate action should be taken to reestablish the airway. The neck should be supported while the head is tilted back. If this maneuver does not work, the mandible should be grasped and firmly pulled forward with the head tilted backward. Care should be taken not to forcibly manipulate the cervical spine, since cervical spine injury must be considered.

19

*Respiratory failure:* Players with craniocerebral injuries may have apneic episodes complicated by obstruction of the airway from transient paralysis of the oropharyngeal musculature. Oral airways and Ambu bags should be available. Because of the fear of cervical spine injury, the helmet of an injured player who is unconscious should not be removed because of the manipulation of the cervical region that this would involve. The player with respiratory problems should have his face mask removed, while the helmet is left in place.

*Cardiac arrest:* Arrhythmias are usually the cause of cardiac arrest in the young athlete. Cardiopulmonary resuscitation should be initiated immediately.

*Heat injuries:* Heat exhaustion occurs when an individual is exposed to a high environmental temperature and sweats excessively without salt or fluid replacement. Muscle cramps, excessive fatigue or weakness or both, loss of coordination, slowed reaction time, headache, decreased comprehension, nausea and vomiting, and dizziness may all precede heat exhaustion. Collapse and circulatory failure may follow if treatment with fluids, salt, cooling, and rest is not instituted.

Heat stroke occurs when an unacclimatized individual is suddenly exposed to a high environmental temperature. The thermal regulatory mechanism fails, sweating stops, and body temperature rises. Brain damage and death may follow. The athlete just returning from vacation in a cool climate should be allowed 14 to 21 days of acclimatization before exposure to a competitive situation in warm weather.

To prevent heat injury, players should be allowed unlimited fluids before, during, and after practices and games. In hot weather, players should be given four to eight 10-grain salt tablets daily and allowed liberal use of table salt.

*Intracranial injuries:* These may include concussion, skull fracture, subdural and epidural hematoma, and intracerebral hemorrhage. The high-school player who has any degree of concussion should not be allowed to continue playing. Signs and symptoms that demand emergency action in any athlete who has sustained a blow to the head are increasing headache, nausea and vomiting, inequality of the pupils, disorientation, and progressive impairment of consciousness.

*Cervical spine injuries:* Fracture, dislocation, or fracture-dislocation may occur. Protection of the neural elements from further injury is imperative. Cervical spine injury should be suspected in any unconscious athlete or in those who have severe, unremitting neck pain with or without paralysis. The player should be rolled like a log onto a fracture board, and the head should then be maintained in position by sandbags, wet towels, or traction.

---

Reference: Adamkin, D.H.: Am. J. Dis. Child. (in press).

# THE NEEDLE ASPIRATE AS A DIAGNOSTIC TOOL

The needle aspirate is a valuable, and underutilized, diagnostic aid. The sites that lend themselves to diagnostic needle aspiration in pediatric practice include the following.

*Central nervous system*

Lumbar subarachnoid space
Cisterna magna
Cerebral ventricles
Subdural space

*Cardiorespiratory*

Trachea (percutaneous)
Lung
Pleural cavity
Pericardial cavity
Paranasal sinuses
Middle ear

*Eye*

Anterior chamber

*Digestive system*

Peritoneal cavity

*Hematopoietic system*

Vein
Artery
Bone marrow
Lymph node

*Integument*

Abscess
Pustule
Vesicle
Petechiae
Cellulitis

*Musculoskeletal*

Joint
Subperiosteum

*Genitourinary system*

Urinary bladder (suprapubic)
Amniotic sac

Aspiration of a potential infectious focus should be considered whenever a prompt and specific bacteriologic diagnosis is critical in the management of the patient. The most underutilized procedures include the lung aspirate, the aspirate of the middle ear, the suprapubic aspiration, and the puncture of petechial and vesicular lesions.

## The Lung Puncture

### Indications

1. The critically ill child, with a pulmonary infiltrate, in whom a specific etiologic diagnosis is of importance in guiding therapy.
2. The patient who has not responded appropriately to initial therapy for his pneumonia.
3. The child with pneumonia complicating an underlying disease or receiving medications that compromise normal host defense mechanisms.

### Contraindications

1. Do not attempt needle aspiration when the infiltrate is in close proximity to the heart or great vessels.
2. Do not perform aspiration if patient is receiving positive pressure ventilation.

**19**

### Complications

A very small pneumothorax may occur in 1 to 4 per cent of patients. In most instances, the pneumothorax is asymptomatic and is detectable only by chest roentgenogram.

### Technique

1. The procedure is carried out much in the same manner as a thoracentesis. The child is held in the sitting position.
2. The site of the puncture is defined by physical and x-ray examination.
3. The skin is prepared with iodine and rapidly washed off with 70 per cent alcohol.
4. A 20-gauge needle, 1½ inches in length, is attached to a 10-ml syringe, and the needle is passed through the skin and into the pleural space. Enter the lung over the superior border of the lower rib in an intercostal space in order to avoid the intercostal arteries.
5. If pleural fluid is withdrawn, the needle is removed.
6. If pleural fluid is not present, the lung is entered with gentle withdrawal of the plunger so that negative pressure is maintained, and the needle is passed rapidly into the area of consolidation.
7. Negative pressure is maintained on the syringe as the needle is quickly withdrawn, and the material is discharged into a tube of sterile blood broth.
8. If only a small amount of material is obtained, some of the sterile broth is aspirated into the syringe and emptied back into the tube.
9. Place a few drops of aspirate on glass slides for Ziehl-Neelsen, Gram, and Wright stains.
10. Observe the child. If major changes in vital signs occur, then a repeat chest roentgenogram should be obtained.

### Needle Aspirate in Acute Otitis Media

### Indications

1. The child with recurrent or chronic otitis media.
2. The child who fails to respond adequately to initial therapy for acute otitis media. If the child remains febrile and acutely ill for more than 48 hours after beginning antibiotics, aspiration of the middle ear should be performed.
3. The patient who is critically ill when first seen if otitis media is part of the clinical picture of generalized sepsis. Aspiration in this circumstance may provide a rapid and direct means of obtaining and visualizing the infecting organism.
4. The child with malignancy or altered host defenses who may be infected with an unusual organism.

### Contraindications

1. Patients with a coagulation disturbance.

### Technique

1. Cleanse the external auditory canal with alcohol or sterile saline.

2. Place a speculum in the canal, and under direct vision pierce the tympanic membrane in its posterior inferior quadrant with a 20-gauge needle, 1½ inches long, attached to a 5-ml syringe.

3. Gently aspirate several drops of fluid and place one drop on a clean glass slide for microscopic examination with Gram stain. Inoculate the remainder of the aspirate into a tube containing beef heart broth or some other suitable liquid medium.

### The Suprapubic Aspiration

## Indications

1. In all patients suspected of having a urinary tract infection who cannot provide an adequate voided specimen for culture.

2. In patients with acute sepsis that requires immediate information to guide therapy.

## Contraindications

1. Patients with coagulation disturbances.

## Technique

1. Wait one hour after last voiding. Only aspirate if the bladder can be defined to be present and full by means of palpation or percussion.

2. Compress the male urethra with pressure on the penis.

3. Have the patient supine with the legs in a frog position.

4. Cleanse the suprapubic area with iodine and rinse with alcohol.

5. Pierce the abdominal wall and bladder about 1 to 2 inches above the symphysis pubis, employing a 20-gauge needle, 1½ inches long, attached to a 20-ml syringe.

6. Direct the needle toward fundus of the bladder while aspirating very gently.

7. The aspirated urine may be sent directly to the laboratory in a sealed syringe or discharged into a sterile tube. A portion should be retained for Gram stain and examination of the urinary sediment.

### Aspiration from Petechial and Vesicular Lesions

All such lesions should be examined when the possibility of infection is present.

Aspiration of blood from the center of a petechial lesion may reveal the etiologic agent in a Gram- or Wright-stained smear. Patients with palpable purpura should always be suspected of having meningococcemia.

Aspiration of fluid from vesicles is of value in the diagnosis of herpes zoster, chickenpox, herpes simplex, smallpox, and coxsackie A16 infection (hand, foot, and mouth syndrome). Aspirated fluid can be used for viral cultures.

**19**

In addition to fluid obtained by needle aspiration, material obtained from the base of the lesion can by examined for diagnostic information. For this purpose, a fresh vesicle is selected and the top of the vesicle is removed with a sharp blade. The base of the vesicle should be scraped, but bleeding should be avoided. A portion of this material is placed on a glass slide and Giemsa-stained. Multinucleated giant cells will be seen in patients with chickenpox, herpes simplex, and herpes zoster, but not in smallpox.

Reference: Klein, J.O., and Gellis, S.S.: Pediatr. Clin. North Am., *18*:219, 1971.

## PAINLESS VENIPUNCTURE

Obtaining cooperation of children for procedures can be enhanced by making the procedure less uncomfortable. One simple but often neglected step is that of allowing the isopropyl alcohol on a venipuncture site to dry before puncturing the skin. Your patients will appreciate you for it.

Reference: Phillips, P.J., Pain, R.W., and Brooks, G.E.: N. Engl. J. Med., *294*:116, 1976.

## EXTRAVASATION OF INTRAVENOUS MEDICATIONS

Extravasation (infiltration) of intravenous fluids is the cause of usually transient discomfort for patients. There are some intravenous medications, however, which when extravasated will cause local tissue problems ranging from inflammation to tissue necrosis and sloughing. Some of these medications that demand extra caution are listed below.

| Generic Name | Trade Name |
| --- | --- |
| Levarterenol | Levophed |
| Tromethamine | THAM |
| Thiopental | Pentothal |
| Urea | |
| Calcium salts | |
| Dextrose solutions | |
| Doxorubicin | Adriamycin |
| Dactinomycin | |
| Mithramycin | Mithracin |
| Mechlorethamine | Mustargen |
| Vinblastine | Velban |
| Vincristine | Oncovin |
| 5-Fluorouracil | |
| Daunomycin | |

## mEq/liter and mg %

Confusion often exists in the conversion of mEq/liter to mg % (mg/100 ml). The table below is intended to minimize such confusion.

| ION | IONIC WEIGHT (gm) | EQUIVALENT WEIGHT (gm) | CONVERSION FACTORS mEq/liter | mg % |
|---|---|---|---|---|
| $Na^+$ | 23.0 | 23.0 | mg % × 0.435 | mEq/liter × 2.30 |
| $K^+$ | 39.1 | 39.1 | mg % × 0.256 | mEq/liter × 3.91 |
| $Ca^{++}$ | 40.1 | 20.0 | mg % × 0.498 | mEq/liter × 2.00 |
| $Mg^{++}$ | 24.3 | 12.2 | mg % × 0.823 | mEq/liter × 1.21 |
| $Cl^-$ | 35.5 | 35.5 | mg % × 0.282 | mEq/liter × 3.55 |
| $HCO_3^-$ | 61.0 | 61.0 | vol % ($CO_2$) × 0.45 | mEq/liter × 2.22 (vol %) |
| $HPO_4^{--}$ | 96.0 | 48.0 | mg % (P) × 0.580 | mEq/liter × 1.72 (P) |
| $SO_4^{--}$ | 96.1 | 48.0 | mg % (S) × 0.613 | mEq/liter × 1.60 (S) |

## CONVERSION TABLES

| TEMPERATURE | | | | WEIGHT | | | | LENGTH | | | |
|---|---|---|---|---|---|---|---|---|---|---|---|
| °F | °C | °C | °F | lb | kg | kg | lb | in | cm | cm | in |
| 0 | −17.8 | 0 | 32.0 | 1 | .5 | 1 | 2.2 | 1 | 2.5 | 1 | .4 |
| 95 | 35.0 | 35. | 95.0 | 2 | .9 | 2 | 4.4 | 2 | 5.1 | 2 | .8 |
| 96 | 35.6 | 35.5 | 95.9 | 4 | 1.8 | 3 | 6.6 | 4 | 10.2 | 3 | 1.2 |
| 97 | 36.1 | 36. | 96.8 | 6 | 2.7 | 4 | 8.8 | 6 | 15.2 | 4 | 1.6 |
| 98 | 36.7 | 36.5 | 97.7 | 8 | 3.6 | 5 | 11.0 | 8 | 20.3 | 5 | 2.0 |
| 99 | 37.2 | 37. | 98.6 | 10 | 4.5 | 6 | 13.2 | 12 | 30.5 | 6 | 2.4 |
| 100 | 37.8 | 37.5 | 99.5 | 20 | 9.1 | 8 | 17.6 | 18 | 46 | 8 | 3.1 |
| 101 | 38.3 | 38. | 100.4 | 30 | 13.6 | 10 | 22 | 24 | 61 | 10 | 3.9 |
| 102 | 38.9 | 38.5 | 101.3 | 40 | 18.2 | 20 | 44 | 30 | 76 | 20 | 7.9 |
| 103 | 39.4 | 39. | 102.2 | 50 | 22.7 | 30 | 66 | 36 | 91 | 30 | 11.8 |
| 104 | 40.0 | 39.5 | 103.1 | 60 | 27.3 | 40 | 88 | 42 | 107 | 40 | 15.7 |
| 105 | 40.6 | 40. | 104.0 | 70 | 31.8 | 50 | 110 | 48 | 122 | 50 | 19.7 |
| 106 | 41.1 | 40.5 | 104.9 | 80 | 36.4 | 60 | 132 | 54 | 137 | 60 | 23.6 |
| 107 | 41.7 | 41. | 105.8 | 90 | 40.9 | 70 | 154 | 60 | 152 | 70 | 27.6 |
| 108 | 42.2 | 41.5 | 106.7 | 100 | 45.4 | 80 | 176 | 66 | 168 | 80 | 31.5 |
| 109 | 42.8 | 42. | 107.6 | 150 | 68.2 | 90 | 198 | 72 | 183 | 90 | 35.4 |
| 110 | 43.3 | 100 | 212 | 200 | 90.8 | 100 | 220 | 78 | 198 | 100 | 39.4 |

°F to °C: 5/9 (°F − 32)
°C to °F: (9/5 × °C) + 32

1 lb = 0.454 kg
1 kg = 2.204 lb

1 inch = 2.54 cm
1 cm = 0.3937 inch

**19**

## TEMPERATURE TAKING

The body temperature of a child is an important piece of physical data that is often requested of the parents by nurse or physician. Parents should be carefully instructed in the proper procedure for temperature taking.

1. Studies have shown that a full three minutes is required for the thermometer to reach its final temperature. A falsely low reading may be attained if the thermometer is read before this time, and the temperature will not rise beyond its three-minute reading.

2. The axillary method of temperature taking is useful in infants and young children. The axillary temperature is about 1 degree centigrade lower than the rectal temperature and about 0.5 degree centigrade lower than the oral temperature.

3. If a rectal temperature is to be measured, the thermometer should be lubricated and inserted 3 to 5 cm into the rectum. If this is done hastily, without proper lubrication, or if the child is not properly held, puncture of the rectum may occur.

---

Reference: De Nosaquo, N., Kerlan, I., Knudsen, L.F., et al.: J. Lab. Clin. Med., *29*:179, 1944.

## BLOOD CULTURE TECHNIQUE

Careful attention to the details of collection and incubation of blood facilitates accurate and more rapid identification of the bacteremic patient. The following list includes the important aspects of blood culture technique.

*Collection*

1. Bacteremia usually precedes the onset of fever or chills by approximately one hour. Since it is difficult to predict these events, the patient should be cultured three times in a 24-hour period. One sample may be sufficient in the newborn. The patient who has received antibiotics should have more frequent cultures performed.

2. The site intended for venipuncture should be cleansed with 70 to 90 per cent alcohol as well as an iodine (1 to 2 per cent) solution.

3. At least 10 ml of blood should be collected for each culture. In small children and infants, 1 to 5 ml is sufficient. (The blood sample used for culture should represent 1 per cent of the patient's blood volume.)

4. After replacing the needle used to perform the venipuncture, the blood should be injected into the media bottle. Air should not be introduced into the media bottle, since the unvented bottles allow the growth of both aerobes and anaerobes.

5. Clotted or citrated blood is unsuitable for culture.

*Inoculation of Media and Incubation*

1. Since a high concentration of human serum is bactericidal, the ratio of blood to medium should not exceed 1:10 to 1:20.

2. Two bottles of media should be used — one should be tryptic soy broth and the other thioglycollate.

3. If the patient has been treated with a penicillin or a cephalosporin, penicillinase should be added to the medium.

4. Culture bottles should be examined daily for seven days. Since fastidious organisms may require longer incubation, the bottles should be reexamined after two weeks of incubation.

5. Subculture should be performed within 24 hours of incubation.

Reference: Washington, J.A.: Mayo Clin. Proc., *50*:91, 1975.

# THE NON-THANKSGIVING TURKEY

All of us, as medical students, house officers, or practicing physicians, have at one time or another found ourselves thinking of a certain patient or of certain parents in a less than empathetic manner. The following commentary provides insight to heighten our own awareness of such situations.

The appropriateness of the season lends itself to a few thoughts about a syndrome of considerable importance to physicians, house officers, medical students and nurses: that of the "turkey." Although a term bandied about loosely on most hospital floors, it is a syndrome with a definite symptom complex of a primary and secondary nature. The secondary signs and symptoms are usually readily identified. Typically, it consists of a patient who is uncooperative, gives a poor history, has few findings on physical examination, without any obvious laboratory or radiologic abnormalities, and is admitted to the hospital in the middle of the night with a complaint of being "sick all over" and demanding help from both nurses and doctors. Variations of this secondary symptom complex occur; however, it is the ever present and more subtle primary signs and symptoms that form the core of this "turkey" syndrome and without which indeed there would be no such entity. These symptoms are overworked physicians, house officers, students and nurses whose education and orientation is toward treatment of physical disease, laboratory abnormalities and x-ray anomalies, but who are unable to deal with patients who fail to conform to arbitrary standards of being a "good patient," or who fail to fit readily into a given diagnostic category.

Diagnosing or labeling a patient as a "turkey" is in fact an illness of interaction, with signs and symptoms attributable to both the patients and to the healers involved. Perhaps the cure can only be found in the establishment of mutual rapport between the parties concerned. Nevertheless, the role and responsibility of the healer obliges the medical and nursing professions to examine what is lacking in the education of doctors and nurses and what is faulty in the present system of hospital care that lends itself to the development of this syndrome.

Traditionally, the turkey is a symbol of thanksgiving. It is unfortunate that in present-day medicine there is a situation in which the word engenders such a derogatory connotation.

**19**

Reference: Kaywin, P.R.: N. Engl.. J. Med., *289*:1257, 1973.

# 20
# POTPOURRI

# CAR SEATS FOR CHILDREN

When you discuss safety with parents, do not forget recommendations concerning the purchase of a car seat for their infant or child. Here is some advice taken from the pages of *Consumer's Report*, March 1975.

*Child Seat Restraints*

| | COST | AGE RANGE | WT. RANGE | HT. RANGE | CONVERTIBLE | COMMENTS |
|---|---|---|---|---|---|---|
| **INFANT CARRIERS** | | | | | | |
| *Best* | | | | | | |
| Peterson 75 | $36 | 0–6 months | Up to 18 lb. | — | Yes | Convenient to use. Can be used as infant carrier outside car. Requires long lap belt. Cannot be used in left rear seat. |
| GM Infant Love Seat | $16 | | Up to 20 lb. | — | No | May be used outside car as carrier. Inconvenient to use. |
| *Lower Quality* | | | | | | |
| Bunny Bear Sweetheart Seat II QN97 | $35 | | Up to 15 lb. | To 24" | Yes (see comment) | Child conversion rated tenth in quality. Sits sidewise and bulky between two adults in front seat. |
| Bobby MacCar Seat 4810 | $29 | | Up to 15 lb. | | Yes | Convenient to use. Can be used outside car as carrier. Tall child's head *not* adequately restrained. Child conversion rated ninth. |

*Table continued on following page*

**20**

481

*Child Seat Restraints (Continued)*

| | COST | AGE RANGE | WT. RANGE | HT. RANGE | CONVERTIBLE | COMMENTS |
|---|---|---|---|---|---|---|
| **CHILD RESTRAINTS** | | | | | | |
| *Best* | | | | | | |
| Strolee Wee Carseat 597 | $41 | | 18–43 lb. | 30–42″ | No | Reclines but not recommended as such. More comfortable than most. Top tether cannot be used with bucket seat. |
| Peterson 74 | $29 | Shield: 7 months–2 years / Harness: 2–4 years | 18–30 lb. / 25–40 lb. | To 35″ / To 40″ | Yes | Not to be used in front center or left rear. |
| *Lower Quality* | | | | | | |
| Century Motor Toter | $30 | | 15–40 lb. | To 40″ | No | Not with bucket seat. |
| Teddy Tot Aeroseat V | $30 | Seat and harness | To 40 lb. | 15–42″ | Yes | Not with bucket seat. |
| Ford Tot Guard | $30 | To 5 years | To 50 lb. | 18–28″ seated | No | Long lap belt, child can get out easily. |
| GM Love Seat | $33 | | 20–40 lb. | To 40″ | No | Essentially same as Century Motor Toter. |

# RED HERRING

During hunts in the seventeenth century, the challenge to the hunting dogs was sometimes increased by dragging a red herring (i.e., a cured or smoked herring or other dead animal) across the quarry's track in an attempt to throw the dogs off the scent. Thus, the term has come to mean any subject that diverts attention from the question at hand.

Reference: Oxford English Dictionary. New York, Oxford University Press, 1971.

# INCIDENCE OR PREVALENCE

"It has been said that the easiest way to distinguish a clinician from an epidemiologist is by the clinician's incorrect use of the term 'incidence.' " It is unfortunate, both for interpretation of facts and figures, as well as for personal expression, to be unaware of the difference between incidence and prevalence. The correct definitions are:

$$\text{Incidence rate} = \frac{\text{number of new cases of a disease}}{\text{total population at risk}} \text{ per unit of time}$$

$$\text{Prevalence rate} = \frac{\text{number of existing cases}}{\text{total population}}$$

Reference: Friedman, G.D.: Ann. Intern. Med., *84*:502, 1976.

# REGIMEN NOT REGIME

These two words are often confused and used improperly.

A *regimen* refers to a systematic course or program, while a *regime* is defined as a mode of rule or management such as the prevailing governmental or social system. Patients are placed on therapeutic *regimens*.

# ILLINGWORTH'S LIST OF POPULAR FALLACIES

Professor Illingworth has selected a group of common errors that are made when interpreting symptoms. They are worth remembering.

1. [In the young infant,] vomiting, crying, green stools, or diarrhea are *not* due to breast-feeding not suiting the baby. The only exceptions to this are the exceedingly rare conditions of galactosemia or lactose intolerance . . . . Green stools in fully breast-fed babies do not suggest an abnormality.

20

2. Vomiting, crying, or diarrhea are not due to the breast milk being too strong for the baby — or not strong enough.

3. Vomiting, crying, or diarrhea in a full-term breast-fed or bottle-fed baby are not due to overfeeding. Babies know when to stop and do not take too much.

4. Infrequent stools in the well breast-fed baby are not due to constipation. They are normal.

5. True constipation in an artificially fed baby is not due to insufficiency of roughage in the diet. It may be due to inadequate fluid, inadequate sugar (when the baby is having nothing but milk) or to other factors.

6. Crying at night in the older baby is not due to indigestion or wind. It is almost certainly due to mismanagement and habit formation.

7. A poor appetite in a well child is almost certainly not due to disease — though routine physical and urine examination should be carried out; it is almost certainly due to food forcing. [Or eating between meals — Ed.]

8. Bedwetting after the age of three, when it has always occurred, is certainly not merely psychological in origin, or due to jealousy or faulty management — though psychological problems can readily be added to the basic problem of delayed maturation.

9. Constant dribbling incontinence is not due to delayed maturation; in the boy it is usually due to urethral valves, and in the girl to an ectopic ureter in the vagina.

10. Delayed walking is not a problem for the orthopedic specialist. It is not due to congenital dislocation of the hip.

11. Teething does not cause bronchitis, convulsions, fever, or diarrhea.

12. Delayed talking is not due to tongue-tie, laziness, 'everything being done for him,' and certainly not to jealousy. If the child is mentally normal, it is usually a familial feature, but may be due to deafness.

---

Reference: Illingworth, R.S.: *In* Common Symptoms of Disease in Children. 3rd Ed. Oxford, Blackwell Scientific Publications Ltd., 1971, p. 310.

## BOOKS FOR CHILDREN ABOUT DEATH

Books can be used in a constructive fashion to help familiarize children with the concepts of death. The list below may help you advise parents about appropriate books for their children.

*Books for Preschool Children*

*The Dead Bird*, by Margeret Wise
*About Dying*, by Sara Bonnet Stein
*The Tenth Good Thing about Barney*, by Judith Viorst

*Books for Children 5 to 8 Years of Age*

*Annie and the Old One*, by Miska Miles

*Books for Children 8 to 11 Years of Age*

*A Taste of Blackberries*, by Doris B. Smith
*Charlotte's Web*, by Elwyn B. White
*The Birds' Christmas Carol*, by Kate Douglas Wiggin
*The Magic Moth*, by Virginia Lee
*The Thanksgiving Treasure*, by Gail Rock

*For the Young Adolescent*

*Little Women*, by Louisa May Alcott

You may wish to read these books yourself before recommending them to your patients and their families. A brief description of each book is provided in the reference listed below.

Reference: Aradine, C.R.: Pediatrics, 57:372, 1976.

## WHO INVENTED THE POPSICLE?

Frank Epperson was the inventor who made lemonade from a specially prepared powder that he sold at an Oakland, California, amusement park. While visiting friends in New Jersey, he prepared a batch of special lemonade and inadvertently left a glass of it on a windowsill with a spoon in it. The temperature went down below zero during the night, and in the morning Epperson saw the glass. He picked it up by the spoon handle and ran hot water over the glass, releasing the frozen mass. In his hand was the first Epsicle, later to be known as the Popsicle. Epperson saw immediately the potential of what he held in his hand and applied for a patent, which was granted in 1924. He was fortunate, because research conducted by *The Ice Cream Review*, in 1925 revealed that a major ice cream company was experimenting with "frozen suckers" at the time of the windowsill incident, and as far back as 1872 two men doing business as Ross and Robbins sold a frozen-fruit confection on a stick, which they called the Hokey-Pokey.

Reference: Dickson, P.: *In* The Great American Ice Cream Book. New York, Atheneum, 1973. (Reprinted in Pediatrics, 55:29, 1975.)

**20**

# RELIGIOUS RITES

On occasion we may forget about our own religion, but we should never lose sight of its importance to our patients and their families. The table below provides some guidelines for the physician when dealing with the birth, death, and special dietary customs of the three major faiths.

| OCCASION | JEWISH | PROTESTANT | ROMAN CATHOLIC |
|---|---|---|---|
| **Birth** | | | |
| General precepts | Jewish infants are not baptized. It is a basic ritual among all Jews that male babies be circumcised on the eighth day after birth. (Circumcision of an infant in poor health may be postponed.) There is no special rite for Jewish girl babies. | Emergency baptism should be performed on all Protestant infants in danger of death, with the exception of Baptists and Disciples of Christ. If possible, a baptized person should be present as sponsor. If none is available, anyone present may serve as a witness. | Emergency baptism must be conferred on every Catholic infant in probable danger of death; on every monstrosity; on every stillborn and aborted fetus, whatever its stage of development, unless it is certainly dead. *For purposes of baptism,* the only certain sign of death is noticeable corruption. |
| What to do | Nothing. | Call a minister. But if there is danger of death and the minister may not arrive in time, anyone may baptize. Pour water on the infant's head (not merely on the hair), saying simultaneously: "(Name). I baptize you in the name of the Father and of the Son and of the Holy Spirit. Amen." If the child has not yet been named, use the equivalent of "Baby Boy Smith." Excess water must be poured off onto the ground. If cotton was used to wipe baby's head, it must be burned. Later, report all available information about the infant to a clergyman of his denomination. | Call a priest. But if there is danger the infant will die before the priest arrives, anyone may and should baptize. Pour water on the infant's head (*not* merely on the hair), saying simultaneously: "I baptize you in the name of the Father and of the Son and of the Holy Spirit." Water must flow on the skin. Giving a name is not essential. If it is a medically dead fetus still enclosed in membranes, immerse it in a basin of water, break the membranes, and pronounce the words while moving the fetus about in the water. If the infant is likely to die in utero, a medically qualified person should attempt baptism in utero with a sterile syringe containing sterile water; the membranes must be pierced before the water is released; after delivery, the baptism should be repeated. Following such a baptism, report all available information about the infant to the priest. |

### Death

| | Jewish | Protestant | Roman Catholic |
|---|---|---|---|
| **General precepts** | When a Jewish patient dies in the hospital, a rabbi, or some responsible member of the Jewish community, will make proper arrangements for burial. Since many Jews are opposed to autopsy for religious persons, a rabbi, or some responsible member of the Jewish community, should discuss the matter of autopsy with the deceased's family. | Most Protestant denominations do not observe last sacraments. Those that do administer them before death. There is no moral objection to autopsy among most Protestants. | Every Roman Catholic should receive the last sacraments (penance, Communion, and extreme unction) before death. But penance and extreme unction can be administered conditionally up to several hours after medical death has occurred. The patient's body should not be wrapped in a shroud until after the last rites have been administered. There is no moral objection to autopsy performed in accordance with the provision of civil law. |
| **What to do** | Notify a rabbi or some responsible member of the Jewish community. Follow routine care for the body after death. | Call a minister. Follow routine care for the body after death. Place arms at the sides, or fold them; close eyes. | Call a priest. When he's finished his ministrations, follow routine care for the body after death. |
| **Dietary Rules** | Observant Jews eat only kosher (permissible) meat, fish, and dairy products. These are prepared in utensils and served in dishes that have been cleaned and kept separate in a ritually prescribed manner; and they are eaten in a prescribed sequence. If the patient's medical diet requires him to have milk and meat products at the same meal, the milk products should be served *first*. During Passover, the observant Jews will not eat leavened products or drink liquids containing grain alcohol. | Many Protestants observe rules of fasting (only one full meal a day) and abstinence (no meat). It is wise to ask the patient about special dietary rules he prefers to follow. | On weekdays of Lent and on certain other days, Catholics between the ages of 21 and 59 are subject to the law of fasting. This law does not apply to the genuinely sick for whom fasting would be detrimental or exceptionally difficult. |
| **How to Address Clergy** | Rabbi | Mister or Doctor. When in doubt, Mister (never Reverend). Lutheran ministers are usually called Pastor. Many Episcopal priests are called Father. | Father. |

Reference: Medical Economics, June 1959.

**20**

## A QUOTE ON QUOTATIONS

If you quote from one person
    it is plagiarism;
If you quote from two it
    is considered research;
When you quote from six or more,
    then you are a professor.

---

Reference: Weisberg, H.F.: Nutrition Today, *10*:55, 1975.

# AUTHOR INDEX

# SUBJECT INDEX

Note: Page numbers in *italics* refer to illustrations.